BIOMECHATRONICS in Medicine and Health Care

RAYMOND TONG

PAN STANFORD PUBLISHING

BIOMECHATRONICS in Medicine and Health Care

Published by

Pan Stanford Publishing Pte. Ltd.
Penthouse Level, Suntec Tower 3
8 Temasek Boulevard
Singapore 038988

E-mail: editorial@panstanford.com
Web: www.panstanford.com

British Library Cataloguing-in-Publication Data
A catalogue record for this book is available from the British Library.

Biomechatronics in Medicine and Healthcare

ISBN: 978-981-4241-61-8 (Hardcover)
ISBN: 978-981-4303-51-4 (eBook)

Printed in Singapore.

Preface

Being multidisciplinary involving subjects such as electronics, mechanics, medicine and health care, this book provides a fundamental concept as well as a comprehensive discussion on the field of *Biomechatronics*. The book is the result of several years of research work by many groups on the development and application of biomechatronics on human subjects. Basic information is provided in the beginning of each chapter to facilitate clinicians, engineers and students to have background knowledge and then appreciate the application of the technical as well as clinical aspect at the latter part of the chapter. There is a growing need for biomechatronic device in medical field hence more research groups are developing different systems in this area. The new development can support the medical profession to have better health care.

The aim of the book is to present the insights of experts on emerging technology and development that are or will be applied in medical professions on a variety of clinical challenges and then demonstrate how to apply biomechatronic in providing better care and service. It also incorporates new and exciting multidisciplinary areas of research across the medical field and engineering field, such as robotic therapeutic training system for stroke rehabilitation, exoskeletons for daily activities on persons with disability, Functional Electrical Stimulation (FES) and Wireless Active Capsule Endoscopy. Each chapter provides substantial background materials relevant to the particular subject. This can be a primary reference for students and researchers in the field of *Biomechatronics*.

The book is enriched by the contribution of outstanding scientists and experts worldwide in different topics addressed here. This book would not have been possible without help and contributions from them and I wish to express my gratitude to all of them for their efforts.

The research group from Arizona State University (USA), consisting of Sivakumar Balasubramanian and Jiping He, have contributed to Chapter 2 with new concepts for a wearable exoskeletal system for interactive therapy on upper extremity for persons after stroke.

Olivier Lambercy and his collaborators, of the ETH Zurich (Switzerland), National University of Singapore, Simon Fraser University, McGill University and Imperial College London, have contributed to Chapter 4 with the robot-assisted rehabilitation of hand function after stroke with the Haptic Knob and the HandCARE. The introduction part of neurological basic knowledge of stroke and hand function after stroke provide a good background information for stroke rehabilitation.

The book also reflects Japan's place at the forefront of robotics research. Toru Suzuki and Eiichi Saitoh from Fujita Health University, Aichi (Japan), have provided valuable contribution to Chapter 3 about a wearable exoskeletal robot WPAL using in assisting gait for paraplegia. Research group of Kunihiko Oda, Takehito Kikuchi, Shiro Isozumi and Junji Furusho, of the Osaka Electro-Communication University (Japan) and Osaka University (Japan), introduced their isokinetic exercise machine using high performance magnetorheological (MR) fluid brake and iso-contraction exercise in Chapter 11. The third group is Jorge Solis and Atsuo Takanishi from Waseda University (Japan). They have contributed to Chapter 12 with robotic-assisted technology of dental and skin surgery simulation for medical training purposes.

A very special contribution of researchers from University of Sydney (Australia), Nur Azah Hamzaid, Che Fornusek and Glen M. Davis, provided a clear introduction of functional electrical stimulation (FES) which is a kind of technology integrated in biomechatronics in Chapter 7 for FES's application in leg exercise of stroke therapy.

I would like to thank the contributions from research groups in Taiwan and Hong Kong. Chou-Ching K. Lin, Ming-Shaung Ju, Pin-Cheng Kung, Shu-Min Chen, of the National Cheng Kung University Hospital and National Cheng Kung University (Taiwan), contributed to Chapter 9 with robots for active rehabilitation of the upper limbs on the transverse plan for stroke patients. Xiaona Wang and Max Q.-H. Meng, of the Chinese University of Hong Kong China, contributed to Chapter 13 with wireless active capsule endoscope.

There is also a contribution from the Netherlands research group, Birgit I. Molier, Gerdienke B. Prange, Thijs Krabben, Michiel J. A. Jannink, Jaap H. Buurke, Hermie J. Hermens, of the Roessingh Research and Development (the Netherlands), University of Twente and Rehabilitation Centre 'the Roessingh' to Chapter 10 with upper extremity rehabilitation systems and augmented feedback.

In writing this book I have received the unstinting support of my colleagues and students in the Department of Health Technology and Informatics, the Hong Kong Polytechnic University (PolyU) (Hong Kong). The build-up of a robotic system is a team work from my graduate students, research staff, colleagues in PolyU and clinical partners. I would to thank all of them, in particular Le Li, Xiaoling Hu, and Newmen S. K. Ho for their contribution in the introduction to *Biomechatronics* (Chapter 1), our intention-driven rehabilitation robotic system PolyJbot (Chapter 5), hand robotic system (Chapter 6) and a robotic system combined with FES for wrist training (Chapter 8). Persons after stroke gave us a lot of constructive comments during the experimental setup and system design. I would like to express my gratitude to their support and feedback. They are the driving force and I want to do more for them.

Most of the work presented in this book has been developed as part of the product ready for clinicians to apply on persons with disability:

- Robotic upper-extremity repetitive trainer (Arizona State University, USA)
- WPAL — Wearable Power-Assisted Locomotor, (Fujita Health University, Aichi, Japan)
- HAPTIC KNOB and HandCARE — (ETH Zurich, National University of Singapore, Simon Fraser University, McGill University and Imperial College London)
- PolyJbot — an interactive robotic system using EMG (PolyU, Hong Kong)

I am very grateful for all the contributors and their strong support.

Finally, many thanks to my wife, Wai-nga Lam, and our daughter and son, Lok-ching Tong and Lok-tin Tong, for their support, encouragement, and patience. They have been my driving source.

Raymond Kai-Yu Tong
Associate Professor
The Hong Kong Polytechnic University
Hong Kong

Contents

Chapter One

An Introduction to Biomechatronics

Le Li and Raymond Kai-Yu Tong
Department of Health Technology and Informatics,
The Hong Kong Polytechnic University, Hung Hom, Hong Kong, China

In this book, research groups across the world interested in the state of the art in the biomechatronics, including wearable exoskeletal rehabilitation robots for upper limb and lower limb; intention-driven robot for stroke rehabilitation at hand, wrist and elbow joints, as well as robot-assistant method in medical training and capsule endoscope. The promising technology integrated in biomechatronics such as functional electrical stimulation (FES) and augmented feedback control are also covered in this book.

1.1 WHAT IS BIOMECHATRONICS?

Biomechatronics is a recently defined research area, aiming at the development of assistive systems for human rehabilitation and mobility improvement. This multidisciplinary field combines the intelligence and efforts of engineers, researchers and clinicians from many disciplines including biology, biomedical and biomechanical engineering, Human-machine interaction, rehabilitation medicine, prosthetics and orthotics.

The term *mechatronics* was introduced in Japan in the mid 1970s and has been defined as the engineering discipline dealing with the research, design and implementation of hybrid systems comprising mechanical, electrical and intelligent components or subsystems (Pons, (2008)).

The scope of biomechatronics is broader than mechatronics in aspects such as biomechatronics intrinsically includes the development of mechatronics systems, e.g. (control structures and actuators) and biomechatronics uses biologically inspired design to integrate the mechanical parts with biological system, e.g. robot fish.

Biomechatronics in Medicine and Healthcare by Le Li and Raymond Kai-Yu Tong

www.panstanford.com
978-981-4241-61-8

1.2 WHY STUDY BIOMECHATRONICS?

Biomechatronics in health care and medicine covers the interdisciplinary field of interaction with the human neuromusculoskeletal (NMS) system with the objective to assist impaired human motor control. In this field technology is developed that integrates neuroscience, robotics, sensor technology, electronics and control theory together to improvement human motor performance or regain the ability.

1.2.1 An Overview of the Neuromusculoskeletal System

The neuromusculoskeletal (NMS) system can be considered as a controlled motion system within the body. The NMS is composed of nervous control systems (central nervous system and peripheral nervous system), the muscular and skeletal systems. The central nervous system (CNS) processes the sensory information, generates the motor commands, and sends the motor commands to skeletal muscle via the efferent division to execute the effectors (Martini, (1995)). Millions of nerves, hundreds of muscles and bones are delicately integrated within the human body to react together and form the functional chain of human biomechanics. A schematic diagram of the neuromusculoskeletal system is shown in Fig. 1.1. There is also a feedback mechanism in the NMS system. The sensory information from muscle spindles and tendons will feedback to CNS and regulate the central descending commands. This system can be impaired because of disease or trauma, which can affect several parts of the motor system. For example, the mechanical system is affected in the case of amputations, and actuators are affected in the case of muscular dystrophy, and sensors may be affected as a result of long term diabetes. Spinal cord injury (SCI) affects the control part of spinal circuits by the brain, while stroke, Parkinson and cerebral palsy (CP) directly affect the brain.

1.2.2 The Role of Biomechatronics

Biomechatronincs could be used in rehabilitation and one successful example is the assisted-robotic training in stroke.

Rehabilitation after stroke is important for releasing the uncomfortable symptoms and partially restoring motor functions. Traditionally, physical training programs in poststroke rehabilitation are usually time consuming and labor demanding to both therapist and patient with one-to-one manual interaction. The controversy in the current rehabilitation treatments implies that conventional rehabilitation approaches need to be improved for better outcome and the improvement should depend on increased understanding of brain plasticity and also on the development of rehabilitation devices. It is important to enhance motor function in the early rehabilitation period (Langhammer and Stanghelle (2003)). On the other hand, long term regular physical training is also needed in order to maintain the function improvement after hospitalization. Therefore, the two important issues that we should focus are how to help the patients after stroke

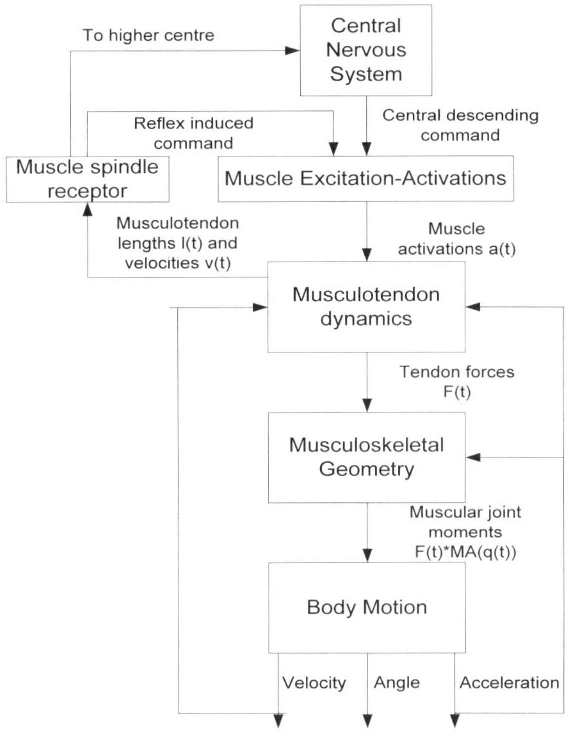

Figure 1.1 Scheme of the nervous system showing the different parts involved in motor control. Relationships are marked by arrows.

to perform rehabilitation training after discharge from hospital and how to find a better way for them to relearn motor functions.

Recent technologies have made it possible to use robotic devices as the assistance to the therapist, providing safe and intensive rehabilitation with repeated motions to persons after stroke (Colombo *et al.* (2005); Lum *et al.* (2002)). One of the primary benefits of robotic technology is that the robot can assist the human therapists to conduct rehabilitation programs with more quantitative and reproducible training motions. Secondly, a rehabilitation robot could not only share a large portion of the repeated labor work in a long-term physical training program but could also be a platform for continuous and quantitative monitoring of the performance during training, which may provide further understanding on the recovery mechanism due to the standardized experimental setup and the high repeatability of motion tasks. Positive effects on motor recovery have been reported in many studies on robot-assisted poststroke trainings when compared with conventional treatments. For example, robot-assisted gait training and robot-assisted gait treatment augmented with FES on subacute stroke subjects (<6 weeks poststroke) had better improvement on walking speed and more independent walking ability than subjects receiving conventional gait therapy (Tong *et al.* (2006)). In comparing the effectiveness of robot-assisted training with active-assisted mode and continuous passive movement (CPM) mode, it was reported that the motor improvements by the active-assisted robot treatments were better than those with CPM by retraining and posttraining evaluations (Volpe *et al.* (2000)).

Therefore, the robots providing active-assisted treatments will usually follow a user's intention to complete a desired task. In robot-assisted physical training with active-assisted movements, voluntary efforts from a patient are involved, which could result in more significant motor improvements in stroke rehabilitation when compared with a continuous passive movement.

1.2.3 What would be a Biomechatronic System Look Like?

Biomechatronics can be analyzed by analogy to biological systems integrating a musculoskeletal apparatus with a nervous system (Bar-Cohen, (2006)). Biomechatronic systems integrate mechanics, embedded control and human-machine interaction (HMI), sensor, actuators and energy supply in such a way that each of these components, and the whole biomechatronic system, is interacted with the user (Fig. 1.2). Van der Helm (1994) reported that a model structure of a robotic system could be divided into four blocks:

(1) The linkage system is the mechanical structure of the robot like the human bones, intermediate joints and ligaments.
(2) The actuator system by the electrical motor is used to generate forces and power the same as the function of muscles.
(3) The sensory system adopts the transducer such as potentiometer and force sensor to measure the position, velocity and force. It is similar to the function of muscle spindles and Golgi tendon organ.
(4) The control system is applied to the motor controller such as PID control and Fuzzy logic to control the movement of the robot like the function of central nervous system.

Biofeedback involves translating the physiologic activity of a patient's muscular response into a visual or auditory signal which allows him/her to be aware of the volitional changes in motor unit activity. The subject can facilitate or inhibit the muscular activity depending on the guide. The mechanism by which biofeedback can help to improve the outcome in the rehabilitation may be the reasons that the subjects can gain conscious control over undamaged upper neuron pathways which are in turn able to promote the restoration of missing functions. In practice, biofeedback is often combined with traditional physiotherapy as a useful complementary unit. EMG biofeedback has been applied on the recovery of upper limb (Basmajian *et al.* (1982)) and lower limb (Bradley *et al.* (1998)). Stein, (2004) expected that robotic and sophisticated biofeedback technologies for motor relearning after stroke might converge into combined training systems (Stein, (2004)).

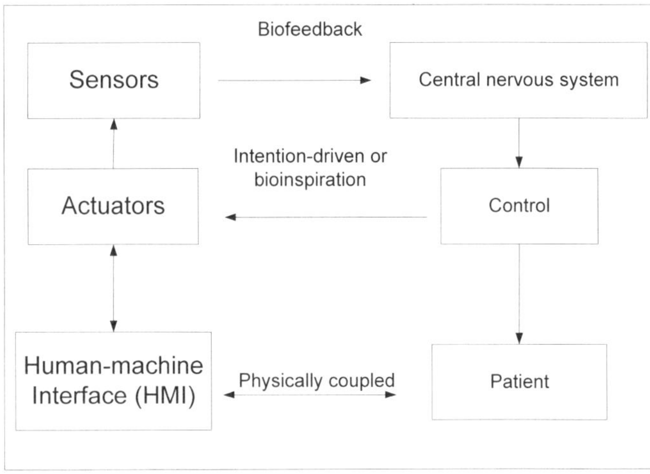

Figure 1.2 Diagram of a typical biomechatronic system.

One of the commonly used biofeedback methods is using the electromyography (EMG) signal from the muscle to control the actuator. Myoelectric control is related to the subject's intention and can be used as a control variable since EMG signals reflect the activities of the muscles. EMG signals have been frequently applied in the control of prosthetics for more than forty years. Myoelectrical control has also been reported for the control of functional electrical stimulation systems in rehabilitation, since voluntary physical exercise is important to promote the recovery of brain function in patients after stroke. Recently, many researchers have used EMG signals to continuously control exoskeleton robots that can be worn by human subjects as an assistive device. The researchers used EMG signals of selective muscles to estimate the joint torque, and applied the assistive torque to the joint to provide additional power (Rosen *et al.* (2001)). Recently, another promising technology called brain-control interface (BCI), using electroencephalography (EEG) as control signal, provides new approach to learn the mechanism of cerebral plasticity as well as to assist the rehabilitation process (Meng *et al.* (2009)).

This book reviews the various aspects of biomachtronics from mechanism to applications as well as various scales of the field in medicine and healthcare. Chapter 1 provides an overview of the field of biomachronics addressing technologies that adapt its principles using biology, mechanics and electronics. Chapter 2 describes one of the important aspects of biomachatronic, wearable exoskeletal robot, and also introduces the application of the technology in stroke rehabilitation. Another example of wearable robot is covered in Chapter 3, where evolutionary development of gait assisted robot—a wearable power-assisted locomotor for paraplegia are described. Chapter 4 covers the mechanization of the stroke rehabilitation and provides the introduction of interactive robot-assisted rehabilitation for hand function after stroke. Chapter 5 describes the intention-driven control method used in interactive robotic training in stroke. The development of the robot is introduced first then followed by the evaluation of the effectiveness of the robot used in elbow training in stroke. Chapter 6 follows the interactive robot design, with especially used for hand function improvement for stroke patients. The next two chapters deal with one of the new technology of functional electrical stimulation (FES) with Chapter 7 describing basic knowledge of FES and then its application in leg exercise and therapy, where Chapter 8 covering the topic of FES combined with robot system for poststroke wrist training. Chapter 9 covers the development of robots for active rehabilitation of the upper limbs on the transverse plan for stroke patients. Chapter 10 describes a novel control method with augmented feedback in upper extremity rehabilitation for stroke and Chapter 11 describes an application of magnetorheological fluid brake used in isokinetic and iso-contraction exercise machine. Besides the application of the biomechatronic robot in rehabilitation training, Chapter 12 describes this kind of robotic-assisted technology could also be applied in medical training purposes. Last but not least, Chapter 13 covers another application example of biomechatronic devices with a wireless active capsule endoscope application in medicine and health care.

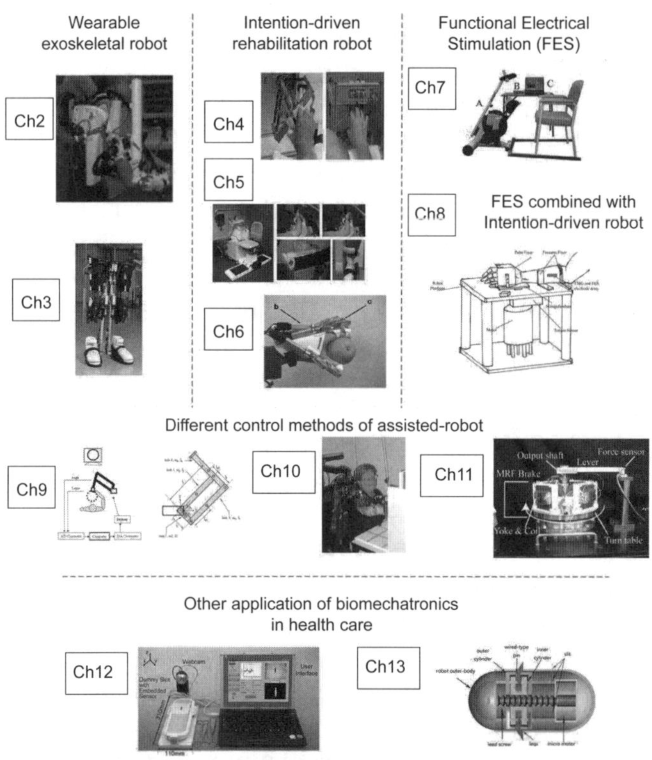

Figure 1.3 Structure of the book. For color reference, see page 209.

1.3 CONCLUSIONS

Biomechanics application, especially the robot-assisted rehabilitation is a promising area where engineering technology is combined and applied in rehabilitation medicine. The close cognitive and physical interaction between robots, a systemic biomechatrionic approach is required in order to develop this scientific area fully. The trend of modern biomechatronics will increase miniaturization in component design and increase intelligence which mainly in the areas of intelligent cognitive and physical human-machine interaction. Furthermore, more compact solutions based on multifunctional components are developed continuously with the integration of hybrid systems.

References

Bar-Cohen Y. (2006). *Biommimetics-biologically Inspired Technologies*, CRC Press, Taylor & Francis Group. USA

Bradley L, Hart BB, Mandana S, Flowers K, Riches M, Sanderson P. (1998). Electromyographic biofeedback for gait training after stroke, *Clin. Rehab.*; **12**: 11–22.

Basmajian JV, Gowland C, Brandstater ME, Swanson L, Trotter J. (1982). EMG feedback treatment of upper limb in hemiplegic stroke patients: a pilot study. *Arch. Phys. Med. Rehabil.*, **63**: 613–616.

Colombo R, Pisano F, Micera S, Mazzone A, Delconte C, Carrozza MC, Dario P, Minuco G, (2005). Robotic techniques for upper limb evaluation and rehabilitation of stroke patients. *IEEE Trans. Neural Syst. Rehabil. Eng.*, **13**: 311–323.

Fugl-Meyer A, Jaasko L, Leyman I, Olsson S, and Seglind S. (1975). The post-stroke hemiplegic patient method for evalustion of physical performance. *Scand. J. Rehabil. Med.*, **7**: 13–31.

Langhammer B, Stanghelle JK. (2003). Bobath or Motor Relearning Programme? A follow-up one and four years post stroke. *Clin. Rehabil.*, **17**(4): 731–734.

Lum RS, Burgar CG, and Shor PC. (2004). Evidence for improved muscle activation patterns after retraining of reaching movements with the MIME robotic system in subjects with post-stroke hemiparesis. *IEEE Trans. Neural Syst. Rehabil. Eng.*, **12**: 186–194.

Martini FH. (1995). *Fundamentals of Anatomy and Physiology*, New Jersey: Prentice Hall.

Meng F, Tong KY, Chan ST, Wong WW, Lui KH, Tang KW, Gao XR, Gao SK, (2009), Cerebral plasticity after subcortical stroke as revealed by cortico-muscular coherence, *IEEE Trans. Neural Syst. Rehabil. Eng.*, **17**(3): 234–43.

Pons JL (2008). *Wearable Robots: Biomechatronic Exoskeletons*, Wiley, NJ, USA.

Rosen J, Brand M, Fuchs MB, and Arcan M.(2001). A myosignal-based powered exoskeleton system. *IEEE Trans. Syst. Man. Cybern. A*, **31**: 210–212.

Song R, Tong KY, Hu XL, and Li L, (2008). Assistive control system using continuous myoelectric signal in robot-aided arm training for patients after stroke. *IEEE Trans. Neural Syst. Rehabil. Eng.*, **16**(4): 371–379.

Stein J. Motor recovery strategies after stroke, (2004). *Top Stroke Rehabil.*, **11**(2): 12–22.

Tong KY, Ng MF, Li LS, (2006). Effectiveness of gait training using an electromechanical gait trainer, with and without functional electric stimulation, in subacute stroke: A randomized controlled trial. *Archives of Physical Medicine and Rehabilitation*, **87**(10): 1298–1304.

Van del Helm FCT. Large-Scale Musculoskeletal System: Sensorimotor Integration and Optimization, (1994). *Biomechanics and Neural Control of Posture and Movement*, **32**: 407–424.

Veltink PH, Koopman HFJM, Van der helm F CT, Nene AV, (2001). Biomechatronics–assisting the impaired motor system. *Arch. Physiol. Biochem.*, **109**: 1–9.

Volpe BT, Krebs HI, Hogan N, Edelstein OTR, Diels C, Aisen M, (2000). A novel approach to stroke rehabilitation: Robot-aided sensorimotor stimulation. *Neurology*, **54**: 1938–1944.

Chapter Two

A Wearable Exoskeletal Rehabilitation Robot for Interactive Therapy

Sivakumar Balasubramanian and Jiping He
School of Biological and Health Systems Engineering, Arizona State University, Tempe, Arizona 85287-9309, USA

2.1 INTRODUCTION

One of the important requirements for achieving functional independence in day-to-day life is one's ability to use his/her upper-extremity (UE) dexterously. The upper-extremity plays a crucial role in our ability to interact with our environment, and also in performing other less obvious functions such as balance, protection against a fall etc. Given the importance of the UE in our daily life, any interruption of its normal motor control can possibly result in functional motor deficits of the UE. Central nervous system (CNS) lesion caused by stroke is one of the common conditions that interrupts normal motor control. Since, currently there is no cure for conditions such as stroke, rehabilitation therapy is a crucial step in the process of recovering lost motor abilities, at least partially if not fully.

Traditional rehabilitation techniques are strongly based on the neurophysiological studies carried by Sherrington early in the 20th century. These traditional techniques, that include the works of Bobath, Brunnstrom, Kabat and many others, are referred to as neurophysiologic approaches. These techniques place a lot of emphasis on reflexes, joint synergies, and the modulation of sensory input to the CNS. These approaches rely on utilizing sensory stimuli and reflexes to facilitate/inhibit muscle tone and movement patterns, and quite often focus on individual muscles or sensory pathways. Although the neurophysiologic methods have been around for a long time and have received considerable attention, their effectiveness has been controversial. One of the major shortcomings of the neurophysiologic approach is the lack of carry over into functional activities (Carr (1987)). Also, controlled studies comparing the different neurophysiologic

Biomechatronics in Medicine and Healthcare by Le Li and Raymond Kai-Yu Tong

www.panstanford.com
978-981-4241-61-8

techniques have failed to detect any difference in the general outcomes and in upper-limb function (Feys *et al.* (1998)).

In recent years, various novel therapeutic interventions, based on the current theories of motor control, have been developed. Some of these novel techniques include — task oriented therapy (Page (2003)), constraint induced movement therapy (CIMT) (Taub *et al.* (2002)), virtual rehabilitation (Huang *et al.* (2006)), functional electrical therapy (Popovic *et al.* (2002)), and robot-assisted rehabilitation. However, not all these techniques can be used effectively on all stroke survivors. For example, the first three techniques require some level of residual motor ability for subjects to actively train under these techniques, which makes them unsuitable for patients with low motor ability. The latter two therapy techniques, however, are suitable even for subjects with very low motor functionality because they provide movement assistance while performing therapy tasks. Over the last couple of decades there has been a significant growth of interest among the rehabilitation community in robot-assisted rehabilitation.

2.2 WHAT IS ROBOT-ASSISTED REHABILITATION?

Robot-assisted rehabilitation is a novel approach towards stroke rehabilitation where robotic devices are used to administer task-oriented motor training to subjects with movement disorders. Although the idea of using robots as assistive devices has existed for quite some time, the use of these device for therapeutic purposes is relatively new. The main purpose of these devices is to provide mechanical assistance/support while subjects perform various tasks during therapy. Additionally, these devices also quantify movement related variables that are useful for both diagnosis and clinical assessment.

2.2.1 *Why is it Used?*

Over the last 10–15 years there has been an increased amount of interest in the use of robotic devices for motor rehabilitation of stroke survivors. The strong interest is driven by multiple inter-related factors,

- *Increasing stroke population that is in need of therapy* – Rehabilitation therapy is the main form of treatment available to stroke survivors. With a constantly increasing stroke population, there is an ever increasing need for more resources for the rehabilitation of these patients. Because of the limited availability of resources, the average length of stay of stroke survivors as an inpatient has been on the decline over the past decade in the US; currently, this average length of stay is about 20 to 23 days (Fasoli *et al.* (2004)). Because of this there is more focus on teaching these subjects compensatory movements for the benefit of a quicker path to reduce motor disability, and improve motor function. But this is at the expense of possibly developing abnormal motor control patterns. Additionally, long-term therapy outside of the initial acute inpatient rehabilitation is rarely provided. However, with the availability of devices that can be controlled (directly or remotely) by therapists, subjects can receive meaningful therapy long after the initial acute rehabilitation therapy.

- *Repetitive task-oriented therapy can be labor intensive and time consuming* – Repetitive movement therapy has been observed to produce positive clinical outcomes by several studies. A meta-analysis of 9 controlled clinical studies revealed that training intensity has a significant effect on improving motor outcomes (Kwakkel *et al.* (1997)). In addition to high intensity, practicing movements that are task-oriented and functionally meaningful to the patient can result in better motor outcomes than that of conventional therapeutic techniques (Page (2003)). This type of therapy, however, is labor intensive and time consuming. But with the use of programmable robotic devices, some of the aspects of this therapy can be automated to relieve some burden off the therapist and expanding their ability to provide more efficient service.
- *Robots can provide unparalleled objective measurement of patient's movement* – Current evaluation techniques used in rehabilitation clinics can be very subjective. Although the reliability of some of these evaluation methods have been demonstrated, there is still a lot of room for subjective interpretation of a person's movement ability. Additionally, the use of ordinal scales to rate movement performances is not optimal because such a scale lacks the sensitivity to measure small but significant changes that might occur with therapy. Thus, objective measures of subject performance with good sensitivity are very important for the therapy process. These measures will not only enable us to keep track of a subject's progress during therapy but will also be useful in evaluating the efficacy of newly developed therapy techniques.
- *Robots can provide novel sensorimotor stimulation to the patient, which would be impossible for a therapist to simulate* – The sensorimotor stimuli that can be provided by a human therapist are often highly variable and limited in variety when compared to that of a robotic device. A robot can be easily programmed to provide various force fields in which the patient can train movements.
- *Robots can be easily combined with other rehabilitation technologies such as virtual-reality and haptic technology.*
- *Robots can also serve as tools for studying motor control* – Due to its intrinsic precision and the built-in actuating and sensing abilities, robotic devices can generate/simulate controlled motor conditions and provide real-time assessment of motor function performance and learning process.

2.3 REVIEW OF REHABILITATION ROBOTS FOR THE UPPER-EXTREMITY

Ever since the first report about the MIT MANUS therapy robot (Krebs *et al.* (1998)), there has been an explosive growth in the number of robotic devices developed for the therapeutic training of the upper-extremity. The earlier devices had mainly focused on training simple reaching movements that use the shoulder and elbow joints. However, the later ones had incorporated additional degrees-of-freedom (DOFs) in the robotic structure to include the training of the wrist/hand as well; there are also devices that are purely used for training the hand and the wrist. Each of these devices varies in terms of the exact mechanical design of the robot, the number of DOFs, the type of actuators and instrumentation used in these devices, and the types of movements supported by the robot etc. These rehabilitation robots can be classified into different types based on their interaction with user, and their engineering details. One of the possible schemes for classifying these devices was proposed by (Micera *et al.* (2005a)). We have added an extra category to this (Micera *et al.* (2005a)) classification scheme to make it more general (Table 2.1), which results in a scheme with two levels of classification – the first level is based on the nature of the mechanical structure of the robot, which differentiates rehabilitation robots into two major categories,

- Operational machines – These are robotic devices with an end-effector that is in physical contact with either the subject's hand or the forearm. The distal part of the upper-extremity is the only part of the subject's body that is in contact with the robot. This means that the subject is free to utilize their own joint movements to execute the tasks that are programmed in the operational space of the robot. These devices are also relatively easy to design and implement, as the mechanical structure of the device is mostly unaffected by the mechanical structure of the subject's upper-extremity. The only requirement for these devices is that they should have enough DOFs to sufficiently cover the subject's workspace for training different types of movements. Additionally, these devices can be operated by users either with their right or left arm, without requiring any change to the device.

Table 2.1 Classification of Rehabilitation Robots.

Category	DOF Control[a]	Backdrivabe	Complexity	Cost
Operational Class I	No	Yes	High	Moderate
Operational Class II	No	No	Low	Low
Exoskeleton I	Yes	Yes	High	High
Exoskeleton II[b]	Yes	No	Moderate	Low

[a]This indicates if the different DOFs of a human UE can be controlled independently by the robot.
[b]This is the additional category not included in the (Micera *et al.* (2005a)) classification scheme.

- Exoskeleton machines – Exoskeleton robots, unlike the operational machines, follow the anatomy of subject's UE; the device is attached to the subject's UE at different point, the humerus and the forearm etc. The number of DOFs of the robot is at least equal to the number of joints in the subject's UE that are targeted for robot-assisted therapy. The design of these devices is more involved because of the need to align the subject's joint rotation axis with the rotational axis of the robot's joint mechanism; this is a non-trivial problem for complex human joints such as the shoulder joint (Nef and Riener (2008)). Additionally, the need to fit subjects of different body types compounds the complexity of the design. Exoskeletons, in general, are specific to a particular side of the arm i.e. a device designed for the right arm, in most cases, cannot be used for the left arm and vice versa. The major advantage of exoskeletons, however, is that they allow for the possibility to measure and control individual joint movements, which is not possible with operational machines. Also, the static arm posture of the patient's arm is fully determined with an exoskeleton, but not with an operational machine. Exoskeleton might be more suitable for subjects with low levels of residual motor control, as the joint synergies of these subjects are usually altered by stroke (Micera *et al.* (2005a)).

The second level of classification of these devices further divides the two categories from the first level into two sub-categories, class I and class II. The distinction between these two sub-categories is based on the engineering details/complexity of the robotic devices in the operational and exoskeleton categories. Class I devices are characterized by low mechanical impedance, high backdrivability, use of advanced controllers such as impedance controllers, ability to generate finely controlled force fields and quantify mechanical properties of the arm, and high cost. Class II devices are in general relatively simpler devices. They have a simple mechanical structure, no backdrivability, some of these devices have active friction and inertia compensation, and low cost.

Some of the existing robots for training the UE are the MIT MANUS (planar module (Krebs *et al.* (1998)), wrist module (Krebs *et al.* (2007)) and hand module (Masia *et al.* (2007))), Mirror Image Motion Enabler (MIME) (Burgar *et al.* (2000)), Assisted Rehabilitation and Measurement (ARM) Guide (Reinkensmeyer *et al.* (2000)), Arm In (Nef and Riener (2008)), Gentle/S (Loureiro *et al.* (2004)), Pneu-WREX (Sanchez *et al.* (2005)), MEMOS (Micera *et al.* (2005b)), NeRebot (Rosati *et al.* (2007)), HWARD (Takahashi *et al.* (2008)), and Hand Mentor™ (Koeneman *et al.* (2004)). The details of these rehabiliation robots are summarized in Table 2.2.

The details summarized in Table 2.2 are mainly concerned with the engineering aspects of the robotic devices that determine a device's range of motion, its workspace, and the different movements supported the robot. In addition to this, the other crucial aspect of rehabiliation robots is the role played by the robot during therapy. This is termed as the "mode of therapy" in the rehabilitation robotics literature. The mode of therapy is mainly determined by the hardware

Table 2.2 Details of Some of the Current Upper-Extremity Rehabilitation Robots

Name	Type [a]	DOF [b]	Movements [c]	Actuators	Sensors	Clinical Study
MIT MANUS (Planar module)	OC I	2	2D planar reaching	Brushless DC motors	Position, velocity & Force	Yes
MIT MANUS (Wrist module)	OC I	3	Wrist FE Wrist yaw Wrist SP	Brushless DC motors	Position & Force	Yes
MIT MANUS (Hand module)	OC I	1	Hand opening/closing	Brushless DC motors	Position, velocity & Force*	No
MIME	OC II	3	3D reaching	DC motors	Position & Force	Yes
ARM Guide	OC II	1	Reaching along a straight line	DC motor	Position & Force	Yes
Arm In (II)	Ex I	6	3D reaching Eblow SP Wrist FE	DC motors & harmonic drives	Position & Force	No
Gentle/S	OC I	3	3D reaching	3 DOF Haptic Master (FCS Robotics)	Position	Yes
Pneu-WREX	OC I	4	3D reaching	Pneumatic pistons	Position, Velocity & Pressure	No
MEMOS	OC II	2	2D planar reaching	DC motors	Positon & Force	Yes
NeReBot	OC II	3	3D reaching	Cables driven by DC motors	Position & Force*	Yes
HWARD	Ex II	3	Wrist FE Finger/thumb FE	Pneumatic pistons	Position & Force*	Yes
Hand Mentor™	Ex II	1	Wrist FE(coupled with finger FE)	Pneumatic muscle actuator	Position & Force*	Yes

[a]Robot classification (Table 2.1) (OC - Operational Class, Ex - Exoskeleton).
[b]Indicates the number of actuated degrees of freedom.
[c]The different movements supported by the robot (FE - Felxion/Extension, SP - Supination/Pronation, AbAd - Abduction/Adduction)
*Force is measured indirectly through the inputs to the actuators (eg. motor current, pressure etc.)

specifications of the robot, and the type of controller used to control the kinematics and dynamics of the robot. In general, the control achitecture of a rehabilitation robot consists of two levels of control, a low-level control and a high-level control. The low-level control schemes are usually implemented using traditional position or hybrid force controllers. The low-level controller peforms the task of acheiving the desired kinematic and dynamic behavior demanded from the robot. On the other hand, the high-level control scheme deals with the robot-user interaction; this is usually implemented using a rule-base. A detailed review of the different types of robot therapy modes for rehabiliation robotcs can be found in (Marchal-Crespo and Reinkensmeyer (2009)).

2.4 ROBOTIC UPPER-EXTREMITY REPETITIVE TRAINER–RUPERT

Robotic upper-extremity repetitive trainer or RUPERT is a wearable exoskeleton robot developed by Kinetic Muscles Inc. (Tempe, AZ) in collaboration with the Arizona State University. The main motivation behind the development of this device was to have a simple, low cost device targeted for clinical and home use. The very first prototype of the robot was reported in 2005 (He *et al.* (2005)), and its mechanical structure and technical specifications have gone through an evolutionary process since the first design (Sugar *et al.* (2005)). The pictures of the different versions of RUPERT are shown in Fig. 2.1. The first three versions of the robot (RUPERT, RUPERT II, and RUPERT III) had four DOFs, shoulder flexion/extension, elbow flexion extension, forearm supination/pronation, and wrist flexion/extension. The current version of the robot (RUPERT IV) has an additional DOF at the shoulder the humeral internal/external rotation; this added DOF gives the robot a 3D workspace, which is useful for practicing tasks related to ADL.

The first working prototype of the robot was designed after verifying that the design of the robot would have the required range of motion in all the DOFs, and the pneumatic muscle actuators used for actuating the different DOFs could acheive the required range of motions for assisting ADL related tasks such as reaching, washing and self-feeding. The second version of the robot resulted from the modification of the previous design to accomodate for subjects of varying body types and shapes. In this version, the center of rotation of each joint and the length of each segment of the robot were made adjustable, which resulted in increasing the device complexity, number of components on the robot, and also its final weight. Version III was developed (Fig. 2.1(c)) based on the fitting evaluations from a range of statures of able-bodied and stroke subjects, and device testing of Version I (Fig. 2.1(a)) and II (Fig. 2.1(b)) at Banner good Samaritan Regional Medical Center. The robotic components of RUPERT III were built from a composite material that helped reduce the overall weight of the robot. All these three versions of the robot had four DOFs with two DOF controlling reaching and other two controlling the orientation of the hand. This meant that the reaching workspace of these robots was a 2D surface. Although this is suitable for training

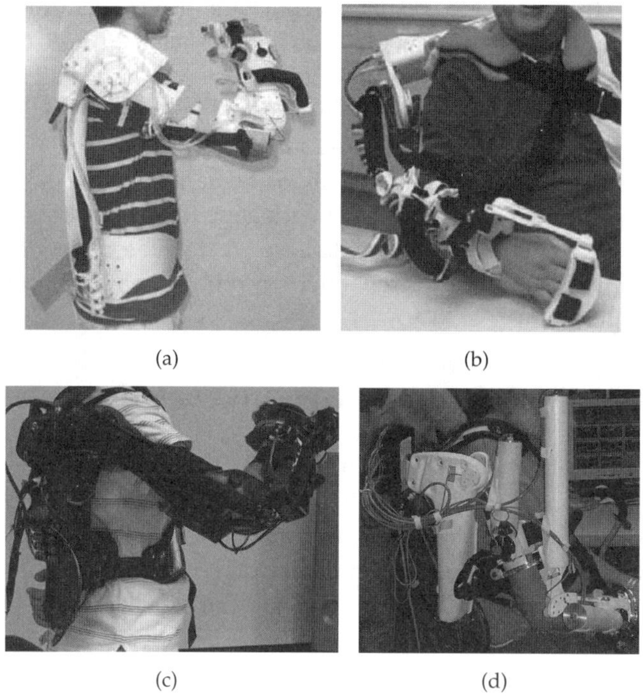

Figure 2.1 Pictures of the four versions of RUPERT depicting the changes in the device over the years. (a) RUPERT; (b) RUPERT II; (c) RUPERT III; (d) RUPERT IV. For color reference, see page 210.

simple reaching movements involving shoulder and elbow flexion/extension, it does not reflect the natural movements made in real life situations. Thus, an additional DOF was added at the shoulder to increase the workspace of the robot to a 3D space. The DOF added at the shoulder was the humeral internal/external rotation, increasing the total number of DOFs of the robot to five.

Each one of the DOFs of RUPERT is actuated using a single Mckibben-type pneumatic muscle actuator (PMA) . Since PMAs are unidirectional actuators, the use of single PMA in each DOF results in a robot that is unidirectionally actuated in each DOF. The different DOFs of the robot and the direction of actuation in each of these DOFs is listed in Table 2.3. The choice of pneumatic muscles as the robotic actuators was motivated by the following features of these actuators,

- *Light weight of the actuator* – The exoskeleton nature of the robot demands that the overall weigth of the robot be a low as possible. And, PMAs are very light weight actuators, and offer a superior power/force-to-weight (or volume) ratio (Davis *et al.* (2003)).
- *Compliant nature of the actuator* – PMAs are also, by nature, compliant. Thus, the use of these actuators will ensure some level of compliance in the robot used for human interaction (Davis *et al.* (2003)).

Table 2.3 Degrees of Freedom of RUPERT and their Direction of Actuation.

Degree-Of-Freedom	Direction of Actuation	Actuation in the other direction
Shoulder Flexion/ Extension	Shoulder Flexion	Gravitational pull on the arm
Elbow Flexion/ Extension	Elbow Extension	Subject's motor control
Elbow Supination/ Pronation	Elbow Supination	Subject's motor control
Wrist Flexion/ Extension	Wrist Extension	Subject's motor control
Humeral Internal/ External Rotation*	Humeral External Rotaiton	Subject's motor control

*Additional DOF present in RUPERT IV.

- *Low Cost* – These actuators can be easily built using parts that can be obtained off-the-shelf, which lowering the cost of the acuator.

These features of the PMA fit very well with the primary goal which is to develop a simple, light-weight and low cost rehabiliation robot.

All versions of RUPERT are instrumented with two types of sensors – (a) joint angle sensors to sense the angular position of each DOF, and (b) pressure sensors to monitor the pressure inside the PMA actuating each DOF. The joint angle data provides the joint space kinematics of the movement performed with RUPERT, which can be used for deriving other kinematic variables. The pressure sensor data, on the other hand, can be used for obtaining some very basic and crude information about some variables related to movement kinetics. RUPERT IV uses non-contact magnetic angle sensors (Ametes 360 ASMC-01, GWM Assosciates) and peizoelectic pressure sensors (MPX5700GP, Freescale) for sensing the angular position of the joints and the pressure in the PMAs respectively.

RUEPRT has two unique features that distinguish it from the other therapy robots currently available for the upper-extremity. The first and most important feature of RUPERT is that it is a wearable exoskeleton robot that allows a greater degree of mobility to the patient. There are a few exoskeleton rehabilitation robots used in various research labs (Nef and Riener (2008), Sanchez *et al.* (2005), Carignan *et al.* (2005)). All these robots, however, are grounded i.e. they are fixed to a static structure. The wearablity of RUPERT, on the other hand, allows it to be used for training tasks in different settings, sitting or standing etc., which is important from a task-oriented training perspective. For example, a simple reaching task might involve the same set of UE muscles both in a standing or a seated position; while, the postural control muscles will be drastically different in these two cases. Thus the availability of a wearable robot makes it possible to practice tasks in all these different settings that mimic real life activities. The second unique feature of RUPERT is its unidirectional actuation. Each DOF of RUPERT is actuated by a single PMA, thus resulting in unidirectional actuation in the different DOFs. The actuation in the other direction is achieved either through gravitational pull on the different segments of the robot or through the patient's existing motor control. This particular design of the robot was based on two factors -

(1) Most stroke patients have difficulty moving in one direction (for example, difficulty in extending the elbow) because of a weak agonist or hyperactive antagonist. In a majority of stroke patients the stroke affected UE assumes a pose with flexed and supinated elbow, along with flexed wrist and fingers. The direction of actuation in each DOF of RUPERT (Table 2.3) was thus chosen based on this pattern of motor disability seen in a large section of the stroke population.
(2) When a patient wears the robot, it is basically mounted on the patient's torso through a patient fixation system. Thus, a light weight exoskeleton is crucial for the comfortable use of the device. The use of single PMA to actuate each DOF, instead of two, helps reduce the weight and size of the robot. Additionally, this design also reduces the other required components of the system (such as air regulators, pressure sensors, and analog and digital IO channels on the computer interface board) by half, which can lower the overall cost of the device.

However, in some of the DOFs such as the elbow flexion/extension and elbow supination/pronation a passive elastic element (bungee cord) was introduced in order to provide some assistive force in elbow flexion and elbow pronation respectively. This was done mainly for subjects who have a weakness in directions such as elbow flexion and pronation, when their corresponding PMAs are not activated. Although these elastic elements will help assist the subject in elbow flexion and pronation, their inclusion does require additional force from the PMA to overcome its resistance in addition to the force required for providing active assistance in elbow extension extension.

The under-actuated design of RUPERT is an important issue to consider from an engineering point-of-view. Such designs are not very common in engineering systems because of the lack of controllability that results from these designs. This lack of controllability could also be therapeutically disadvantageous because of limited repertoire of sensorimotor stimulation that can possibly be provided by the robot.

Additionally, the use of unidirectional actuation will also encourage a greater level of volutnary participation from the subject while using the robot for training assisted therapy tasks. Although this might not be a good approach for subjects with very weak muscle control, the under-actuated design can potentially keep the subject engaged in therapy and reduce "slacking behavior" when the subject lets the robot take over and do the work for them (Wolbrecht *et al.* (2008)).

2.5 ROBOT CONTROLLER AND THERAPY MODES

In addition to the mechanical hardware of the robot, the RUPERT system consists of other components that are required for using the robot to administer robot-assisted therapy. The schematic diagram of the overall RUPERT system is shown in Fig. 2.2. The PC104 single board computer (Advantech PCM-3370) houses the controller software that senses the state of the robot (joint and pressure signals) and modulates its output to the electronic pressure reagulators (E22 series, Numatics, Inc.), which in turn control the air pressure inside

the PMAs actuating the robot. The maximum input pressue to these pressure regulators is set to 80 psi. The box housing the single board computer and the pressure regulators (control box) is connected to a host PC through an Ethernet cable. The communication between these two computers is achevied through the TCP/IP and UDP protocols. The host PC houses a GUI that the therapist/physician uses to set up the robot and the biofeedback interface for administering therapy.

2.5.1 *RUPERT Controller Overview*

The RUPERT controller was developed and tested in a Matlab/Simulink environment using the xPC toolbox. The overall structure of the controller for RUPERT, as shown in Fig. 2.3, consists of two feedback loops, the Inner-Loop (IL) and the Outer-Loop (OL), each with its own controller. The IL controller works at the level of the individual joints. It consists of five independent PID-based joint position controllers, corresponding to each DOF in RUPERT. These controllers are basically PID controllers with some structural modifications, such as

(1) Saturation limit for the integrator.
(2) Saturation limit and a rate limit for the output from the controller. The saturation limits on the output restricts the control output between $[0, 5]$, where 0 corresponds to $0psi$ (relative to the atmospheric pressure) and 5 corresponds to maximum pressure limit set for a given PMA.

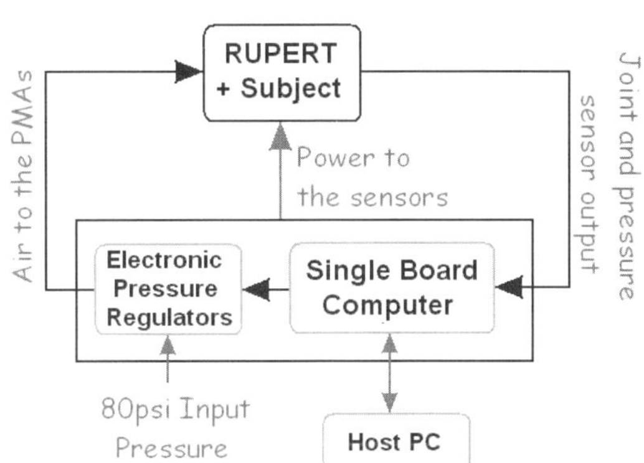

Figure 2.2 Schematic of the overall RUPERT system.

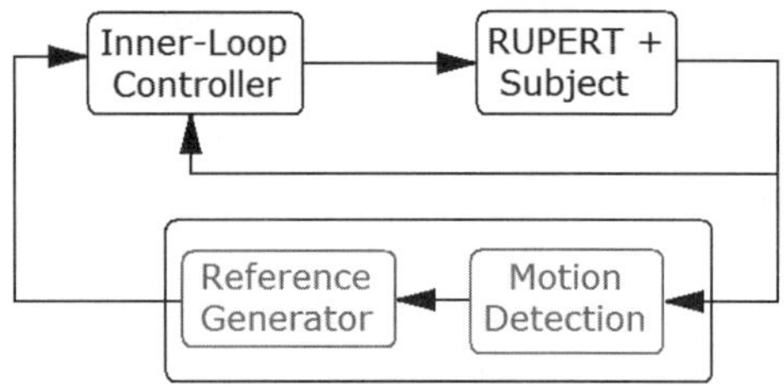

Figure 2.3 Schematic of the RUPERT controller structure.

(3) The derivative part of the feedback controller is implemented as a high-pass filter. A high-pass filter can be regarded of as a differentiator and a low-pass fiter in series. The low-pass filter attenuates the high frequency noise, and thus reducing the amplification of high frequency noise by the differentiator. This will reduce the effect of high frequency noise from corrupting the control signal, and will ensure a quiet operation from the pressure regulator.

The gains for these IL controllers need to be selected to provide a robust performance on stability applicable to users of different body sizes and builds with a large range of parameters and variable impairments. They were obtained experimentally by trial-and-error through testing the robot on different able-bodied subjects. Since the application does not demand very accurate control performance, a common set of gains that provides a smooth assistance for overcoming spasticity, and driving the arm to reach the desired location for different subjects was taken to be sufficient.

The outer-loop controller consists of two blocks, the 'reference generator' and the 'motion detection' block (Fig. 2.3). The outer-loop controller is a higher level controller that contains the logic for the different therapy modes, and also the reference generator block that generates the reference signals for the inner-loop position controllers. The 'motion detection' block contains the logic for the different therapy modes, which enables/disables the 'reference generator' and the inner-loop controller, thus controlling the activation/deactivation of robotic assistance. The reference generator when enabled by the 'motion detection' block generates a smooth reference signals for the inner-loop controller using the minimum jerk equation.

$$\theta_j^{ref}(t) = \begin{cases} \theta_j^{act}(t), & t < t_0 \\ \left(\theta_j^{Tgt} - \theta_j^{act}(t_0)\right) \times \left(6\tau^5 - 15\tau^4 + 10\tau^3\right) + \theta_j^{act}(t_0), & t \geq t_0 \end{cases} \tag{2.1}$$

$$\tau = \min\left(1, \frac{t - t_0}{T_{dur}}\right).$$

where,

t_0 is the time when the reference generator is enabled by the motion detection block (i.e. output of motion detection block changes from 0 to 1).

$\theta_j^{act}(t)$ is the actual joint angle for the joint j measured by the joint sensor in the robot at time t.
θ_j^{Tgt} is the target angle for the joint j.
T_{dur} is the task duration, i.e. the time taken by the reference signal to reach the target value (θ_j^{Tgt}) from the initial value ($\theta_j^{act}(t_0)$).

2.5.2 Robot Therapy Modes

The controller shown in Fig. 2.3 can be used to practice therapy tasks in three different modes *passive mode, co-operative mode,* and *active-assist mode.*

(1) **Passive Mode** – In this mode of therapy the subject is relaxed and the robot does all the work in driving the arm to the target location. The output of the motion detection block is set to 1 from the start of the therapy task (i.e. $t_0 = 0$). Thus, robotic assistance is always enabled. The passive therapy mode helps to stretch soft tissues to improve range of motion, keep soft tissue compliant, reduce tone (Reinkensmeyer *et al.* (2001)), preventing contractures (Hogan *et al.* (2006)) and conditioning for further therapy.
(2) **Co-operative Mode** – The co-operative mode stands for a therapy mode where both the robot and the subject work together to achieve a particular therapy task. The different blocks of the RUPERT controller function the same in this mode as they do in the passive mode. However, there is voluntary participation from the subject in this mode to complete the given therapy task. The unidirectional actuation of the robot becomes a very useful feature for this particular therapy mode. In a fully actuated robot, the robot controller will resist movements from the subject that are faster than the desired movement of the robot. However, because RUPERT is unidirectionally actuated in each DOF, the subject will not feel any resistive force from the robot, when his/her movement is faster than the desired movement of the robot in the direction of actuation. However, if the subject's movement lags behind the desired movement, the subject will feel an assistive force from the robot. This type of a therapy mode was implemented in the MIT MANUS robot where the subject feels no force if he/she is able to move ahead of the desired trajectory, but feel an impedance from the robot when his/her movement lags behind the desired movement (Krebs *et al.* (2003)). The co-operative therapy mode can be summarized by the following set of equations,

$$\tau_j(t) = \begin{cases} 0, & k_j^d \times \theta_j^{error}(t) < 0 \\ C_j^{IL}\left(k_j^d \times \theta_j^{error}\right), & k_j^d \times \theta_j^{error}(t) \geq 0 \end{cases} \tag{2.2}$$

where,

$\tau_j(t)$ is the torque applied to the joint j.
$\theta_j^{error}(t) = \theta_j^{ref}(t) - \theta_j^{act}(t)$ is the error between the reference angle (θ_j^{ref}) and its corresponding actual angle (θ_j^{act}) for the joint j at time t.

k_j^d indicates whether the angle at the joint j increases or decrease in the direction of actuation in joint j. For example, the shoulder flexion/extension (SFE) angle increases from 0 deg to 90 deg when the shoulder is flexed. So, $k_{SFE}^d = +1$ for the shoulder. While for the elbow flexion/extension (EFE) joint, the joint angle decreases from about 110 deg to 0 deg when the elbow is extended, thus $k_{EFE}^d = -1$.

$C_j^{IL}(\bullet)$ is a function that combines the inner-loop control law and actuator dynamics for the joint j.

(3) **Active-Assist Mode** – The active-assist therapy mode is implemented in the form of a triggered assistance mode. When a reaching task is presented to the subject, the subject starts the task by making a voluntary effort to reach the target. The output of the motion detection block is 0 at the start of the therapy task, thus allowing the subject to start the task voluntarily. During this period of voluntary movement, the motion detection block monitors the distance between the endpoint of the subject's arm and the target location ($r_{EP}(t)$). The robotic assistance remains disabled as long as the rate of change of $r_{EP}(t)$ is less than a particular threshold i.e. $dr_{EP}/dt(t) < v_{EP}^{th}$ (This is so, because when the subject is moving towards the target $dr_{EP}/dt(t)$ will be negative). The value of v_{EP}^{th} will determine the sensitivity of the algorithm to either stops in the subject's movement or a movement away from the target. Once the value of $dr_{EP}/dt(t)$ crosses the threshold (v_{EP}^{th}), the output of the motion detection block is changed to 1, thus initiating robotic assistance to assist the subject's arm towards the target. It should be noted that after the initiation of assistance, the functioning of the robot will be similar to the co-operative mode if the subject continues to make any voluntary contribution to the movement.

The use of these three therapy modes for performing reaching movements by a stroke subject is demonstrated in Fig. 2.4. This figure displays the temporal plots of the three DOFs of the robot involved in reaching movements, shoulder flexion/extension, elbow flexion/extension and humeral rotation. The figure consists of a 9 plots arranged in three rows and columns, which correspond to the three therapy modes, and the three DOFs respectively. In the passive mode (row 1) the subject was relaxed and the position controller of the robot drives the three DOFs to their corresponding target angles. While in the co-operative mode (row 2), the subject provided voluntary contribution to the movement which can be seen in the section of the movement where the actual angle (blue trace) leads the corresponding reference angle (red trace). In the active-assist mode, the subject starts the movement voluntarily, and the robotic assistance is initiated later when the 'motion detection' block detects either a slow movement or a movement away from the target. The difference in the initiation of robotic assistance between the passive and co-operative modes, and the active-assist therapy mode can be seen as a shift in the point-of-assistance (dashed vertical black line), which is defined as the time during the therapy task at which robotic assistance is initiated, between

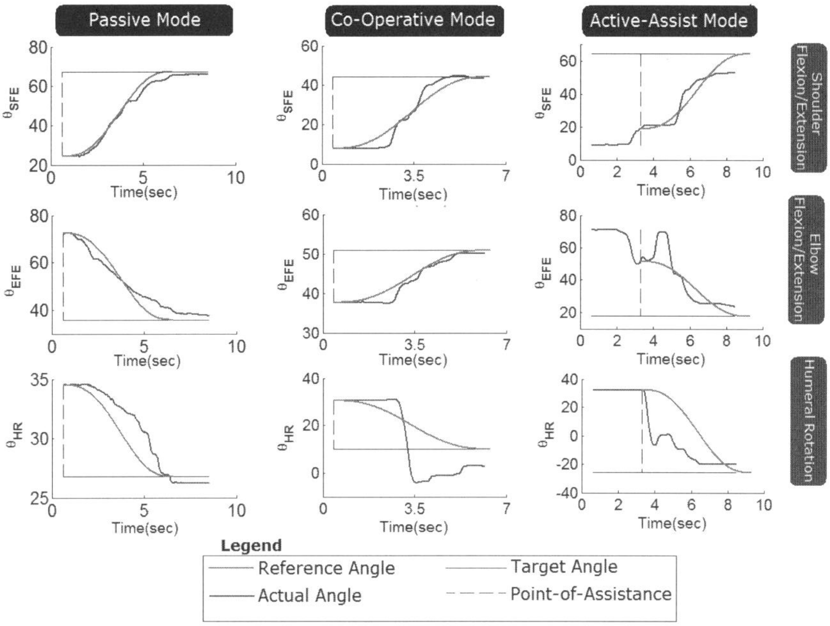

Figure 2.4 Plot of the joint angle profiles of the shoulder flexion/extension, elbow flexion/extension and humeral rotation DOFs for the three therapy modes developed for RUPERT. For color reference, see page 210.

these modes; the point-of-assistance is delayed in the active-assist therapy mode compared to other two modes, where the robotic assistance is present from the start of the therapy task. It is also evident from these plots that when there is voluntary contribution from the subject, the resulting movement's smoothness is reduced (compare row 1 with rows 2 and 3).

2.6 A VIRTUAL REALITY-BASED BIOFEEDBACK INTERFACE

A virtual reality-based biofeedback software interface was developed in our lab using the Panda graphics engine. The software also has the capability to allow a physician/therapist to use the RUPERT system to design and administer robot-assisted therapy. This software is run by the host PC. The screen-shots of the biofeedback interface for practicing reaching movements is shown Fig. 2.5. The interface consists of a virtual model of the human arm that is driven by the joint sensors in RUPERT. The data recorded from these sensors are streamed by the single board computer to the host PC through an UDP interface. In addition to the visual stimuli provided through the virtual environment, the program also provides suitable audio cues about the therapy task to the subject. Since the virtual environment is driven by the joint angles sensed using robot that is worn by the stroke subject, the effect of trunk movement is completely eliminated; pure trunk movements without any movement of the arm relative to the trunk will not change

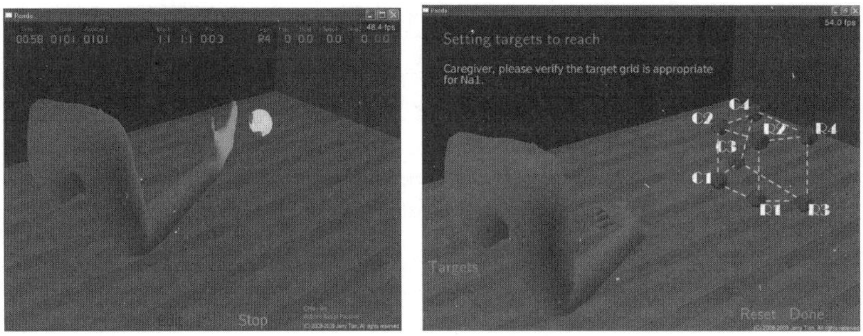

(a) (b)

Figure 2.5 Screen-shot of the virtual reality environment of the biofeedback interface (a) Screen short of subject performing a reaching task. (b) Screen-shot of the different targets used to practice reaching tasks. For color reference, see page 211.

joint angles sensed by the robot, thus force the subject to move his/her arm to achieve tasks in the virtual environment.

2.7 CLINICAL STUDY

The RUPERT system described above is currently being used in a small clinical study to test the capability of the device for therapeutic use in a clinical environment. The study consists of 12 stroke subjects who are at least 6-months post stroke; the twelve subjects are divided into an experimental group and a control group with 6 subjects each. The experimental group undergoes robot-assisted therapy using RUPERT, and the control group practices exercises at home that are prescribed by the therapist at the start of their course of therapy. Each subject in the experimental group undergoes 12 therapy sessions (each session lasts for about one hour) over a period of 4 weeks with 3 sessions per week. All subjects are evaluated by another therapist that is blinded to the subject's group (experimental or control). The evaluation is performed both pre- and post-therapy, and the subjects are evaluated using the Fugl-Meyer Scale, the Wolf Motor Function Test, the Stroke Impact Scale, and the Motor Activity Log.

The therapy protocol used for the experimental group follows the HIFUS principle, where the therapy progresses from easy to difficult tasks. The therapy tasks for the experimental group involves performing reaching movements to a set of 8 targets, which are the combinations of different targets location at two different reaching distances (Near and Far), two different reaching directions (Center and Right), and two different reaching heights (Low and High) as shown in Fig. 2.5(b). Each therapy session mainly consists of two types of movements, voluntary movements, and robot-assisted movements with the robot functioning in the co-operative mode. Each therapy session starts with the subject performing voluntary reaching movements to these 8 targets. Based on their performance, the targets that could not be reached by the subject voluntarily are ordered according

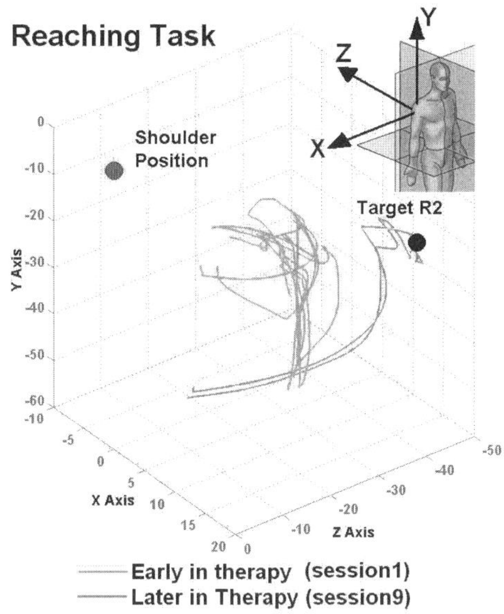

Figure 2.6 Endpoint trajectories of voluntary reaching movements to target R2. The figure shows the endpoint trajectories early (red trace) and late (blue trace) in therapy. For color reference, see page 211.

to their level of difficulty. Subsequently, this order of targets is used as the order in which the subjects will practice robot-assisted movements in the co-operative mode.

2.7.1 Preliminary Results

At the moment, three of the six stroke subjects in the experimental group have completed the study. This section presents some of the preliminary results from the analysis of the data collected during therapy from one of the subjects. The results presented here are only preliminary results, as we are yet to perform any analysis on the data collected from the study. The kinematic data collected from the voluntary movements performed during therapy was used to calculate two performance measures related to movement performance.

- **Accuracy** is the measure of how close the subject can get to a target while reaching to this target. This is measured as the minimum distance between the endpoint of the arm and the target location during the reaching movement. In addition to the magnitude of the distance we also calculate the direction of this error in term of the direction cosine.
- **Smoothness** is a measure of temporal coordination in a movement. Many different techniques for quantifying movement smoothness can be found in the current rehabilitation robotics literature. In our analysis we used five different metrics to calculate the smoothness of a movement -
  (1) Mean Jerk Metric (Rohrer *et al.* (2002))

Table 2.4 Comparison of movement accuracy and smoothness at early (therapy session 1) and late (therapy session 9) in therapy

Target	Movement Accuracy (%) [a]		Movement Smoothness[b]	
	Early in Therapy	Late in Therapy	Early in Therapy	Late in Therapy
C1	7	5	−2.39	−1.10
C2	4	0	−2.11	−1.11
C3	18	27	−3.15	−1.13
C4	19	12	−2.87	−1.13
R1	8	3	−3.2	−2.95
R2	13	5	−2.92	−1.74
R3	27	20	−2.75	−4.47
R4	32	14	−2.92	−3.60

[a]The best value of accuracy is 0. The values in the table are rounded off to the nearest integer.
[b]The best value of smoothness is −1.

(2) Speed Metric (Rohrer *et al.* (2002))
(3) Peaks Metric (Rohrer *et al.* (2002))
(4) Mean Arrest Period Ratio Metric (Rohrer *et al.* (2002))
(5) Spectral Metric (Balasubramanian *et al.* (2009))

A summary of the changes that occurred in one of the subject's movement kinematics towards the end of the study relative to the start of the therapy is shown in Fig. 2.6; this figure shows the qualitative change in the subject's endpoint trajectory while performing a voluntary reaching movement to target R2 (Fig. 2.5(b)). The corresponding quantitative changes in the movement accuracy and movement smoothness for the 8 targets used in the therapy are summarized in Table 2.4. It is evident from Fig. 2.6 and Table 2.4 that the reaching ability of the subject to the different targets had improved the subject was able to reach further away from the body, and the reaching movement was much smoother than at the start of the therapy.

2.8 CONCLUSION

A wearable exoskeleton robot for upper-extremity stroke rehabilitation, its associated controller and therapy modes, and a virtual reality based biofeedback system were described. The system described above is currently being used in a clinical study to test the device's capability for therapeutic training in a clinical setting.

Our current work is focused towards developing adaptive robotic therapy modes that modulate the robotic assistance according to the subject's motor ability. The robotic therapy modes developed for RUPERT are still very basic in nature, and do not account for the differences in motor abilities between different subjects. One of the important factors for driving motor learning is active voluntary participation (Hogan *et al.* (2006)). By having an adaptive therapy mode, the robotic assistance is modulated based on the subjects motor ability, and thus encouraging maximim voluntary participation from the subject.

References

Balasubramanian, S., Wei, R., Herman, R. and He, J. (2009). Robot-measured performance metrics in stroke rehabilitation, in *Complex Medical Engineering, 2009. CME. ICME International Conference on*, pp. 1–6, doi:10.1109/ICCME.2009.4906654.

Burgar, C. G., Lum, P. S., Shor, P. C. and Machiel Van der Loos, H. F. (2000). Development of robots for rehabilitation therapy: The Palo Alto va/Stanford experience, *Journal of Rehabilitation Research and Development* **37**, 6, pp. 663–673.

Carignan, C., Liszka, M. and Roderick, S. (2005). Design of an arm exoskeleton with scapula motion for shoulder rehabilitation, in *Advanced Robotics, 2005. ICAR '05. Proceedings 12th International Conference on*, pp. 524–531.

Carr, J. H. (1987). *Movement Science: Foundations for Physical Therapy in Rehabilitation* (Aspen Publishers, Rockville, Md.).

Davis, S., Tsagarakis, N., Canderle, J. and Caldwell, D. G. (2003). Enhanced modelling and performance in braided pneumatic muscle actuators, *The International Journal of Robotics Research* **22**, 3-4, pp. 213–227.

Fasoli, S. E., Krebs, H. I., Ferraro, M., Hogan, N. and Volpe, B. T. (2004). Does shorter rehabilitation limit potential recovery poststroke? *Neurorehabil. Neural Repair* **18**, 2, pp. 88–94.

Feys, H. M., De Weerdt, W. J., Selz, B. E., Cox Steck, G. A., Spichiger, R., Vereeck, L. E., Putman, K. D. and Van Hoydonck, G. A. (1998). Effect of a therapeutic intervention for the hemiplegic upper limb in the acute phase after stroke: A single-blind, randomized, controlled multicenter trial, *Stroke* **29**, 4, pp. 785–92.

He, J., Koeneman, E. J., Schultz, R. S., Huang, H., Wanberg, J., Herring, D. E., Sugar, T., Herman, R. and Koeneman, J. B. (2005). Design of a robotic upper extremity repetitive therapy device, in *Rehabilitation Robotics, 2005. ICORR 2005. 9th International Conference on*, pp. 95–98.

Hogan, N., Krebs, H. I., Rohrer, B., Palazzolo, J. J., Dipietro, L., Fasoli, S. E., Stein, J., Hughes, R., Frontera, W. R., Lynch, D. and Volpe, B. T. (2006). Motions or muscles? some behavioral factors underlying robotic assistance of motor recovery, *Journal of Rehabilitation Research and Development* **43**, 5, pp. 605–618.

Huang, H., Wolf, S. L. and He, J. (2006). Recent developments in biofeedback for neuromotor rehabilitation, *J. Neuroeng. Rehabil.* **3**, p. 11.

Koeneman, E., Schultz, R., Wolf, S., Herring, D. and Koeneman, J. (2004). A pneumatic muscle hand therapy device, in *Engineering in Medicine and Biology Society, 2004. IEMBS '04. 26th Annual International Conference of the IEEE*, Vol. 1, pp. 2711–2713, doi:10.1109/IEMBS.2004.1403777.

Krebs, H. I., Hogan, N., Aisen, M. L. and Volpe, B. T. (1998). Robot-aided neurorehabilitation, *Rehabilitation Engineering, IEEE Transactions on [see also IEEE Trans. on Neural Systems and Rehabilitation]* **6**, 1, pp. 75–87.

Krebs, H. I., Palazzolo, J. J., Dipietro, L., Ferraro, M., Krol, J., Rannekleiv, K., Volpe, B. T. and Hogan, N. (2003). Rehabilitation robotics: Performance-based progressive robot-assisted therapy, *Autonomous Robots* **15**, pp. 7–20.

Krebs, H. I., Volpe, B. T., Williams, D., Celestino, J., Charles, S. K., Lynch, D. and Hogan, N. (2007). Robot-aided neurorehabilitation: A robot for wrist rehabilitation, *Neural Systems and Rehabilitation Engineering, IEEE Transactions on* **15**, 3, pp. 327–335.

Kwakkel, G., Wagenaar, R. C., Koelman, T. W., Lankhorst, G. J. and Koetsier, J. C. (1997). Effects of intensity of rehabilitation after stroke. A research synthesis, *Stroke* **28**, 8, pp. 1550–6.

Loureiro, R., Amirabdollahian, F. and Harwin, W. (2004). *A Gentle/S Approach to Robot Assisted Neuro-Rehabilitation*, pp. 347–363, *http://dx.doi.org/10.1007/10946978_22*

Marchal-Crespo, L. and Reinkensmeyer, D. (2009). Review of control strategies for robotic movement training after neurologic injury, *Journal of NeuroEngineering and Rehabilitation* **6**, 1, p. 20.

Masia, L., Krebs, H. I., Cappa, P. and Hogan, N. (2007). Design and characterization of hand module for whole-arm rehabilitation following stroke, *Mechatronics, IEEE/ASME Transactions on* **12**, 4, pp. 399–407.

Micera, S., Carpaneto, J., Posteraro, F., Cenciotti, L., Popovic, M. and Dario, P. (2005a). Characterization of upper arm synergies during reaching tasks in able-bodied and hemiparetic subjects, *Clin. Biomech. (Bristol, Avon)* **20**, 9, pp. 939–46.

Micera, S., Carrozza, M., Guglielmelli, E., Cappiello, G., Zaccone, F., Freschi, C., Colombo, R., Mazzone, A., Delconte, C., Pisano, F., Minuco, G. and Dario, P. (2005b). A simple robotic system for neurorehabilitation, *Autonomous Robots* **19**, pp. 271–284.

Nef, T. and Riener, R. (2008). Shoulder actuation mechanisms for arm rehabilitation exoskeletons, pp. 862–868, doi:10.1109/BIOROB.2008.4762794.

Page, S. J. (2003). Intensity versus task-specificity after stroke: How important is intensity? *Am. J. Phys. Med. Rehabil.* **82**, 9, pp. 730–2.

Popovic, M. B., Popovic, D. B., Sinkjaer, T., Stefanovic, A. and Schwirtlich, L. (2002). Restitution of reaching and grasping promoted by functional electrical therapy, *Artif Organs* **26**, 3, pp. 271–5.

Reinkensmeyer, D. J., Kahn, L. E., Averbuch, M., McKenna-Cole, A., Schmit, B. D. and Rymer, W. Z. (2000). Understanding and treating arm movement impairment after chronic brain injury: Progress with the arm guide, *J. Rehabil. Res. Dev.* **37**, 6, pp. 653–62.

Reinkensmeyer, D. J., Takahashi, C. D., Timoszyk, W. K., Reinkensmeyer, A. N. and Kahn, L. E. (2001). Design of robot assistance for arm movement therapy following stroke, *Advanced Robotics* **14**, 7, pp. 625–637.

Rohrer, B., Fasoli, S., Krebs, H. I., Hughes, R., Volpe, B., Frontera, W. R., Stein, J. and Hogan, N. (2002). Movement smoothness changes during stroke recovery, *J. Neurosci.* **22**, 18, pp. 8297–304.

Rosati, G., Gallina, P. and Masiero, S. (2007). Design, implementation and clinical tests of a wire-based robot for neurorehabilitation, *Neural Systems and Rehabilitation Engineering, IEEE Transactions on* **15**, 4, pp. 560–569, doi:10.1109/TNSRE.2007.908560.

Sanchez, J., R.J., Wolbrecht, E., Smith, R., Liu, J., Rao, S., Cramer, S., Rahman, T., Bobrow, J. and Reinkensmeyer, D. (2005). A pneumatic robot for re-training arm movement after stroke: rationale and mechanical design, in *Rehabilitation Robotics, 2005. ICORR 2005. 9th International Conference on*, pp. 500–504, doi:10.1109/ICORR.2005.1501151.

Sugar, T. G., Jiping, H., Koeneman, E. J., Koeneman, J. B., Herman, R., Huang, H., Schultz, R. S., Herring, D. E., Wanberg, J., Balasubramanian, S., Swenson, P. and Ward, J. A. (2007). Design and control of rupert: A device for robotic upper extremity repetitive therapy, *Neural Systems and Rehabilitation Engineering, IEEE Transactions on see also IEEE Trans.on Rehabilitation Engineering* **15**, 3, pp. 336–346, Journal Article.

Takahashi, C. D., Der-Yeghiaian, L., Le, V., Motiwala, R. R. and Cramer, S. C. (2008). Robot-based hand motor therapy after stroke, *Brain* **131**, Pt 2, pp. 425–37.

Taub, E., Uswatte, G. and Elbert, T. (2002). New treatments in neurorehabilitation founded on basic research, *Nature Reviews. Neuroscience* **3**, 3, pp. 228–236.

Wolbrecht, E. T., Chan, V., Reinkensmeyer, D. J. and Bobrow, J. E. (2008). Optimizing compliant, model-based robotic assistance to promote neurorehabilitation, *Neural Systems and Rehabilitation Engineering, IEEE Transactions on* **16**, 3, pp. 286–297.

Chapter Three

Development of Gait-Assisted Robot WPAL (Wearable Power-Assist Locomotor) for Paraplegia

Toru Suzuki* and Eiichi Saitoh†
*Faculty of Rehabilitation, School of Health Sciences, Fujita Health University, Aichi, Japan
†Department of Rehabilitation Medicine, School of Medicine, Fujita Health University, Aichi, Japan

3.1 INTRODUCTION

Patients with complete paraplegia, the main etiology of which is spinal cord injury, are unable to stand or walk and are forced to depend solely on a wheelchair. Restoration of gait in patients with spinal cord injuries (SCIs) has several advantages. Life in a wheelchair is likely to result in a variety of medical problems such as osteoporosis, contracture, constipation, and obesity (Kunkel, (1993); Kaplan, (1978); Messenger, (1989)). From the psychological viewpoint, advantages such as increased self-esteem through standing and being at eye level with others as well as through walking, even if only a little, can not be neglected (Cybulski, (1986); Stallard, (1989)). It is a matter of fact that most paraplegic patients want to walk on their own legs (Subbarao, (1991)).

To restore gait in patients with SCI, orthoses are available until today. Today, with advance in robotic technology, gait reconstruction for SCI changes to new frontiers. In this chapter, we overview gait reconstruction with orthosis, and introduce our newly robot for SCI.

3.2 OVERVIEW OF GAIT RECONSTRUCTION OF SCI WITH ORTHOSES

Orthoses are classified as the bilateral external joint type and the medial single hip joint type according to the position of the orthotic hip joint.

Biomechatronics in Medicine and Healthcare by Le Li and Raymond Kai-Yu Tong

www.panstanford.com
978-981-4241-61-8

The hip-knee-ankle-foot orthosis (HKAFO) has been used for reconstruction of paraplegic gait. In Western countries, reconstruction of paraplegic gait with the HKAFO equipped with bilateral lateral-sided hip joints and hard pelvic support, such as the hip guidance orthosis (HGO: Fig. 3.1) and the reciprocating gait orthosis (RGO: Fig. 3.2), has been the mainstream appliance (Major, (1981); Douglas,

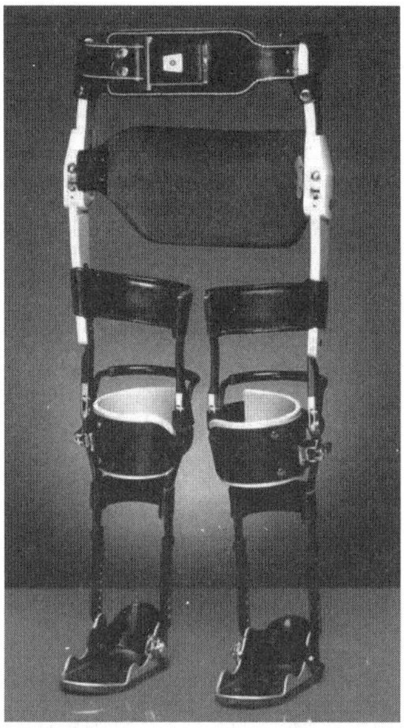

Figure 3.1 Hip Guidance Orthosis.

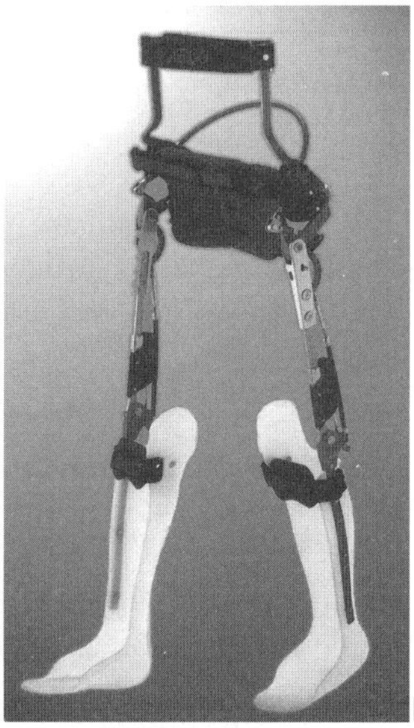

Figure 3.2 Reciprocating Gait Orthosis.

(1983); Jefferson; (1990)). We have termed this the "lateral system" (Saitoh; (1996)). With the lateral system, the positional gap between the anatomical and orthotic hip joints is small and the motion of the orthosis during the gait is similar to a anatomical motion.

On other hand, in the RGO, the hard pelvic support that links the hip joints is not rigid enough to achieve good stability during standing and walking. The very rigid pelvic band in the HGO greatly restricts trunk movement. In addition, the structure of these orthoses, i.e., lateral-sided hip joints and hard pelvic support, makes it difficult to use a wheelchair while wearing them.

To address these issues, a new unique system, which we call the "medial system", has become available in medical practice. It is characterized by a medial single hip joint located between the thighs of KAFOs under the perineum (Saitoh; (1996), Saitoh; (1997)).The medial system, introduced as the Walkabout in 1992, had excellent standing stability and wheelchair compatibility. However, there was a height gap in the position between the orthotic hip joint and the anatomical hip joint, as well as the problem of a short stride in walking. Therefore, Primewalk, which has a sliding hip joint with a virtual axis to reduce the height gap problem, was developed and put into use (Saitoh; (1997), Suzuki; (2007)).The Primewalk system is shown in Fig. 3.3, example of walking is shown in Fig. 3.4.

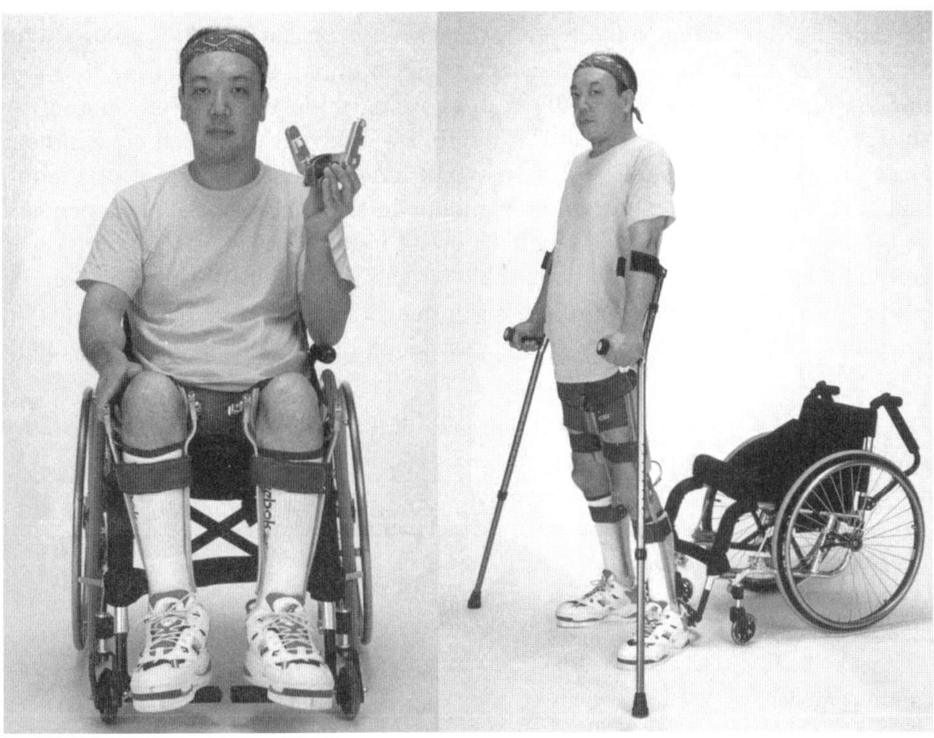

Figure 3.3 Primewalk System. For color reference, see page 212.

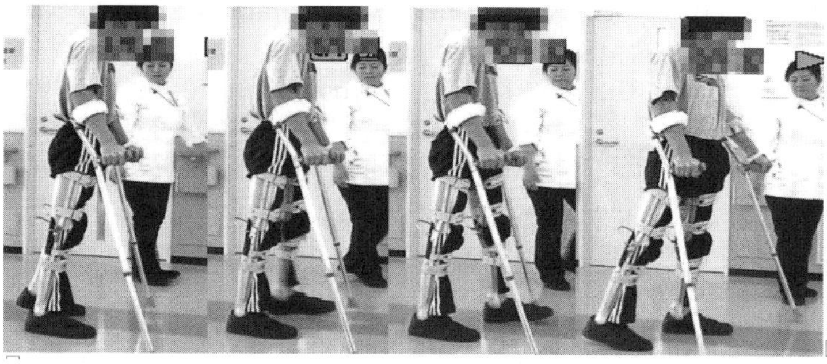

Figure 3.4 Gait with Primewalk.

3.3 INTRODUCTION OF WALKING ABILITY AND PREDICTION OF WALKING ABILITY OF PRIMEWALK

We surveyed walking abilities and walking independence with Primewalk (Suzuki; (2007)).

Walking abilities were determined with 45 patients with SCI. All the subjects were fulfill following criteria: (1) ASIA Impairment Scale grades A, B, or C and wheelchair-dependent in daily living, (2) training periods of at least 1 month for orthotic gait as an in-patient, (3) completion of gait training during in-patient rehabilitation and, (4) the presence of no comorbidity that forced patients to lessen the training dose. The subject group consisted of 36 men and 9 women with a mean age of 34.0 years. Level of neurological impairment was classified into three groups: a cervical group (C) with neurological levels between C6 and C8; an upper-middle thoracic group (UT) with T4–T10 levels, and a thoracolumbar group(TL)(T12-L1 levels). The degree of gait independence was rated by the following five-point scale: outdoor independent gait (5 points), indoor independent gait (4 points), indoor supervised gait (3 points), indoor assisted gait (2 points), and gait within parallel bars (1 points). Table 3.1 shows the relationship between the neurological level and the degree of gait independence. Five of 10 patients (50%) in group C were able to walk without assistance, but only one was independent

Table 3.1 Degree of Independence of Gait Gccording to Neurological Level with Primewalk.

Level of injury	C6	C7	C8	T4	T5	T6	T7	T8	T9	T10	T12	L1
Degree of independence of gait												
Outdoor independent											1	4
Indoor independent	2	2		2	2	3	2			1	3	3
Indoor assited	2	1			1					2		1
within parallel bar	1	1		1			1					

45 cases, 34.0 ± 13.2 yo male/female: 36/9

Table 3.2 Walking Parameters According to Neurological Level and Goals of Gait with Primewalk.

Level of paresis	Gait speed (m/min)	Step length (cm)	cadence
Cervical injury ($n = 3$)	7.6 ± 7.5	15.8 ±7.6	44.5±12.5
Thoracic injury ($n = 13$)	11.3 ± 7.5	23.7 ± 12.2	47.0 ± 16.5
Thoracolumbar injury ($n = 10$)	18.0 ± 8.8	31.2 ± 12.8	57.7 ± 16.9

indoors without supervision. In the UT group, the majority of patients (75%) did not require any assistance and as the thoracic level moved caudally more patients became independent indoors without supervision. In the TL group, only one out of 15 required any assistance with less than half of remaining 14 requiring supervision, and 5 of 15 achieving independence outdoors. For patients able to walk in orthosis without any assistance, the lower the level of neurological impairment and the higher the degree of gait independence, the greater were walking speed, step length, and cadence (Table 3.2). The walking speed of the subject was almost comparable with that of patients using HKAFO such as RGO (Suzuki; (2007)).

We made decision tree to predict gait independence with Primewalk with following procedure. Inhibitory factors that could interfere with achievement of gait independence were spasticity, involuntary spasms, pain, contracture, weakness of the upper extremities, and decreased motivation for performing gait exercise. The effect of each was evaluated as 'present' when it inhibits walking exercise and as 'absent' when it did not inhibit walking exercise. Recursive partitioning was used to predict the final status of gait expected at the end of walking training in the basis of age, sex, neurological level, and inhibitory factors. The decision tree for goals of gait constructed for the subjects is shown in Fig. 3.5. The neurological level was the first decisive factor. In the second step, age was extracted in group C and UT, whereas decreased motivation was extracted in group TL. In this group, five of 10 patients with high motivation attained the outdoor-independent level, where all patients with decreased motivation remained at the level of indoor-supervision or less. The remaining patient stayed at the indoor-assisted level. Among patients in groups C and UT and under the age of 50, weakness of upper extremities was a decisive factor in gait independence in addition to the neurological level and the presence/absence of spasiticity. The coincident ratio between the value predicted from the decision tree of gait and the value actually observed was 68.9%. These results provide useful information to medical teams that prescribe orthoses to SCI.

3.4 LIMITATION OF ORTHOSIS AND FUTURE OF ROBOTICS

In the case of any brace, whether a medial or lateral system, the orthotic gait eliminates the degree of freedom (DOF) of the knee and ankle joints and achieves

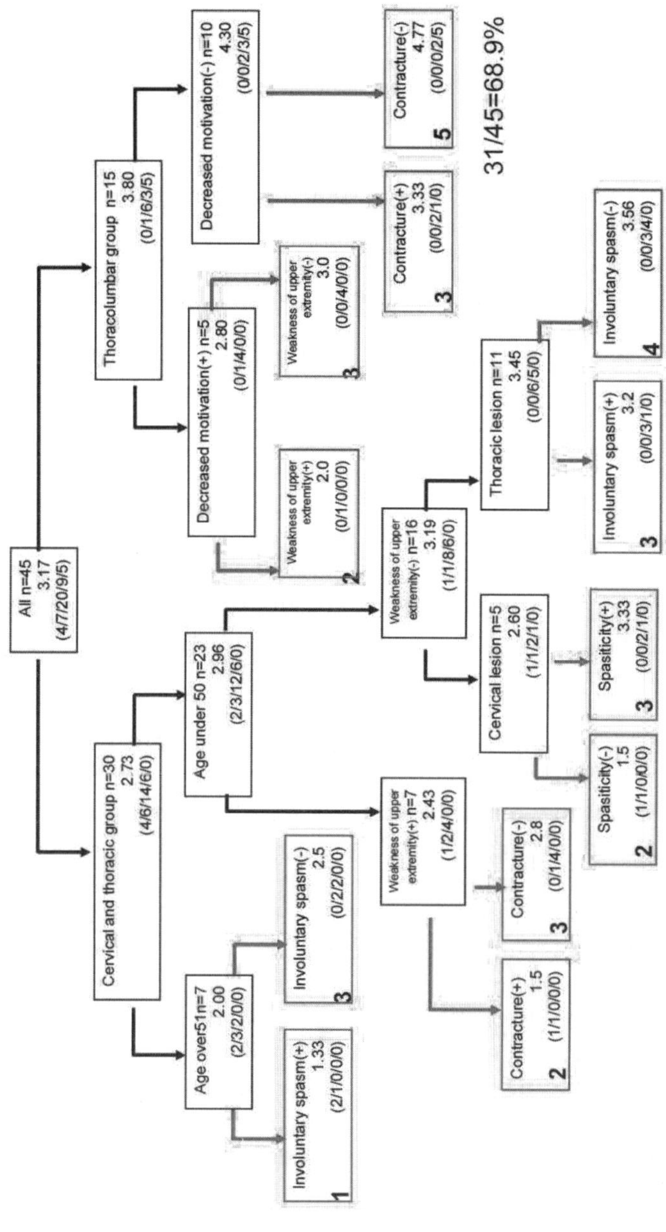

Figure 3.5 Gait with Primewalk.

walking by simplifying the range of motion (ROM) of the hip joint to only one direction of flexion and extension (limiting the DOF). In addition, the system has no power source, and power exerted by the upper extremities is mostly used for progression and lateral motion of the body during walking. Therefore, problems have arisen that are related to the large burden placed on the upper extremities and high energy consumption in walking, making practical use of these orthoses difficult (Suzuki; (2007), Greene; (2003), Greene; (2000)). In addition, standing-up and sitting-down motions with the fixed knee extension position of KAFOs are difficult tasks for paraplegic patients.

As a method to overcome the limitation of the orthoses described above, it is conceivable that actuators, power sources for movement of the lower extremities, could be attached to orthoses and control movement. In other words, gait reconstruction would take place through use of a wearable robot as an evolutional development in the design of orthoses. Nevertheless, considering the actual life of paraplegic patients, wheelchair compatibility with a wearable robot is an essential prerequisite for use of the orthosis. For these reasons, a medial system should be adopted for a wearable robot.

We developed a wearable robot (Wearable Power-Assist Locomotor: WPAL) that adopts a medial system and has 6 motors equipped at the bilateral hip, knee, and ankle joints.

3.4.1 Basic Information of WPAL

Figure 3.6 shows the WPAL, as well as the hip, knee and ankle joints. Also shown is a full frontal view of the orthosis. The WPAL is comprised of a robotic part and an orthotic part. The robotic part is modular to enable mass production,

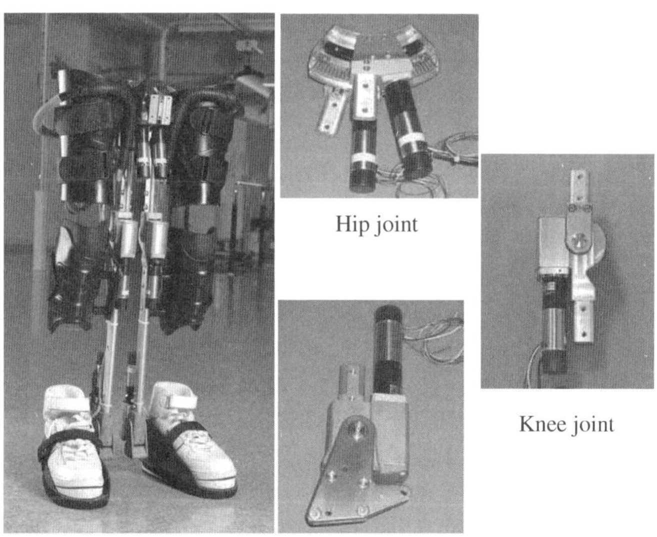

Figure 3.6 (WPAL) Wearable Power-Assist Locomotor. For color reference, see page 212.

while the orthotic part is composed of shoes, calf cuffs, and thigh cuffs, which are customized to fit the lower extremities of individual patients. While wearing part of the orthosis, users are able to completely combine the robotic and orthotic parts while still in the wheelchair, and then stand and begin walking. (see Figs. 3.7–3.9)

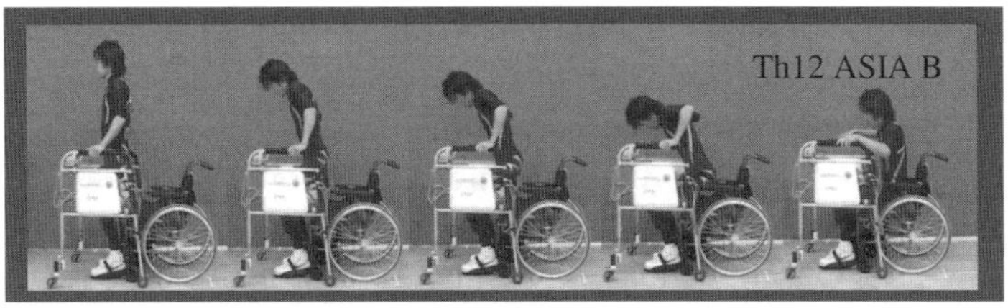

Figure 3.7 Standing up with WPAL. For color reference, see page 213.

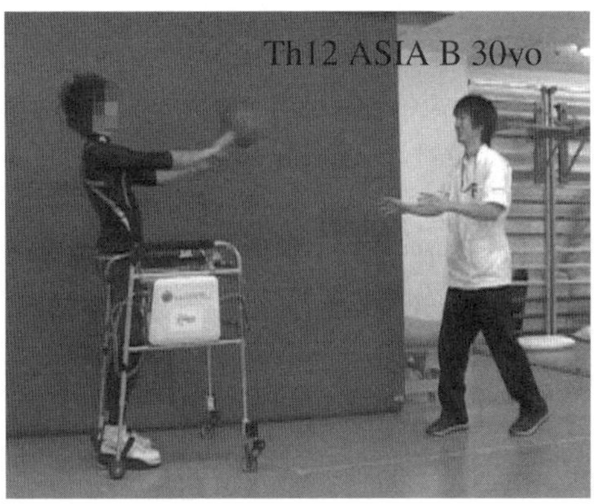

Figure 3.8 Standing balance with WPAL Th12 ASIA B 30 yo. For color reference, see page 213.

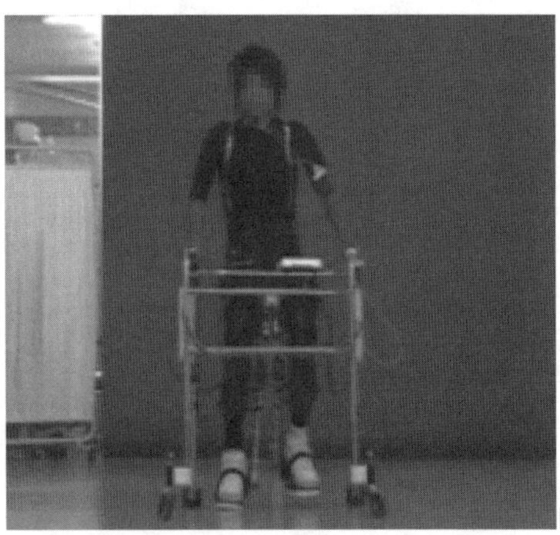

Figure 3.9 Gait with WPAL. For color reference, see page 213.

The robotic part consists of hip, knee, and ankle joints, which independently performed flexion-extension movements. The bilateral robotic hip joints located between the bilateral thighs under the perineum moved independently. The maximal ROM of each joint was hip, 40 degrees; knee, 120 degrees; and ankle, 50 degrees.

The total weight of the robotic part, depending on the length of the upright strut according to the height of the user, was about 12 kg. The orthotic part was mostly made of carbon fibers and polypropylene and weighed about 1.5 kg. The main controller, remote controller, and battery were built into the custom-made reciprocal walking frame (total weight of the walker, 10 kg). WPAL was designed to allow the user to stand up and sit down as well to walk with the walking frame.

Safety was a critical challenge in the development of the wearable robot. The basic safety concept with the WPAL was "to stop when unwanted or accidental motion occurred". Additionally, it was equipped with a stop switch of the pull-out type to enable emergency shut down by the user or others in case of unexpected motion. When an emergency shutdown occurs, the WPAL assumes a standing position so that the user will not fall. After an emergency stop, function can be restarted with the user in a standing position by push-up switch.

Movement patterns of the robotic joint angles in walking were constructed based on the results of walking of health subjects with orthosis by the three-dimensional analyzer. A template of combination of joint angles was made from orthotic walking of healthy volunteers with the Primewalk system. For practical use, precise adjustment of movement pattern was made in actual trial of each patient.

In addition, to control the gait mode, an automatic mode and a feedback mode based on detection of motion of the upper extremities were prepared. The specific step length and cadence appropriate for the user were decided upon in advance in the automatic mode, while timing of starting the lower extremity swing and size of the swing (stride) were determined by sensing the distance of the walker's movement in the feedback mode (Kagawa, (2007)).

3.4.2 Abilities of WPAL

We introduce WPAL to SCI who were dependent on a wheelchair in daily life and had experience with Primewalk walking. The subject was male, aged 30 years old. Spinal cord functional levels was T-12, according to the Impairment Scale of the American Spinal Cord Injury Association (ASIA AIS) Grade B.

Standing-up, sitting-down and level-ground walking with a reciprocal walking frame were performed with both the Primewalk and WPAL.

For standing-up and sitting-down, the patient required assistance with Primewalk while he was independent in the use of WPAL. Consecutive walking with WPAL was lasted for 40 min and 580 m. Consecutive walking distance and time were several-fold longer with WPAL compared with Primewalk.

3.5 ADVANTAGES TO INTRODUCE ROBOTICS TO SCI GAIT RECONSTRUCTION

As trials for gait reconstruction in paraplegics, orthoses, functional electrical stimulation (FES) (CS; (2005)), or hybrid assistive systems (HAS), which combine FES and an orthosis (Popovic; (1989)), have been used. An orthosis, providing standing stability, maintains stance stability in the stance phase and smooth clearance in the swing phase by restriction of the DOF in the lower extremities. However, restriction of the DOF to fix the knee in an extension position causes difficulties in standing up and sitting down.

Since paraplegics lack power in the lower extremities, the upper extremities are mostly used for progression and lateral motion of the body in orthotic walking, which places a large burden on the upper extremities and high energy consumption in walking (Suzuki; (2007)) making it difficult to continue walking for a long distance without rest.

Subject was able to stand and walk independently with the WPAL that we developed. The sit-to-stand motion requires the largest torque for knee joint movement, and it has been postulated that torque of 12–50 N is required for one knee to achieve standing from a seated position on a regular height chair. (Yoshioka; (2007)) Since design of the WPAL was focused on small size, light weighted and ability to be used with a wheelchair, the largest torque of the developed knee joint motor produced 33 N, which was not considered sufficient. However, standing from a wheelchair with the support of the upper extremities with a walker was smoothly achieved, and the subject felt that the burden on the upper extremities was not large.

Recently, as a trial to apply robotic engineering for reconstruction of paraplegic gait, a system to control knee and hip joints with a motor (RGO) (Ohta; (2007)) and a robot to regulate hip and knee joints (ReWalk) (Medgadget; (2008)) have been developed. However, taking into account compatibility with a wheelchair, it would be necessary to develop a robot adopting the medial system.

Consecutive walking distance and time was lengthened several-fold with WPAL compared with Primewalk. It was presumed that a reduced burden on the upper extremities during walking enabled continuous walking. Swinging lower extremities in walking with an orthosis becomes a pendulum movement due to gravity. Therefore, it is necessary to keep the trunk ahead of the lower extremities and support most of the weight of the trunk tilted to the anterior side with the upper extremities using a cane or an orthosis. (Saitoh; (1997)) The addition of power to the lower extremities can reduce the anterior tilting of the trunk and the burden on the upper extremities.

Walking with an orthosis without free ROM in knee and foot joints presented a large problem. Toe clearance can be obtained by knee flexion and ankle dorsiflexion at the initial stage of the swing phase in the normal gait. Sufficient clearance has not been obtained during the swing because of the extended knee and fixed ankle joints with an orthosis, making the length of the swing phase equal to that of the stance leg. Therefore, as compensatory movement, it is necessary to elevate the trunk on the swing side by bending the trunk toward the stance leg. This movement uses muscles of the upper extremities and places a large burden on the upper extremities. In walking, this is the state where pushing-up is repeated for lateral bending of the trunk.

This problem has been addressed through the design of the WPAL. The functional length of the lower extremities in the swing phase was shortened by adding the free ROM and power source to the knees and feet as a robot, which enabled swinging without large lateral bending of the trunk.

3.6 CONCLUSION

We reviewed orthotic gait reconstruction for SCI. We introduced Primewalk orthosis that widely used in Japan. Primewalk has benefit in standing stability and wheelchair compatibility. Also we are now introducing a robot WPAL.

Consecutive walking distance with WPAL was increased several-fold compared with Primewalk. These results suggested the possibility that walking with WPAL placed a lower burden on the upper extremities. In further development of the WPAL, we would like to focus on patients' practical use by enabling them to accomplish comfortable walking patterns safely. Further work will include reducing the weight of the product including control unit; elaborating the sensor system; and adding a stair-climbing function. We will also attempt to develop trunk supporting unit adapted for patients with high-thoracic lesions as well as cervical lesions.

ACKNOWLEDGMENT

This work was partially supported by the Grant-in-Aid 2005–2007 (P. 05026) and 2008-2009 (No. 04010065) of New Energy and Industrial Technology Development Organization (NEDO), Japan.

We extend our thanks profoundly to all of the members of WPAL projects including participants.

References

Kunkel CF, Scremin AME, Eisenberg B, Gracia JF, Roberts S, Martinez S (1993). Effect of standing on spasiticity, contracture, and osteoporosis in paralysed males. Arch Phys Med Rehab 74: 73–78.

Kaplan P, Gandhabadi B, Goldschmidt L (1978). Calcium balance in paraplegic patients: influence of injury duration and ambulation. Arch Phys Med Rehab 59: 447–450.

Messenger N, Rithalia SVS, Bowker P, Ogilvie C (1989). Effect of ambulation on the blood flow in paralysed limbs. J Biomed Eng 27: 70–75.

Cybulski GR , Jeager RJ. Standing performance of persons with paraplegia (1986). Arch Phys Med Rehab 67: 103-108.

Stallard J, Major RE, Patrick JH (1989). A review of the fundamental design problem of providing ambulation for paraplegic patients. Paraplegia 27: 70–75.

Subbarao JV (1991). Walking after spinal cord injury- Goal or wish? West J Med 154: 612–614.

Major RE, Stallard J, Rose GK (1981). The dynamics of walking using the hip guidance orthosis (HGO) with crutches. Prosthet Orthot Int 5:19–22.

Douglas R, Larson PF, D'Ambrosia R, McCall RE (1983). The LSU reciprocation gait orthosis. Orthopedics 6:834–9.

Jefferson RJ, Whittle MW (1990). Performance of three walking orthoses for the paralyzed: a case study using gait analysis. Prosthet Orthot Int 14:103–110.

Saitoh E, Sonoda S, Imahori R, Sarai S, Suzuki M, Baba M, Domen K, Tomita Y, Hayashi M, Tatematsu K (1992). A Power-Assisted Modified Medial Single Hip Joint for Paraplegic Walking. IXth World Congress of International Society for Prosthetics and Orthotics; 1998 June; Amsterdam: North-Holland p355–6.

Saitoh E, Suzuki T, Sonoda S, Fujitani J, Tomita Y, Chino N (1996). Clinical experience with a new hip-knee-ankle-foot orthotic system using a medial single hip joint for paraplegic standing and walking. Am J Phys Med Rehabil 75: 198–203.

Saitoh E, Baba M, Sonoda S, Tomita Y, Suzuki M, Hayashi M (1997). A New Medial Single Hip Joint for Paraplegic Walkers. In: Ueda S, Nakmura R, Ishigami N, editors. 8th World Congress of International Rehabilitation Medicine Association. Bologna: Italy, p1299–1305.

Suzuki T, Sonoda S, Saitoh E, Onogi K, Fujino H, Teranishi T, Oyobe T, Katoh M, Ohtsuka K (2007). Prediction of gait outcome with the knee-ankle-foot orthosis with medial hip joint in patients with spinal cord injuries: a study using recursive partitioning analysis. Spinal Cord. 45:57–63.

Greene PJ, Granat MH (2003). A knee and ankle flexing hybrid orthosis for paraplegic ambulation. Med Eng Phys. 25:539–45.

Greene PJ, Granat MH(2000). The effects of knee and ankle flexion on ground clearance in paraplegic gait. Clin Biomech. 15:536–40.

Kagawa T. Uno Y. Muraoka Y. Saitoh E (2007). A human interface predicting intended strides for a paraplegic locomotor device. The 3rd International Symposium on Measurement, Analysis and Modeling of Human Functions. Lisbon: Portogal; 2007, p189–196.

To CS, Kirsch RF, Kobetic R, Triolo RJ (2005). Simulation of a functional neuromuscular stimulation powered mechanical gait orthosis with coordinated joint locking. IEEE Trans Neural Syst Rehabil Eng. 13:227–35.

Popovic D, Tomovic R, Schwirtlich L (1989). Hybrid assistive system–the motor neuroprosthesis. IEEE Trans Biomed Eng. 36:729–37.

Yoshioka S, Nagano A, Himeno R, Fukashiro S (2007). Computation of the kinematics and the minimum peak joint moments of sit-to-stand movements. Biomed Eng Online. 3; 6:26, 2007. Available from: URL: http://www.pubmedcentral.nih.gov/ articlerender.fcgi?tool=pubmed&pubmedid=17608922

Ohta Y, Yano H, Suzuki R, Yoshida M, Kawashima N, Nakazawa K (2007). A two-degree-of-freedom motor-powered gait orthosis for spinal cord injury patients. Proc Inst Mech Eng H. 221:629–39. http://medgadget.com/archives/2008/03/rewalk_exoskeleton.html

Chapter Four

Robot-Assisted Rehabilitation of Hand Function After Stroke with the HapticKnob and the HandCARE

Olivier Lambercy[*,†], Ludovic Dovat[†], Berna Salman[‡], Roger Gassert[*], Theodore E. Milner[§], Etienne Burdet[**] and Chee Leong Teo[†]

[*] *Rehabilitation Engineering Lab, ETH Zurich, Switzerland*
[†] *Department of Mechanical Engineering, National University of Singapore, Singapore*
[‡] *Department of Biomedical Physiology and Kinesiology, Simon Fraser University, Canada*
[§] *Department of Kinesiology and Physical Education, McGill University, Canada*
[**] *Department of Bioengineering, Imperial College London, UK*

4.1 INTRODUCTION

Robot-assisted rehabilitation is one of the most promising approaches to complement current clinical strategies for stroke rehabilitation. It could increase the intensity of therapy with affordable costs, and offer advantages such as (i) precisely controllable assistance/resistance during movements, (ii) good repeatability, (iii) objective and quantifiable measures of subject performance, and (iv) increased training motivation through the use of interactive feedback, such as virtual reality environments and stimulation of afferent pathways.

Over the last decades, upper limb robot-assisted rehabilitation after stroke has focused mainly on restoring arm function, yielding promising results that illustrate the potential of robots to complement traditional therapies and support stroke rehabilitation (Prange *et al.* (2006), Kwakkel *et al.* (2008)). However, arm function alone is not sufficient to perform most activities of daily living (ADL), such as eating/drinking, writing/typing and personal hygiene. In fact, hand function is fundamental to all these daily activities. These observations motivated us to develop robot-assisted rehabilitation strategies focusing on the distal parts of the upper extremity, i.e. the wrist, hand and fingers.

Biomechatronics in Medicine and Healthcare by Le Li and Raymond Kai-Yu Tong

www.panstanford.com
978-981-4241-61-8

A questionnaire given to a population of 27 stroke subjects illustrated that hand tasks such as handwriting, typing, and operating knobs and buttons are activities that stroke survivors find difficult and would like to recover most (Dovat *et al.* (2006)). This prompted us to develop robotic devices to train similar functional tasks. However, such hand activities are complex, require precise control and/or coordination of the forearm, wrist and fingers and involve a large number of joints. Further, hand activities also require contribution of the elbow and shoulder to support the weight and properly position the hand.

A possible approach is to decompose complex hand tasks into a combination of simple subtasks to be trained individually. For example, the task of operating a door knob can be decomposed into a series of subtasks (i) reaching for the knob, (ii) grasping the knob, (iii) turning the knob, and (iv) releasing the knob. These subtasks can be trained separately with dedicated interfaces and exercises (Fig. 4.1). Recent studies on rehabilitation of arm function in stroke patients did not yield better results in terms of motor improvement compared to complex tasks were trained directly (Krebs *et al.* (2008)); however, this presents the advantage of simplifying both the robot design and the implementation of exercises.

In order to optimize rehabilitation of hand function, patients should be able to train at home or in decentralized centers, in the context of their daily activities. Because this would limit transportation costs, be less disruptive to the patient and require only minimal (or remote) supervision from a therapist, it might allow the intensity and duration of therapy to be increased without increasing the costs. To facilitate their acceptance, rehabilitation robots should be designed with a human centered approach, focusing on stroke patients' needs and desires. They should

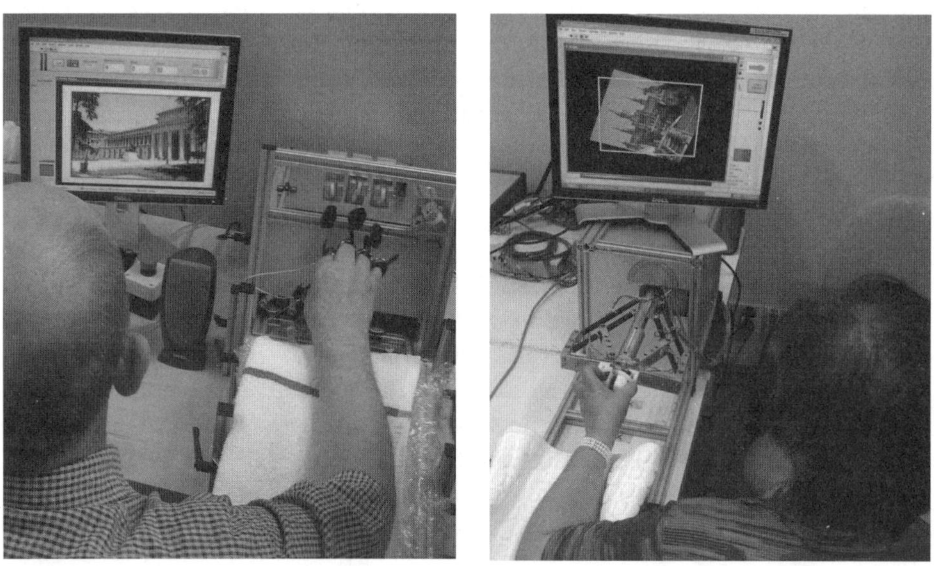

Figure 4.1 The *HandCARE* and the *HapticKnob*, two complementary robotic systems for rehabilitation of hand function.

also be compact, safe when used by the patient alone, "plug and play" on a personal computer, simple to use, adaptable to the user, and relatively inexpensive for patients or rehabilitation centers to buy or rent.

This chapter gives an overview of the challenges of robot-assisted rehabilitation of hand function after stroke. Two robotic devices we have designed for rehabilitation of hand function, the HapticKnob and the HandCARE, are then presented, and strategies for hand rehabilitation using such devices are discussed. Finally, the principal findings of clinical studies with the two systems are presented to illustrate the potential and future challenges of robot-assisted rehabilitation of hand function after stroke.

4.2 HAND FUNCTION AFTER STROKE

The hand is a fascinating neuromechanical system and a defining characteristic of humans. The ability to position the thumb in opposition to the other fingers in order to grasp objects is a unique characteristic of the human species, which is believed to have played a decisive role in our evolution. *Precision grip*, employed where fine motion and force are required, and *power grip*, employed to generate high force, provide the basis for almost all prehensile tasks used in ADL, such as eating, manipulating tools or enabling communication with each other, for example through gestures and writing. In addition to its motor function, the human hand acts as a sensory organ during tactile exploration of the environment, which is possible because of the high density of cutaneous sensory receptors in the fingertips. Tactile sensation is capable of replacing vision when this sense is impaired or unreliable. The hand is central to human psychology, as it is used in executive, perceptual and expressive activities (Valero-Cuevas (2009)).

Because of its direct control by the motor cortex, the hand is usually impaired after a stroke. Different dysfunctions such as muscle weakness, spasticity and compulsory co-activation of anatomical muscles at multiple joints contribute to impairment of finger and hand function after stroke (Fugl-Meyer *et al.* (1975)). Extension, abduction, and adduction of the fingers are particularly impaired, leaving the fingers in a flexed finger posture (Hunter and Crome (2002)).

In terms of function, damage to the sensorimotor system leads to specific impairments of the hand that include (i) limited ability to open the hand or position the thumb in opposition to the other fingers, which is the basis for all types of grasp (Kamper *et al.* (2006), Cruz *et al.* (2005), Dovat *et al.* (2007)), (ii) loss of finger independence, limiting the ability to move and generate force independently with individual fingers (Lang and Schieber (2004), Raghavan *et al.* (2006), Schieber *et al.* (2009)) and (iii) inability to control finger force and explore the environment, due to insufficient tactile sensation and impaired sensorimotor translation. These impairments result in difficulties in grasping and manipulating objects, leading to slow and uncoordinated movements.

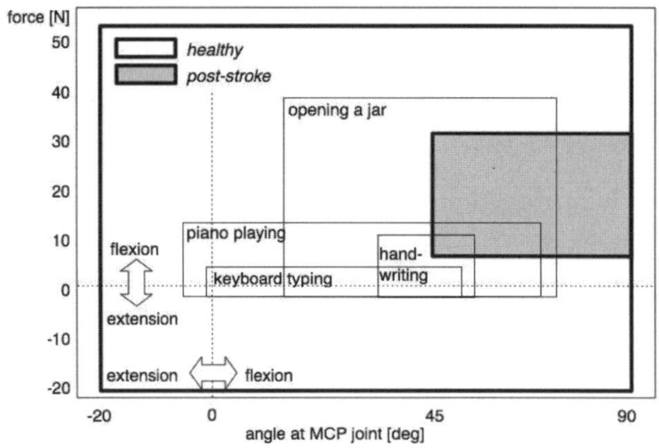

Figure 4.2 Finger range of motion (x-axis: angle at the Metacarpophalangeal (MCP) joint) and force (y- axis: force at the fingertips) required to complete typical ADL. The white square (thick outline) represents the performances of healthy subjects, in terms of maximal extension/flexion movement and force, while the black square represents the limited performances of poststroke subjects with mild impairments. Performances are based on actual data from the participants of the research study presented in this chapter (7 chronic stroke patients), while the range of motion and force required to complete the ADL are empirical. Post-stroke subjects are unable to completely perform the selected activities.

These impairments are often linked and severely limit stroke survivors' ability to perform ADL. Figure 4.2 summarizes data from stroke patients to illustrate how limited they are in performing typical activities requiring hand movements such as in typing, writing or opening a jar.

The principal challenge of hand rehabilitation after stroke is thus to restore grasping function and hand-wrist coordination, which are required to manipulate objects and essential for ADL. In addition, fine finger control should be addressed as it plays a crucial role in tactile exploration, manipulation of small objects and fine motor tasks such as handwriting. However, for the more severely impaired subjects, hand rehabilitation has to begin by training hand opening and working on overcoming flexor muscle synergies that prevent subjects from performing almost any type of activity with their hand.

4.3 ROBOT-ASSISTED REHABILITATION OF HAND FUNCTION

Robotic devices developed for arm and, more recently, for wrist rehabilitation, obtained promising results, suggesting that robot-assisted treatment may lead to increased gain relative to traditional therapy, which motivates the development of new devices dedicated to hand rehabilitation (Takahashi *et al.* (2008), Hesse *et al.* (2003), Lambercy *et al.* (2009)) (Fig. 4.3).

The HWARD (Takahashi *et al.* (2005)) and the GENTLE/G (Loureiro and Harwin (2007)) are examples of actuated exoskeletons designed to train grasping and releasing of objects, while the Gifu Haptic Interface (Kawasaki *et al.* (2007)) is

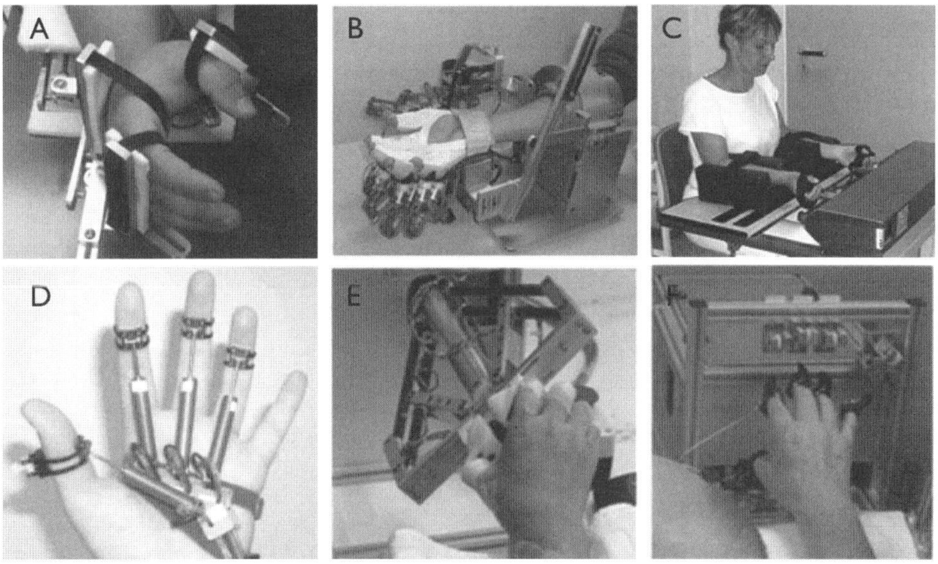

Figure 4.3 Hand rehabilitation robots. UC Irvine's HWARD (A) (Takahashi *et al.* (2005)), Gifu Haptic Interface (B) (Kawasaki *et al.* (2007)), BiManuTrack (C) (Hesse *et al.* (2003)), the Rutgers Master II (D) (Bouzit *et al.* (2002)), as well as our HapticKnob (E) (Lambercy *et al.* (2007)) and HandCARE (F) (Dovat *et al.* (2008)).

an exoskeleton designed to train movement of each finger individually. Exoskeleton devices usually are complex mechanical structures with multiple degrees-of-freedom (DOF), controlling several joints. Such systems have the advantage of precisely controlling subjects' movements and providing assistance in performing complex tasks, but it is difficult to adapt them to stroke patients with different hand sizes and impairments, and they suffer from inertia and friction due to the large number of joints.

On the other hand, end-effector robots such as the BiManuTrack (Hesse *et al.* (2003)), or the Rutgers Master II (Bouzit *et al.* (2002)) interact with the user only at the level of the hand or fingers. This may offer a more flexible solution with fewer mechanical constraints on how the movement is performed, corresponding better to manipulation of real objects in everyday life. Furthermore, end-effector devices are usually mechanically simpler, easier to use and more compact, which are important considerations for the deployment of robotic devices in rehabilitation centers or patients' homes. Following such an approach, we have developed and clinically evaluated the HapticKnob, and the HandCARE, two complementary end-effector based rehabilitation devices to train hand and finger function.

4.3.1 The HapticKnob

The HapticKnob is a 2 DOF robotic device for training grasping in coordination with pronation and supination of the forearm. A linear DOF enables opening and closing of the hand, and a rotational DOF provides pronation and supination around the long axis of the forearm. The HapticKnob uses two moving parallelograms similar to an umbrella, on which the user places the fingers (Fig. 4.3E). Fixtures of different size and shape can be attached to train various functionally relevant grips such as power grasp, precision grip or lateral pinch. The device can generate forces of up to 50 N in both opening and closing directions and torques of up to 1.5 Nm in pronation and supination.

Four force sensors are incorporated into the structure to measure grasping forces of up to 30 N applied by the subject. Various force effects can be implemented, e.g. to resist or assist movement as a function of the user's impairment in an assist-as-needed manner. This robot has dimensions of $60\times30\times25$ cm^3 and can easily be transported and set up in minimal time. Further information on the HapticKnob can be found in (Lambercy *et al.* (2007)).

4.3.2 The HandCARE

The HandCARE is a cable driven robotic device, where each fingertip is attached to a cable loop, connected to a single motor, allowing predominantly linear displacement corresponding to finger flexion/extension (Fig. 4.3(F)). The interface can thus assist the subject in hand opening and closing movements. Instead of using five actuators, a clutch system has been developed, which simplifies the control of the robotic device and reduces the cost. The clutch allows switching between three modes, (i) active, where the torque generated by the motor is transmitted to the finger, (ii) fixed, where no finger movement is possible and force control can be trained isometrically, and (iii) free, where the finger can be moved freely along the path of the cable. This clutch system makes training of different movements possible with only one actuator and one clutch per finger. It is thus possible to train grasping and precision grip as well as fractionation, i.e. independent movement or isometric force training of each finger, thereby increasing strength in individual muscles and coordination between fingers.

The active workspace consists of five linear paths of 8 cm length corresponding to a finger extension/flexion angle range of $0 - 70^\circ$ at the metacarpophalangeal (MCP) joint. The maximal continuous force that can be generated in flexion or extension is 15 N per finger (up to 75 N if only one finger is actuated), while inherent friction is less than 0.8 N in any position of the workspace. Forces applied at the fingertips during the exercises can be recorded by a sensing system measuring the tension in the cable attached to each finger. Further information on the HandCARE can be found in (Dovat *et al.* (2008)).

4.3.3 Rehabilitation Exercises and Strategies

Robotic devices offer a large number of new modalities for the treatment of stroke patients, but interactive, motivating and task oriented exercise programs are critical for subjects to use a rehabilitation robot to its full potential. We review here some concepts that should be considered for the design and implementation of exercises for hand rehabilitation.

Passive and active exercises are currently used in robot-assisted rehabilitation (Marchal-Crespo and Reinkensmeyer (2009)), with robots producing assistive or resistive forces, or more sophisticated assist-as-needed strategies, or event related assistance based on brain or muscle activity. Typically, at an early stage in stroke recovery, movements such as finger extension can only be performed passively, i.e., the robot has to move the fingers in order to compensate for the weakness in finger extensors observed in stroke subjects. In this phase, it is crucial that the robot monitors the interaction forces and gently moves the fingers.

However, passive movements driven by robotic interfaces may not be sufficient for hand rehabilitation; while passive movements contribute to reducing muscle tone and maintaining passive properties of joints and muscles (Hesse *et al.* (2003)), active movements initiated by the subject are required to promote correct patterns of muscle activation and improve strength (Hogan *et al.* (2006), Woldag *et al.* (2007)), which are crucial to dexterous manipulation.

Furthermore, active participation of the subject during training is fundamental to skill acquisition (Winstein *et al.* (2003)). Motor recovery after stroke is considered as a form of motor learning, where undamaged brain regions are recruited to generate motor commands to the same muscles that were used before the injury. It may, therefore, be advantageous to apply the motor learning principles observed in healthy subjects to improve stroke rehabilitation. Note that active participation can also be achieved during passive exercises by giving subjects proper instructions, but movements remain limited by the passive guidance and are thus far from real activities. In this sense, therapy should focus on intensive repetition of active movements where subjects interact with various force fields to help develop strategies that will be optimal for improving hand function in ADL (Krakauer (2006), Reinkensmeyer *et al.* (2004)).

However, intensive repetition of movements involving the impaired limb require considerable effort by the subject and may be painful and tiring. Additionally, after several repetitions, subjects may get bored, leading to decreased concentration and motivation to train, thus affecting the quality of the therapy.

Motivation is important to ensure that subjects are engaged and train at their full potential during therapy sessions, pushing the limits imposed by their impairment. A common way to keep subjects motivated during intense movement repetitions in the use of interactive feedback. Visual feedback is widely used in robot-assisted rehabilitation systems, and is probably the simplest way to interact with a user. Moreover, exercises with visual feedback or virtual environments may help improve the outcome of post-stroke rehabilitation, by augmenting subjects' awareness of their actual performance, and promoting visuomotor coordination (Henderson *et al.* (2007), Holden (2005)).

Robotic devices have the advantage of providing haptic feedback, i.e. specific force and/or torque patterns that can stimulate proprioceptive sensors in skin, joints and muscles to increase subjects' awareness and use of somatosensory information. Similarly, tactile feedback can be used to restore sensation in the impaired limb; typically small vibrator motors can be taped on the subject's hand or arm to stimulate the skin when a task is successfully performed.

Motivating rehabilitation exercises may be implemented as goal-oriented therapeutic games with a score indicative of the performance, and the possibility to choose between different levels of difficulty adapted to the impairment level. Indeed, therapeutic programs that build on a base of successively more demanding performance levels and that promote a sense of personal responsibility for accomplishment is believed to be more successful and motivating (Lewthwaite (1990), Johnson (2006)). It is debatable how sophisticated and complex these virtual reality environments need to be as stroke patients are typically older and do not have previous experience with video games, may suffer from cognitive deficits, and fatigue easily.

Exercises implemented on the HapticKnob and the HandCARE follow this concept, progressively requiring more accuracy or more force for successful completion. Simple and intuitive visual feedback is used, consisting of selected pictures that are visually scaled or rotated as a function of the motor task performed on the robot. Figure 4.4 illustrates the display presented to the subject during an exercise with the HapticKnob, where the objective is to perform pronation and supination movements with the forearm. The orientation and brightness of the picture are modulated as a function of the rotation angle of the robot, such that when the target is reached the picture is oriented normally. In addition to being intuitive, this approach offers subjects the possibility of training with personally selected pictures to further increase motivation and engagement in the therapy, i.e. photo of the family members or of places the patient would like to travel to (Lambercy *et al.* (2007b)).

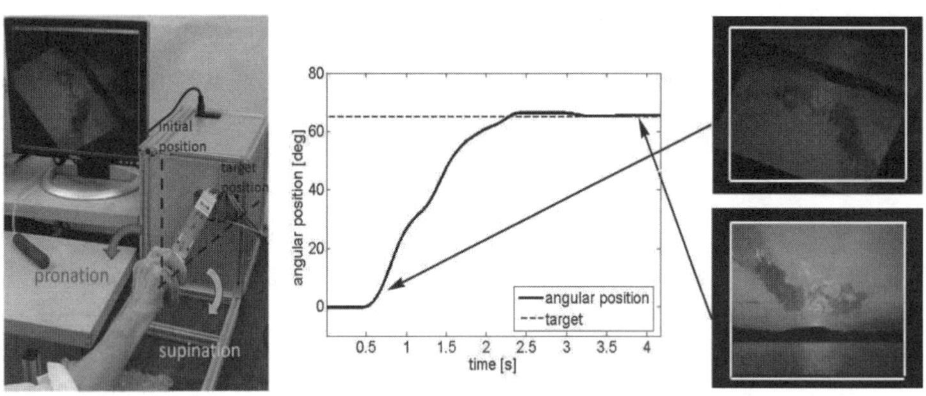

Figure 4.4 Angular position of the HapticKnob during an exercise training pronation/supination movements. Visual feedback is given by means of a picture whose orientation and brightness are modulated as a function of the angular position of the wrist.

4.4 PROMISES OF ROBOT-ASSISTED THERAPY OF HAND FUNCTION

This section presents some of the outcomes of clinical studies performed with the HapticKnob and the HandCARE, and discusses the potential of these robotic devices to restore hand function of chronic stroke survivors.

In a first pilot study, four chronic post-stroke subjects, more than 2 years after stroke (P1-P4, 54–83 years of age, 1 female) participated in an eight-week rehabilitation therapy, training a combination of exercises with the HapticKnob and the HandCARE. All subjects were right-handed and suffered from right hemiparesis. Participants were eligible for the study if they had a minimum manual muscle testing (MMT) level of 3 (i.e. able to move the arm against gravity, but not able to tolerate resistance), no more than level 2 spasticity in hand and arm muscles measured by the Modified Ashworth Scale (MAS, range [0-5], (Bohannon and Smith (1987))) and presented no other neurological disorder such as apraxia or tremor. They were able to move the right arm and hand, but had difficulties in performing many typical ADL.

Therapy sessions were given twice a week, and consisted of 20 minutes of training with the HandCARE followed by 20 minutes of training with the HapticKnob. Therapy was tailored to the subject's level of impairment, and consisted of exercises training sensorimotor function where subjects had to actively perform grasping movements and forearm pronation/supination with the HapticKnob. Exercises with the HandCARE focused on fine motor control by training finger coordination, and generation of independent finger force.

All stroke subjects improved their performance in the different exercises during the robot-assisted therapy, which was accompanied by improved hand motor function and force control.

4.4.1 *Improvement in Motor Function*

In an exercise to train forearm pronation/supination with the HapticKnob, patients were asked to reach a target forearm orientation by turning the knob against a resistive load, simulating the action of turning a door knob. The first movement was always supination, starting from the rest position of the forearm (full pronation). Once the target was reached, the image on the monitor was reoriented to require an identical returning movement in pronation for realignment. Figure 4.5 illustrates the evolution of a pronation movement from beginning to the end of therapy.

Stroke subjects found supination more difficult than pronation, which can be explained by abnormally high elbow flexor muscle activity increasing the difficulty of controlling fine movements in supination. However, significant improvements were found for the supination movement, which was the major goal of the exercise. In average, the time required to perform the "twisting" movement significantly decreased for both supination (−25%) and pronation (−13%) (Fig. 4.5(C)). However,

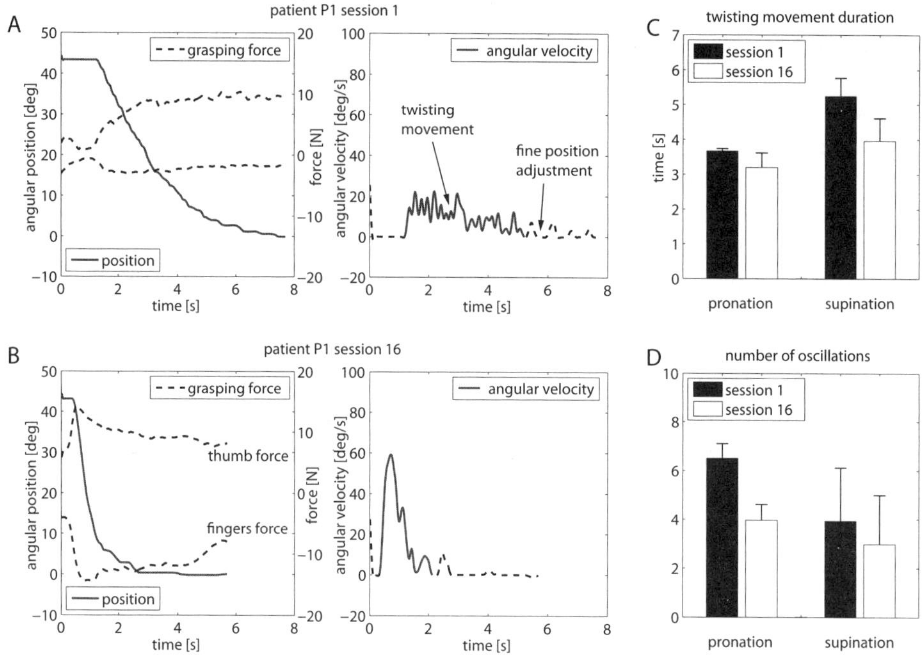

Figure 4.5 Angular position, grasping force and angular velocity during a representative pronation movement with the HapticKnob for stroke subject P1 (male, 63 years old and 2 years post-stroke) in the first (A) and last session of robot-assisted therapy (B). The duration of the twisting movement (C, mean over all patients) as well as the oscillations around the target (D, mean over all patients) decrease for both pronation and supination, while the coordination between forces applied by thumb and fingers increases.

even after training, the movement duration was longer than for healthy subjects of the same age group. In addition to the increase in speed, the number of oscillations to adjust the position around the target orientation decreased (−62% in supination and −24% in pronation, Fig. 4.5(D)). These results illustrate an important improvement in movement precision and control during tasks involving hand and forearm coordination.

Similar results were observed in finger movements trained with the HandCARE. In an exercise where subjects were asked to actively extend and then flex the fingers together, i.e. all fingers moving at the same time, we observed significant improvement in the coordination between the fingers (+31% during extension and +54% during flexion of the fingers). Control of finger motion also improved during the therapy, as we observed smoother movements (+6.2% and +1.4% in extension and flexion respectively).

4.4.2 Improved Force Control

Finger independence and finger force generation were trained with the HandCARE. Subjects were instructed to select different letters on a monitor in order

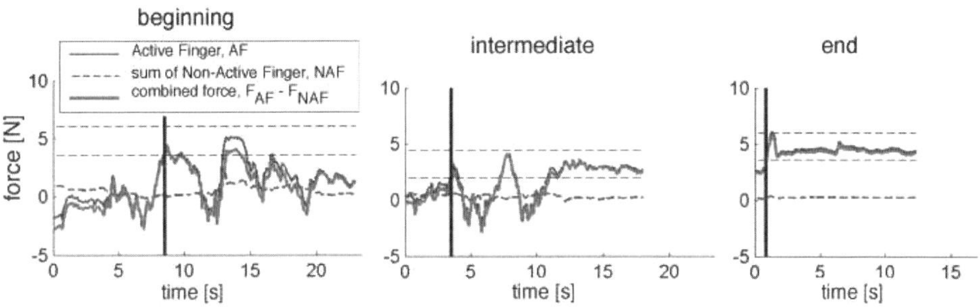

Figure 4.6 Comparison of fingertip force of stroke patient P3 (female, 83 years old and 6 years post-stroke) between the beginning (left), the middle (middle) and the end (right) of the training while the subject had to reach and maintain a target force (between dotted lines) with the index finger (AF in the figure). Forces of the AF and the NAF as well as the combined force are displayed.

to compose a specific word associated with a picture, e.g. the name of a city. While fingers were maintained in a fixed position by the HandCARE, letters were selected by isometrically applying a certain amount of force with a specific finger, i.e. Active Finger (AF), and by minimizing the force applied by the other fingers, i.e. Non- Active Fingers (NAF). The training was focused on the tripod thumb-index-middle as these fingers are most commonly used in ADL.

One stroke subject with limited finger impairment performed this exercise during the entire 8 weeks of therapy. With training, the number of successful trials (i.e. correctly selected letter) increased for these three fingers (+16% for the thumb, +28% for the index, and +29% for the middle finger). The time to perform a successful trial was also significantly reduced (−45%), which indicates that the subject felt more comfortable with the exercise and was able to better control forces generated by these fingers. This suggests that an intense isometric force training promotes recovery of finger function.

Figure 4.6 illustrates how the force applied by the NAF tends to decrease with training when the index finger produces force.

A similar exercise to train the regulation of power grasp force with the HapticKnob illustrated improvement in the ability to generate, quickly adjust and maintain precise grasping force.

4.4.3 Evolution in Muscle Activity Patterns

To determine whether post-stroke subjects were more limited in their ability to modify patterns of muscle activation than age-matched healthy subjects, we computed the principal components of the root-mean-squared (RMS) electromyography (EMG) of 8 muscles of the hand and forearm during the performance of the different exercises. We assumed that greater limitation would be evident as a higher percentage of the variance being accounted for by fewer principal components (PCs). We compared the number of PCs needed to account for at least

95% of the variance in the EMG. We found that in all cases only one or two PCs were needed and that this did not differ between post-stroke and healthy subjects. Therefore, we have no evidence that post-stroke subjects are any more limited in their ability to modify patterns of muscle activation than aged-matched healthy subjects. Because PC1 always accounted for more than 75% of the variance, we concluded that the individual exercises were generally performed using only one predominant pattern of muscle activation, both in the case of healthy and post-stroke subjects.

Although only one PC accounted for most of the variance, the profile of this PC (PC1) was quite different for exercises performed with the HandCARE compared to the HapticKnob (Fig. 4.7(A)) Given that the RMS-EMG was normalized with respect to maximal voluntary contraction prior to conducting the principal component analysis, the weighting coefficients of PC1 represent the relative activation of each muscle in the predominant activation pattern. In the example of Fig. 4.7(A), which represents muscle activity patterns prior to the robot-assisted rehabilitation, the PC1 profile shows that the forearm supinator, biceps (BI), and the finger abductor, first dorsal interosseus (1DI), are the primary muscles contributing to the pattern for the HapticKnob exercises training grasping and pronation/supination. For the HandCARE exercises training finger movement coordination, all of the finger muscles (1DI, FDS, EDC, ADM) contribute relatively equally and their contribution is greater than that of the wrist muscles (ECR and FCU). However, the biceps is the most active muscle, which represents abnormal activation. After the robot-assisted rehabilitation (Fig. 4.7(B)) the activity of the biceps activity in PC1 was the lowest of all the muscles, indicating that this aspect of the abnormal activation patterns had improved with the robot-assisted rehabilitation.

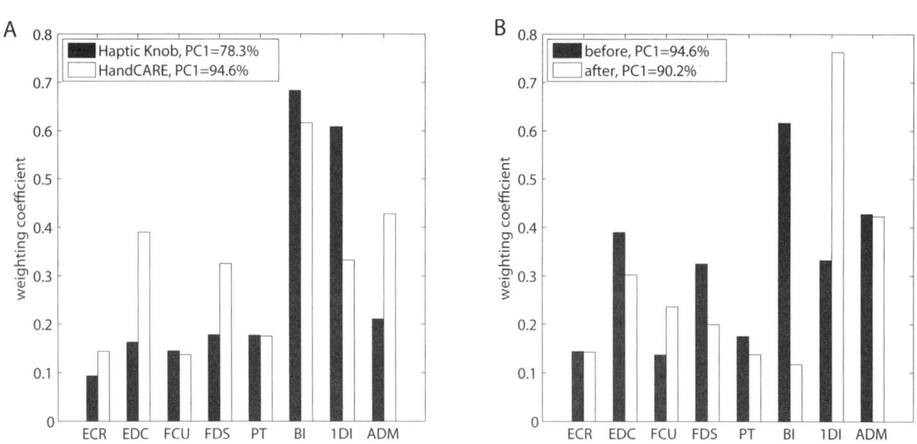

Figure 4.7 PC1 of a stroke patient (P1) pre-rehab muscle activity from PCAs for exercises with the HapticKnob and with the HandCARE (A). Comparison of PC1 of a stroke patient (P1) muscle activity during a grasping exercise with the HandCARE before and after robot-assisted therapy (B).

4.4.4 Improvement in Outcome Measures

Upper limb impairment was assessed before and after the therapy using the Chedoke-McMaster Impairment Inventory (CMMII) (Gowland *et al.* (1993)), where the impairment is scaled from stage 1 (severe impairment) to stage 7 (mild impairment). Robot-assisted training resulted in direct benefits in ADL for the four subjects, and in a reduction of their impairments. A mean improvement of +1.05 stages (+25%) was observed in the four patients who participated to the pilot study. Figure 4.8(A) presents the evolution of CMMII scores for the four stroke patients.

In addition, patients reported improvement in their daily activities at home; they felt more secure in grasping and manipulating objects, more skillful in fine motor tasks such as manipulating buttons or handwriting, and started to use their impaired hand more, which we believe is crucial for further improvement.

These preliminary results motivated a larger clinical study with the HapticKnob. Nine subjects (59.4 ± 12.3 years, 5 females) at the chronic post-stroke stage, 3 right and 6 left hemiparetic, participated in this study. Subjects participated in a one-hour session 3 times a week over a period of 6 weeks, resulting altogether in 18 sessions during which they trained with the HapticKnob. Evolution in arm and hand motor function was assessed using clinical tests including the Fugl-Meyer arm motor scale (FM, range [0-66], (Fugl-Meyer *et al.* (1975))). After 6 weeks of therapy with the HapticKnob, a mean increase of 4.3 points (+14%) was observed in the FM scores, with a maximum improvement of 11 points in one of the patients (Fig. 4.8(B)), which confirmed positive results obtained in the first study with the HandCARE and the HapticKnob (Lambercy *et al.* (2009)).

These results suggest that an intensive and repetitive training program improves motor function in chronic stroke subjects long after completion of con-

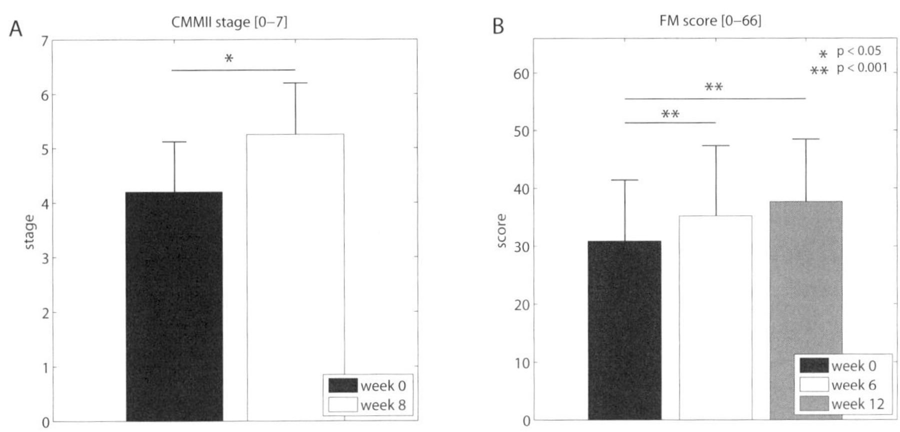

Figure 4.8 Evolution in clinical outcomes after robot-assisted rehabilitation of hand function, during the first clinical study with the HapticKnob and the HandCARE (A) and during the second study with the HapticKnob (B).

ventional therapy. These improvements correspond to a noticeable increase of hand and arm function of stroke survivors, and are in accordance with results obtained in other robot- assisted studies on upper limb rehabilitation of chronic stroke patients. Further, the observed improvements in arm and hand function were found to be maintained after the completion of the therapy, suggesting long term improvement in motor abilities.

4.5 CONCLUSIONS

This chapter offered an overview of the field of robot-assisted rehabilitation of hand function after stroke, by presenting the challenges of restoring fine hand movement and sensation, as well as describing two novel robotic devices developed to train hand and fingers, the HapticKnob and the HandCARE. These robots are based on an end-effector approach, i.e. interacting with the user only at the level of the hand or finger, which we believe provides more freedom and comfort for subjects to perform the required tasks, corresponds better to real interaction with objects during ADL, and also significantly decreases complexity and cost of robotic systems. Two clinical studies have been performed with chronic stroke survivors to determine the potential of our approach and these devices to restore hand sensorimotor function.

First, results of both studies show that robot-assisted rehabilitation with our robots was safe and well accepted by stroke survivors. All patients actively participated in the therapy and completed the study. They found the proposed exercises motivating and useful, eventually asking for more therapy time with the robots. This suggests that the stroke population is ready to accept robot-assisted rehabilitation as a new therapy standard in rehabilitation centers or at home.

Improvements in sensorimotor function of arm and hand were observed in all participants, which illustrates that an intensive and repetitive training program leads to improvement in motor function in chronic stroke subjects even long after completion of conventional therapy, suggesting long term improvement in the motor condition. Although most subjects reached a plateau, several subjects continued to significantly improve their arm and hand motor function after completion of the robot-assisted therapy. This may be due to an increased use of the impaired limb in daily activities at home, mediated by the motor improvements obtained during the therapy, and increased confidence in their motor abilities.

In most robot-assisted studies where only shoulder and elbow were trained, improvement in clinical assessments were mainly observed at the level of the upper arm, and only minimal change was observed in the components relative to the hand (Krebs *et al.* (2007); Volpe *et al.* (2008)). While upper arm training may lead to an increase in arm function, the benefits in subjects' ability to perform ADL may be limited without a similar increase in wrist and hand function. On the other hand, studies on robot- assisted training of hand and wrist function showed an increase in all arm segments (Krebs *et al.* (2007); Takahashi *et al.* (2008)).

Distal arm training involves activation of nerves and muscles in each segment of the upper limb, and consequently results in proximal as well as distal muscle activity. Furthermore, while training with end-effector based robots, subjects used their entire arm to perform the required tasks, thus involving elbow and shoulder, typically to stabilize the arm. Training distal segments of the upper limb may thus help improve arm function in a more homogeneous way and may lead to greater improvement in ADL.

Altogether, our results illustrate the feasibility of improving control of hand and finger motion as well as force control by training with dedicated robotic devices, which are compact, easy to use, and can thus be easily transported and installed. Although training of hand and fingers is limited to stroke subjects with some remaining motor function in these segments, restoring fine hand control, precision and power grip are crucial tasks that could have a significant impact on the quality of life of stroke survivors. In addition, the observed transfer from improvement of hand to arm function opens horizons for the development of new robotic devices focusing on hand and fingers. This could pave the way for a new generation of simple rehabilitation robots to be used as standard therapy and assessment tools in rehabilitation centers or directly in patients' homes.

ACKNOWLEDGMENTS

This work was carried out at the National University of Singapore, Singapore (grant R265-000-168-112) and at Simon Fraser University, Vancouver, Canada. Clinical studies were carried out at Simon Fraser University and at Tan Tock Seng Hospital, Singapore. O. Lambercy and R. Gassert were supported by the NCCR Neural Plasticity and Repair, Swiss National Science Foundation. E. Burdet's involvement was funded in part by the EU FP7 HUMOUR project. The authors thank Vineet B. Jonhson for his help in defining the experimental protocol and recruiting stroke patients.

References

Bohannon, R. and Smith, M. (1987). Interrater reliability of a modified ashworth scale of muscle spasticity, *Physical Therapy* **67(2)**, pp. 206–207.

Bouzit, M., Burdea, G., Popescu, G. and Boian, R. (2002). The Rutgers Master II: New design force-feedback glove, *IEEE/ASME Transactions on Mechatronics* **7(2)**, pp. 256–263.

Cruz, E., Waldinger, H. and Kamper, D. (2005). Kinetic and kinematic workspaces of the index finger following stroke, *Brain* **128**, pp. 1112–1121.

Dovat, L., Lambercy, O., Gassert, R., Maeder, T., Milner, T., Teo, C. and Burdet, E. (2008). HandCARE: A cable-actuated rehabilitation system to train hand function after stroke, *IEEE Transaction in Neural Systems and Rehabilitation Engineering* **16(6)**, pp. 582–591.

Dovat, L., Lambercy, O., Johnson, V., Salman, B., Wong, S., Gassert, R., Burdet, E., Teo, C. and Milner, T. (2007). A cable driven robotic system to train finger function after stroke, *Proc. of the IEEE Int. Conf. on Robotic Rehabilitation (ICORR)*, pp. 222–227.

Dovat, L., Lambercy, O., Ruffieux, Y., Chapuis, D., Gassert, R., Bleuler, H., Teo, C. and Burdet, E. (2006). A haptic knob for rehabilitation of stroke patients, in *2006 IEEE/RSJ International Conference on Intelligent Robots and Systems*, pp. 977–982.

Fugl-Meyer, A. R., Jääskö, L., Leyman, I., Olsson, S. and Steglind, S. (1975). The post-stroke hemiplegic patient. 1. a method for evaluation of physical performance, *Scand. J. Rehabil. Med.* **7**, 1, pp. 13–31.

Gowland, C., Stratford, P., Ward, M., Moreland, J., Torresin, W., Van Hullenaar, S., Sanford, J., Barreca, S., Vanspall, B. and Plews, N. (1993). Measuring physical impairment and disability with the Chedoke-Mcmaster stroke assessment, *Stroke* **24**, pp. 58–63.

Henderson, A., Korner-Bitensky, N. and Levin, M. (2007). Virtual reality in stroke rehabilitation: A systematic review of its effectiveness for upper limb motor recovery. *Top Stroke Rehabil.* **14(2)**, pp. 52–61.

Hesse, S., Schulte-Tigges, G., Konrad, M., Bardeleben, A. and Werner, C. (2003). Robot-assisted arm trainer for the passive and active practive of bilateral forearm and wrist movements in hemiparetic subjects, *Arch. Phys. Med. Rehabil.* **84**, pp. 915–920.

Hogan, N., Krebs, H., Rohrer, B., Palazzolo, J., Dipietro, L., Fasoli, S., Stein, J., Hughes, R., Frontera, W., Lynch, R. and Volpe, B. (2006). Motions or muscles? Some behavioral factors underlying robotic assistance of motor recovery, *Journal of Rehabilitation Research and Development* **45**, pp. 605–618.

Holden, M. (2005). Virtual environment for motor rehabilitation: Review, *Cyber Psychology and Behavior* **8(3)**, pp. 187–211.

Hunter, S. and Crome, P. (2002). Hand function and stroke, *Reviews in Clinical Gerontology* **12**, pp. 68–81.

Johnson, M. (2006). Recent trends in robot-assisted therapy environments to improve real-life functional performance after stroke, *Journal of Neuro-engineering and Rehabilitation* **3**, pp. 29–34.

Kamper, D., Fischer, H., Cruz, E. and Rymer, W. (2006). Weakness is the primary contributor to finger impairment in chronic stroke, *Arch. Phys. Med. Rehabil.* **87**, pp. 1262–1269.

Kawasaki, H., Ito, S., Ishigure, Y., Nishimoto, Y., Aoki, T., Mouri, T., Sakaeda, H. and Abe, M. (2007). Development of a hand motion assist robot for rehabilitation therapy by patient self-motion control, *Proc. of the IEEE Int. Conf. on Robotic Rehabilitation (ICORR)*, pp. 234–240.

Krakauer, J. (2006). Motor learning: its relevance to stroke recovery and neurorehabilitation, *Current Opinion in Neurology* **19**, pp. 84–90.

Krebs, H. I., Mernoff, S., Fasoli, S. E., Hughes, R., Stein, J. and Hogan, N. (2008). A comparison of functional and impairment-based robotic training in severe to moderate chronic stroke: A pilot study, *NeuroRehabilitation* **23**, 1, pp. 81–7.

Krebs, H. I., Volpe, B. T., Williams, D., Celestino, J., Charles, S. K., Lynch, D. and Hogan, N. (2007). Robot-aided neurorehabilitation: A robot for wrist rehabilitation, *IEEE Transactions on Neural Systems and Rehabilitation Engineering* **15(3)**, pp. 327–335.

Kwakkel, G., Kollen, B. J. and Krebs, H. I. (2008). Effects of robot-assisted therapy on upper limb recovery after stroke: a systematic review, *Neurorehabil Neural Repair* **22**, 2, pp. 111–21, doi:10.1177/1545968307305457.

Lambercy, O., Dovat, L., Gassert, R., Burdet, E., Teo, C. and Milner, T. (2007). A haptic knob for rehabilitation of hand function, *IEEE Transactions on Neural Systems and Rehabilitation Engineering* **15**, 3, pp. 356–366.

Lambercy, O., Dovat, L., Johnson, V., Salman, B., Wong, S., Gassert, R., Milner, T., Teo, C. and Burdet, E. (2007b). Development of a robot-assisted rehabilitation therapy to train hand function for activities of daily living, *Proc. of the IEEE Int. Conf. on Robotic Rehabilitation (ICORR)* , pp. 678–682.

Lambercy, O., Dovat, L., Yun, H., Wee, S., Kuah, C., Chua, K., Gassert, R., Milner, T., Teo, C. and Burdet, E. (2009). Rehabilitation of Grasping and Forearm Pronation/Supination with the Haptic Knob, in *IEEE International Conference on Rehabilitation Robotics (ICORR)*, pp. 22–27.

Lang, C. and Schieber, M. (2004). Reduced muscle selectivity during individuated finger movements in humans after damage to the motor cortex or corticospinal tract, *J. Neurophysiol.* **91**, pp. 1722–1733.

Lewthwaite, R. (1990). Motivational considerations in physical activity involvement, *Physical Therapy* **70**, pp. 808–819.

Loureiro, R. and Harwin, W. (2007). Reach & grasp therapy: Design and control of a 9-DOF robotic neuro-rehabilitation system, *Proc. of the 9th IEEE International Conference on Rehabilitation Robotics (ICCOR)* , pp. 757–763.

Marchal-Crespo, L. and Reinkensmeyer, D. J. (2009). Review of control strategies for robotic movement training after neurologic injury, *J. Neuroeng. Rehabil.* **6**, p. 20, doi:10.1186/1743-0003-6-20.

Prange, G. B., Jannink, M. J. A., Groothuis-Oudshoorn, C. G. M., Hermens, H. J. and Ijzerman, M. J. (2006). Systematic review of the effect of robot-aided therapy on recovery of the hemiparetic arm after stroke, *J. Rehabil. Res. Dev.* **43**, 2, pp. 171–84.

Raghavan, P., Petra, E., Krakauer, J. and Gordon, A. (2006). Patterns of impairment in digit independence after stroke, *J. Neurophysiol.* **95**, pp. 369–378.

Reinkensmeyer, D., Emken, J. and Cramer, S. (2004). Robotics, motor learning and neurologic recovery, *Annu. Rev. Biomed. Eng.* **6**, pp. 497–525.

Schieber, M. H., Lang, C. E., Reilly, K. T., McNulty, P. and Sirigu, A. (2009). Selective activation of human finger muscles after stroke or amputation, *Adv. Exp. Med. Biol.* **629**, pp. 559–75, doi:10.1007/978-0-387-77064-2_30.

Takahashi, C., Der-Yeghiaian, L., Le, V. and Cramer, S. (2005). A robotic device for hand motor therapy after stroke, *Proc. of the 9th IEEE International Conference on Rehabilitation Robotics (ICCOR)* , pp. 17–20.

Takahashi, C., Der-Yeghiaian, L., Le, V., Motiwala, R. and Cramer, S. (2008). Robot-based handmotor therapy after stroke, *Brain* **131**, pp. 425–437.

Valero-Cuevas, F. J. (2009). Why the hand? *Adv. Exp. Med. Biol.* **629**, pp. 553–7, doi:10.1007/978-0-387-77064-2_29.

Volpe, B., Lynch, D., Rykman-Berland, A., Ferraro, M., Galgano, M., Hogan, N. and Krebs, H. (2008). Intensive sensorimotor arm training mediated by therapist or robot improves hemiparesis in patients with chronic stroke, *Neurorehabilitation and Neural Repair* **22**, pp. 305–310.

Winstein, C., Wing, A. and Whitall, J. (2003). Motor control and learning principles for rehabilitation of upper limb movements after brain injury, *Handbook of Neuropsychology* **9**, pp. 77–137.

Woldag, H., Renner, C. and Hummelsheim, H. (2007). Immediate effects of therapeutic interventions on the central motor system and their practical consequences, *Rehabilitation (Stuttg)* **46**(4), pp. 228–232.

Chapter Five

A Novel Continuous Intention-Driven Rehabilitation Robot and Its Training Effectiveness

Xiaoling Hu*, Rong Song*, Xiujuan Zheng*, Wallace W. Leung†, Shamay Ng‡, Stephanie S. Au-Yeung‡ and Raymond Kai-yu Tong*

*Department of Health Technology and Informatics, The Hong Kong Polytechnic University, Hung Hom, Kowloon, Hong Kong SAR, China.
†Research Institute of Innovative Products & Technologies, The Hong Kong Polytechnic University, Hung Hom, Kowloon, Hong Kong SAR, China
‡Department of Rehabilitation Sciences, The Hong Kong Polytechnic University, Hung Hom, Kowloon, Hong Kong SAR, China

5.1 INTRODUCTION

Stroke is a main cause of adult disabilities. The extent of restoration of limb functions after stroke is highly associated with the intensive voluntary practice of the affected limbs, which is associated with a motor relearning process to re-establish neuromuscular pathways for desired limb functions (Butefisch *et al.* 1995; Farmer *et al.* 2004). In the absence of direct repair on the damaged brain tissues after stroke, neurological rehabilitation is an arduous process. It is because that poststroke rehabilitation programs are usually time-consuming and labor-intensive for both the therapist and the patient in one-to-one manual interaction. Recent technologies have made it possible to use robotic devices as assistance by the therapist, providing safe and intensive rehabilitation with repeated motions to persons after stroke (Volpe *et al.* 2004; Ng *et al.* 2008). The most commonly reported motion types provided by developed rehabilitation robots are:

(1) continuous passive motion (CPM),
(2) active-assisted movement (Volpe *et al.* 2004), and
(3) challenge-based movement (Marchal-crespo and Reinkensmeyer 2009).

Biomechatronics in Medicine and Healthcare by Le Li and Raymond Kai-Yu Tong

www.panstanford.com
978-981-4241-61-8

In a robot-assisted CPM treatment, there is no voluntary effort required from a patient, and the movements of the patient's limb(s) on the paretic side are dominated by the robot system. This type of intervention was found to be effective in temporarily reducing poststroke hypertonia (Schmit *et al.* 2000). In active-assisted robotic treatment (or interactive robotic treatment), the rehabilitation robot would provide external assisting forces to compensate the weakness in the affected limb when a patient could not complete a desired movement independently. It has been found that with the involvement of voluntary motor efforts of the paretic limbs, the limb functional improvement after interactive robotic treatments were better than those achieved by the CPM treatments (Volpe *et al.* 2004; Tong *et al.* 2006). In a robot-assisted treatment with challenge-based moments, the robot controller will make a training task more difficult or challenging, as opposed to the robotic assistance provided in an interactive robotic treatment. For example, the commonly used challenging control is robotic resistance (Fasoli *et al.* 2003). It has been found that repetitive practice of hand and finger movements against resistive loads resulted in greater improvements in motor performance and functional scales than Bobath-based treatment (Butefisch *et al.* 1995), transcutaneous electric nerve stimulation, and suprathreshold electric stimulation on hand and wrist muscles (Hummelsheim *et al.* 1997).

In recent years, robotic systems developed for stroke rehabilitation have been widely reported in the literatures. Most of these robotic systems can provide all the three motion types mentioned above for poststroke rehabilitation. For example, MIT-MANUS is one of the robotic systems for poststroke upper limb rehabilitation (Hogan *et al.* 1992; Krebs *et al.* 1998). The key feature of MIT-MANUS is its impedance control which could keep a compliant trajectory under perturbation. ARM Guide is a robotic system designed both for training and evaluation of upper limb reaching functions in a linear trajectory (Reinkensmeyer *et al.* 1999; Reinkensmeyer *et al.* 2000). Colombo *et al.* also designed a wrist manipulator with one-degree of freedom and an elbow-shoulder manipulator with two degrees of freedom for the rehabilitation of upper limb movements (Colombo *et al.* 2005). They used admittance control to reduce the inertia and facilitate the movement. Besides, other rehabilitation robots with different mechanical designs also have been well described in other chapters for hand and upper limb trainings (Chapter 2 and 4).

Due to the believed effectiveness in motor improvement by active-assisted robotic treatment (i.e., in comparison with the CPM training mode), the recent developments involving rehabilitation robots has been worked towards the interactive control, which allows the robotic system to react to patients' voluntary intention (Marchal-crespo and Reinkensmeyer 2009). However, most of the interactive controls used in rehabilitation robots are oversimplified on the voluntary inputs from stroke patients and lacking clinical supports on their training effectiveness. The easiest and most commonly used algorithm for the interactive control is the "on/off" strategy, i.e., once the voluntary indicator from a subject is captured or disappears, the assistive function of robotic system will be triggered to help the subject finish the programmed motion (Dipietro *et al.* 2005). Usually the subject only needs to stay passively and have a sensory experience after the assistive function is triggered. According to the sensorimotor integration theory, the voluntary motor efferent and the afferent sensor experiences together are important and helpful to promote the reorganization of the brain (Dipietro *et al.* 2005). A more advanced design in the interactive control requires continuous voluntary motor inputs from a stroke patient to the robot, and the robotic system gives support, or even encourages the output from the motor system of the stroke patient but not to override, during the training. In this chapter, we introduced an interactive robotic system with continuous voluntary intention control developed in our laboratory for poststroke rehabilitation training, and its associated training effects by clinical trial tests.

5.2 REHABILITATION ROBOTIC SYSTEM WITH CONTINUOUS INTENTION DRIVEN CONTROL

Many signals have been used to indicate voluntary intention in the design for rehabilitation devices, such as, limb torque, trajectory, electromyography (EMG), etc. (Hogan *et al.* 1992; Volpe *et al.* 2000; Volpe *et al.* 2004). In the robotic system developed in our study, EMG was selected to reflect the voluntary intention of stroke patients. EMG is the electricity generated in muscles under the control of the nervous system, and it could be detected non-invasively from the skin surface with the amplitude in millivolt. EMG signals have been used as indicators of subjects' voluntary intention in some orthotic and prosthetic devices for paralyzed people (Rosen *et al.* 1999; Rosen *et al.* 2001; Lee and Sankai 2002; Cheng *et al.* 2003), and the trigger signals in some interactive robotic system for stroke rehabilitation training (Dipietro *et al.* 2005). In our works, we developed an interactive robotic system (named PolyJbot) with continuous EMG control (Hu *et al.* 2008; Song *et al.* 2008; Hu *et al.* 2009) for poststroke rehabilitation training on the elbow, wrist, knee, and ankle joints with the attempt to encourage the participants to involve more voluntary efforts during the training (Hu *et al.* 2007; Hu *et al.* 2008; Song *et al.* 2008; Hu *et al.* 2009).

5.2.1 *The Robotic System*

The rehabilitation robot with continuous intention driven control is shown in Fig. 5.1(a). It can be applied for interactive training on the upper and lower limbs with multi-joint configurations. The continuous intention-driven control strategies applied on different joints, i.e., the elbow, the wrist, the knee, and the ankle joints are similar, but with respective limb adapters, range of motions (ROMs), and mechanical setups. In this chapter, the design for the wrist training will be used for illustrating the implementation of the continuous intention-driven control algorithm.

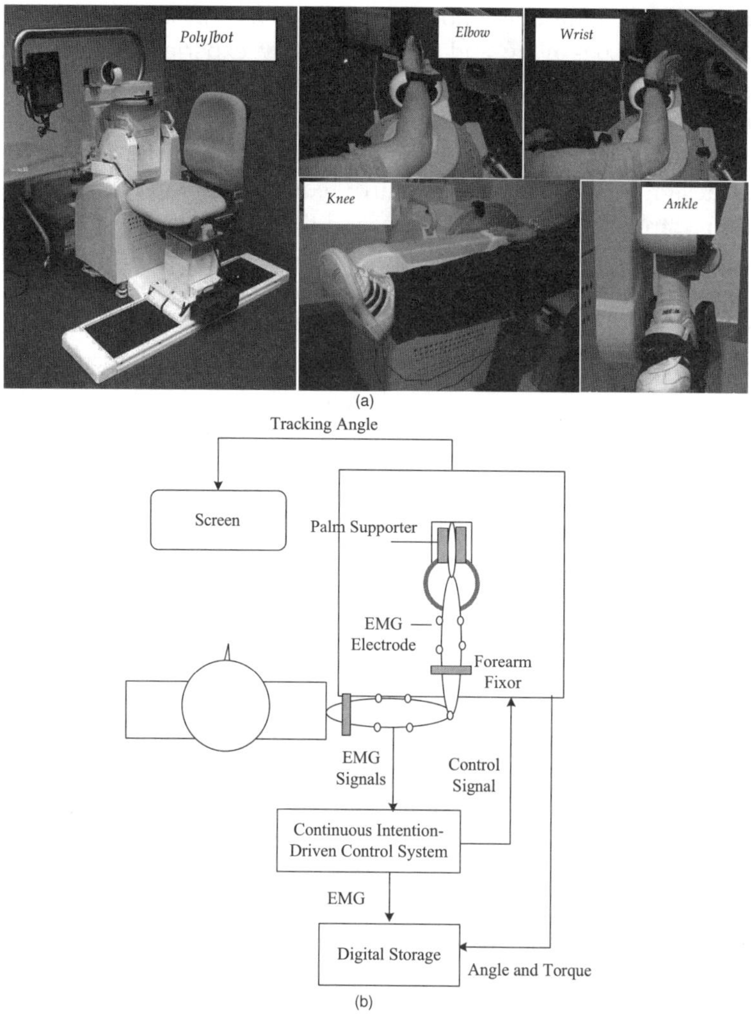

Figure 5.1 The rehabilitation robot (PolyJbot) with continuous intention-driven algorithm for multi-joint training (a), and the schematic diagram of the setup for the wrist training (b). For color reference, see page 214.

During the wrist training, a subject was seated, and the affected upper limb was mounted horizontally on the robotic system, as shown in Fig. 5.1(b). The subject would conduct wrist flexion and extension horizontally with respective limb adapters by tracking a target cursor on a computer screen, moving with an angular velocity at 10°/sec in both extension and flexion directions from −45° (the negative sign represents a extension position) to 60° (the positive sign represents a flexion position) of the wrist angle. Different from other intention-triggered systems, continuous interactive torque associated with the voluntary EMG of the wrist movement would be provided by the robot to help the subject finish the task during tracking on a real-time base.

In the design of the continuous intention-driven control algorithm, EMG signals from the main antagonist muscle pairs related to the wrist flexion and extension was detected, i.e. the flexor carpi radialis (FCR) reflecting the voluntary effort for flexion, and the extensor carpi radialis (ECR) for extension. It was observed clinically that persons after stroke usually had reduced muscle coordinating capability in limb movements (Georgopoulos 1986; Cauraugh *et al.* 2000; Dewald *et al.* 2001; Gribble *et al.* 2003), e.g., when conducting a wrist extension in the paretic upper limb, the muscles related to wrist flexion (FCR) or elbow movements (e.g., biceps brachii (BIC) and triceps brachii (TRI)) may also contract. This is mainly caused by involuntary muscle spasticity and compensatory movements associated with other joints after stroke (Dewald *et al.* 2001). Therefore, in the robot we designed, only the EMG signal from the FCR was used to drive the motor during the wrist flexion phase, and the ECR EMG was applied for the extension phase, to avoid the unnecessary co-contraction from the antagonist muscle (Hu *et al.* 2008).

(1) The raw FCR and ECR EMG signals were first amplified with a gain of 1000 and were band-pass filtered in 10–400 Hz band. Then, the signals were sampled at 1000 Hz through the A/D card and captured by the PC-program. The envelope of the EMG signals was obtained by full-wave rectification and filtering with a moving average window (100 ms). The processed EMG signals from the FCR and ECR muscles at this step were named as, EMG_i, where i represented ECR or FCR.

(2) The EMG signals, EMG_i, were then normalized to the range 0-1, i.e.,

$$M_{\text{Flexion/Extension}} = \frac{EMG_i - EMG_{i,rest}}{EMG_{i,IMVC} - EMG_{i,rest}} \quad \begin{array}{l} \text{i} = \text{FCR in flexion} \\ \text{i} = \text{ECR in extension} \end{array} \tag{5.1}$$

where i represented the FCR or ECR muscle, $EMG_{i,rest}$ was the amplitude of the processed EMG signal of muscle i at rest, and $EMG_{i,IMVC}$ was the maximal amplitude of the processed EMG signal of muscle i during isometric maximum voluntary contraction (IMVC, isometric maximum voluntary flexion for FCR (IMVF) and isometric maximum voluntary extension (IMVE) for ECR) at 0° of the wrist angle, which was detected before the training session.

(3) The assistive torque during tracking was formulated as:

$$T_a = \begin{cases} G \cdot T_{\text{IMVF}} \cdot M_{\text{Flexion}}, & \text{During the flexion tracking phase} \\ G \cdot T_{\text{IMVF}} \cdot M_{\text{Extension}}, & \text{During the extension tracking phase} \end{cases} \tag{5.2}$$

where, T_a represented the motor generated assistive torque in the flexion or extension phase during the tracking, G is a constant gain used to adjust the magnitude of the assistive torque; and T_{IMVE} and T_{IMVF} were the maximal values of the torque during isometric extension and flexion respectively, at the wrist angle of 0° (Hu *et al.* 2008). Figure 5.2 shows the representative EMG and torque signals during isometric maximum voluntary wrist flexion and EMG signals during wrist tracking.

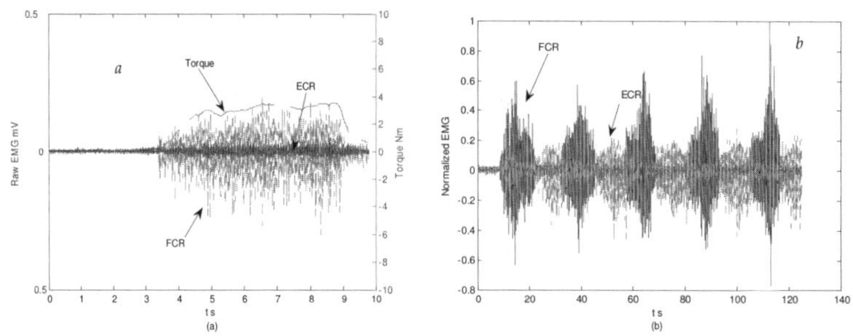

Figure 5.2 The representative EMG signals and torque signal obtained during isometric maximum voluntary flexion at wrist joint of 0° (a), and the representative EMG from the FCR and ECR in a wrist tracking trial (b). For color reference, see page 215.

Besides the assistive torque, the interactive robotic system we developed also could provide optional interactive resistive torque for challenge-based training. The resistive torque could be applied in both flexion and extension directions, that is,

$$T_r = a \cdot T_{MVC,\text{Flexion/Extension}} \tag{5.3}$$

where $T_{r,\text{Flexion/Extension}}$ was the resistive torque, a was the resistive coefficient (e.g., 10% or 20%, alternatively applied to the trials in a session), and $T_{MVC,\text{Flexion/Extension}}$ including two parts, the maximal T_{IMVF}(applied in the flexion phase only) and T_{IMVE} (applied in the extension phase only). The net torque, T_n, provided by the robot during the training would be $T_n = T_a - T_r$, where T_a was assistive torque (Eq. 2) and T_r was resistive torque (Eq. 3), and this net torque was highly adapted to the muscle capability in a training session. It has been found that applying resistance in tracking tasks may improve the muscle strength related to the wrist movements (Hu *et al.* 2009).

5.2.2 Robot as an Evaluation System

Rehabilitation robot could share a large portion of the repeated labor work in a long term physical training program, with the proper administration by a physical therapist. Another advantage of using robot-assisted poststroke rehabilitation training is that the robot could be a platform for quantitative monitoring on the motor recovery process during rehabilitation training, due to the standardized experimental setup and the high repeatability of training motions compared to the modes manually offered. However, in many works on rehabilitation training, only pre- and post-training evaluations were conducted to assess the training effects, even in most of studies related to robot-assisted rehabilitation (Volpe *et al.* 2004). The commonly used clinical scores include the Fugl-Meyer Assessment (FMA) (Fugl-Meyer *et al.* 1975) for assessing voluntary motor functions, the FIM instrument (Keith *et al.* 1987) for evaluating independency in the daily life, the Motor Status Score (MSS) test (Ferraro *et al.* 2002) for voluntary motor assessment in the upper limb, and the Modified Ashworth Scale (MAS) (Ashworth 1964) for measurement on muscle spasticity.

In our previous work on the poststroke wrist training assisted by the interactive robot, several robotic parameters were used to monitor the recovery process during a training program (Hu *et al.* 2008; Hu *et al.* 2009). They were:

(1) **EMG Activation Levels of Muscles**: EMG activation level mainly reflects signal amplitude, and is related to the muscle power, or force, generated in a task. Besides the EMG signals of ECR and FCR muscles, another two muscles related to the elbow joint, i.e. the biceps brachii (BIC) and the triceps brachii (TRI) muscles were also studied in the training program. The raw EMG signals of these four muscles during wrist tracking tasks were recorded and stored in a computer. Then, the linear envelope of the recorded EMG signals was obtained by

   (i) full-wave rectification,
   (ii) low-pass filtering (10Hz cutoff frequency with forth-order, zero-phase forward and reverse Butterworth filter),
   (iii) subtraction of the average EMG activity during the resting state, and
   (iv) normalized to the maximum value of EMG activation in each muscle during either a training session or the IMVE and IMVE of each session. The EMG activation level of a muscle in a tracking trial was calculated by averaging the EMG envelope of the trial.

(2) **Muscle Cocontraction Indexes (CI) of Muscle Pairs**: After obtaining the EMG envelope of the muscles of interest, we also calculated the coactivations between different muscle pairs during the tracking task, which could be expressed by the cocontraction index as introduced in our previous studies (Hu *et al.* 2007; Hu *et al.* 2008; Hu *et al.* 2009), that is,

$$CI = \frac{1}{T}\int_T A_{ij}(t)dt \tag{5.4}$$

where A_{ij}(t) was the overlapping activity of EMG linear envelopes for muscles i and j, and T was the length of the signal. The value of a CI for a muscle pair varied from 0 (no overlapping at all in the signal trial) to 1 (total overlapping of the 2 muscles with both EMG levels kept at 1 during the trial). The representative segments of EMG envelopes obtained in the tracking experiment are shown in Fig. 5.3. The CI value of a muscle pair represents the coordination pattern in a motion task.

(3) **The root-mean-squared-error (RMSE) of tracking trajectories**: The root-mean-squared-error of a trial calculates the difference between the target and the actual elbow angles during the tracking task. This measure represents the performance of a tracking task, i.e. the small the RMSE value, the better the accuracy of performance. An example of the measured actual wrist angle, in comparison with the target angle, is shown in Fig. 5.3.

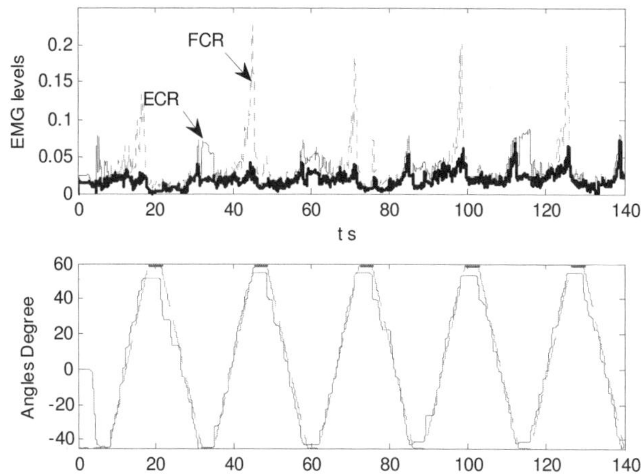

Figure 5.3 A representation of the EMG envelopes of the FCR (doted line), ECR (solid line) muscles, and their overlap (thick solid line) in a tracking trial (upper panel) and the tracking trajectory (lower panel) represented by the actual wrist angle (solid line) and the target angle (dashed line). For color reference, see page 215.

5.3 EVALUATION ON TRAINING EFFECTIVENESS

For evaluation of the effectiveness of the developed continuous intention-driven robot on the wrist joint, we conducted a randomized controlled trial (RCT), which quantitatively compared the training effects of the developed robot with those achieved in a robot-assisted CPM training. After obtaining approval from the Human Subjects Ethics Sub-Committee of the Hong Kong Polytechnic University, we screened voluntarily enrolled persons after stroke coming from local districts. Subjects recruited satisfied the inclusion criteria: 1) had unilateral ischemic brain injury or intracerebral hemorrhage at least 6 months after the onset of single stroke; 2) had moderate level of motor impairment in the affected upper limb, assessed by FMA (9<shoulder/elbow<27, 6<wrist/hand<18); 3) Subjects had to be able to follow the training procedures. Randomization was done by computer-generated random numbers for different groups (i.e., the interactive group and the passive group), assigned according to the order of the recruitment. The study utilized a multiple baseline design, assessed by the clinical scores of the FMA (shoulder/elbow and wrist/hand), and the MAS (wrist and elbow). Each outcome was measured 3 times in two weeks before the training. A total of 86 hemiplegic subjects were screened for the training. Twenty-seven of them met the selection criteria and were recruited for this study. After the randomization, the subjects were divided into the interactive group (n=15) and the passive group (n=12).

5.3.1 Interventions

The subjects received a wrist treatment consisting of 20 sessions, with a training intensity of at least 3 sessions and at most 5 sessions a week. All training sessions were finished in 7 consecutive weeks. For the interactive group in a training session, each subject was seated with the paretic arm mounted on the robotic system as illustrated in Fig. 5.1(b). IMVE and IMVF at 0° of the wrist angle were conducted and repeated 3 times before the training. Then, the subject was required to conduct voluntary wrist tracking tasks. In each session, there were 14 trials, and each trial contained 5 cycles of wrist extension and flexion. During the tracking, interactive assistive torques (according to Eqs. 1 and 2) were provided by the robotic system in both flexion and extension phases. In order to obtain the assistance during tracking, the subjects needed to continuously generate voluntary muscular effort to acquire assistive torque from the robot; otherwise, if no EMG activity from the target muscle, the robot would not generate any assistance. Besides the interactive assistive torque, interactive resistive torques, according to Eq. 3, were also applied in the tracking trials in a session. In the study, 10% and 20% of the maximum wrist torques of IMVE/IMVE were selected for the generation of the interactive resistive torques, which were administrated to all trials alternatively in each session, together with the interactive assistive torques, throughout the training course.

For the passive group, the rehabilitation robotic system (CYBEX and NORM, Computer Sports Medicine, Inc, USA) was used for the training. The standard setup for wrist extension and flexion of the CYBEX and NORM system was adopted for the CPM training (2005). In each session, wrist IMVF and IMVE at the joint angle of 0° were first conducted and repeated 3 times. Then, there were 14 training trials, and each trial contained 5 cycles of passive wrist extension and flexion. The range of motion for the wrist joint was set from −45° to 60°, and the palm was moving passively with an angular velocity of 10°/sec in the range.

5.3.2 Training Effects

After the 20 sessions of wrist training assisted with continuous intention-driven robot on the interactive group, voluntary motor functions for the interactive group on the wrist and elbow joints were improvement as assessed by FMA shoulder/elbow and wrist/hand scores (Fig 5.4). The clinical scores suggested that the interactive wrist training resulted in voluntary motor improvements: not only at the trained joint, i.e., the wrist, but also at the elbow joint. These observations were consistent with previous findings that poststroke training on the distal joints could increase the motor capacity related to the intralimb proximal joint (Krebs *et al.* 1998; Cauraugh *et al.* 2000). Furthermore, the improvement in the FMA shoulder/elbow scores was maintained in the 3-month follow up test for the interactive group. However, for the passive group, no significant changes in the FMA scores after the training. This suggested that the CPM robot-assisted training did not benefit the voluntary motor recovery, consistent with other reports that that CPM did not contribute a lot to the improvement in voluntary motor outcome (Volpe *et al.* 2004). The CPM treatment only released the muscle spasticity at the wrist joint after the training indicated by a reduction in the MAS wrist score

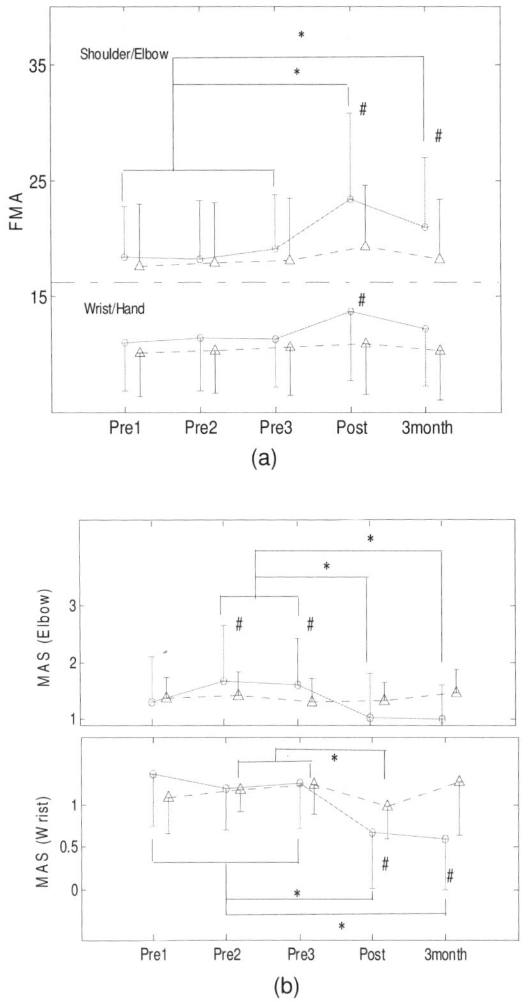

Figure 5.4 Clinical assessments for the interactive (solid lines with circle marks) and the passive groups (dashed lines with delta markers) before and after the robot-assisted wrist training. (a) The FMA shoulder/elbow and wrist/hand scores; and (b) the MAS elbow and wrist scores. The intra-group differences with statistical significance ($P < 0.05$) were marked with "*", and the inter-group differences with statistical significance ($P < 0.05$) were marked with "#".

(Fig. 5.4(b)), whereas this reduction was temporary and could not be maintained after 3 months. Muscle spasticity related to the elbow and wrist joints were both released after the training for the interactive group, and this improvement could be persisted at least for 3 months, as suggested by the MAS scores in Fig. 5.4(b).

In Fig. 5.5, the EMG activation level for the interactive and passive groups and the RMSE for the interactive group were used to describe the motor recovery processes during the training. Decreases in the EMG activation level of the FCR and BIC muscles for the interactive groups and in the FCR of the passive group

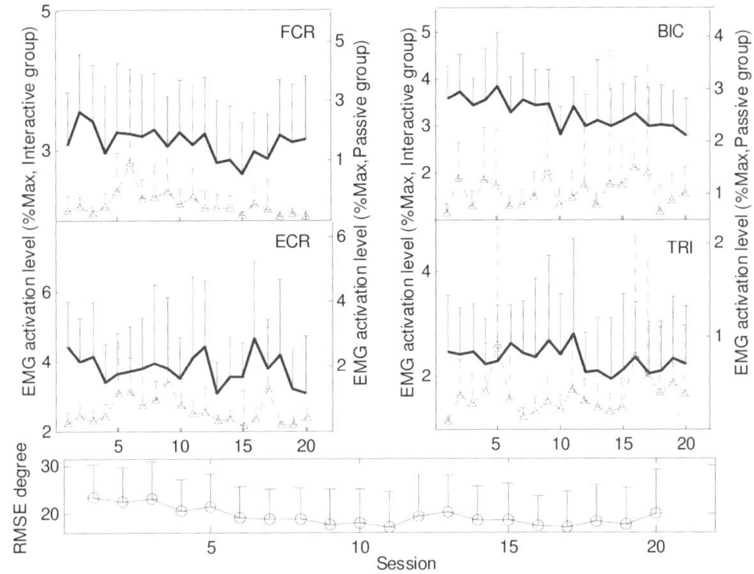

Figure 5.5 The EMG activation levels for the interactive group (solid lines) and the passive group (dashed lines with delta makers) during the robot-assisted wrist training, and the RMSE for the interactive group during the wrist tracking tasks (lower panel, solid line with circle markers).

were found across the training sessions. The RMSE for the interactive group in tracking tasks also demonstrated a decreasing trend before Session 8, and then reached to a steady state in later sessions. The EMG activation levels for all muscles in the interactive group were higher than those for the passive groups. In the interactive group, voluntary muscular efforts were needed when doing the tracking tasks. However, in the passive group, there was no voluntary motor output required during the CPM treatment. Therefore, the EMG activation levels in the interactive group were usually higher than those in the passive group. EMG activities in the passive group during the training were mainly related to the involuntary muscle spasticity. The reduction in the FCR EMG activation level for the passive group suggested a decrease of muscle spasticity of this wrist flexor, which was consistent with the MAS wrist score decrease (Fig. 5.4(b)) after the training. The decreases in the EMG activation levels of FCR and BIC in the interactive group were associated with two factors, i.e., the reduced involuntary muscle spasticity, and the decreased muscle activities during a learning process for a skillful task (Flament *et al.* 1999). A steady state (Georgopoulos 1986) reached by the RMSE after a decreasing phase (Sessions 1–7 in Fig. 5.3) suggested that after Session 7 the wrist tracking skill could be regarded as stably learned by most of the subjects. It also implied that the decreases in FCR and BIC EMG levels after Session 7 could be mainly related to the decrease of muscle spasticity.

Figure 5.6 shows the changes in the muscle CIs for the interactive group across the training sessions. The CIs in a training task, e.g., the wrist tracking tasks

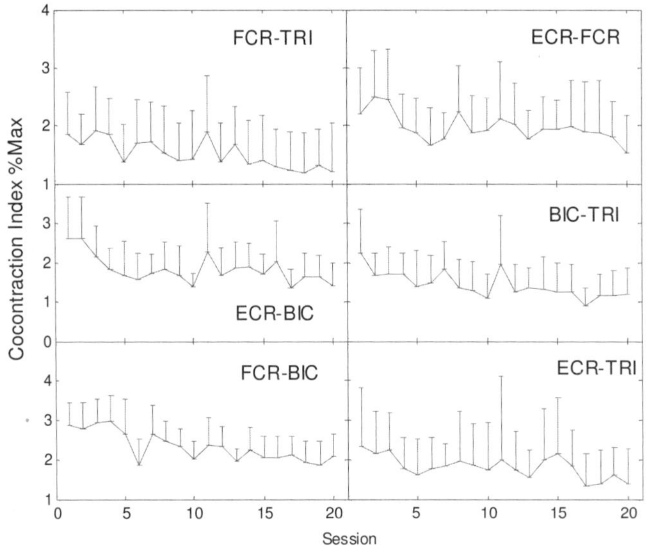

Figure 5.6 The variation of CIs of the different muscle pairs for the interactive group during the training course.

for the interactive group, mainly reflect the muscle co-ordination in voluntary movements. Therefore, there was no CI value for the passive group during CPM wrist movements. We found decreasing trends in CI values of BIC&TRI, FCR&BIC, ECR&BIC, and ECR&FCR for the interactive group. It suggested the reduction in the co-contraction of these muscle pairs. The decreasing CI value of a muscle pair was related to (1) the reduced muscle activation level, and (2) the reduced muscle co-contracting phase. The decreasing CIs involving BIC muscle could be mainly due to the reduced BIC EMG activation level during the training (Fig. 5.5), since the variations of these CIs were consistent with the change in the BIC EMG activation level. It has been often observed clinically that the wrist movements in the paretic side in persons after stroke usually were associated with significant motions of the adjacent joints, such as the elbow. The decrease in CI values related to the BIC muscle also suggested a better isolation of the wrist motions from the elbow movements through the robot-assisted wrist training. The decrease in the CI of ECR&FCR was appeared after Session 13, which is associated with the non-decreasing phase of the FCR EMG level after Session 13 (Fig. 5.5) and the oscillating phase of the overall ECR EMG level. It implied that the decreasing in the CI of ECR&FCR after Session 13 could be mainly related to the reduction of the co-contracting phase of the two muscles during the tracking. It also indicated a better coordinating pattern between this antagonist muscle pair, i.e., the contracting/relaxing pattern, when performing the wrist extension and flexion in tracking tasks. However, this improvement in the coordinating pattern between FCR&ECR appeared in later sessions of the training; and the decrease in the CI of FCR&ECR did not reach a steady state before the end of the training, neither the decreases in the overall CIs related to the BIC muscle. It implied that further improvements in these CIs may be obtained with more training sessions.

5.4 CONCLUSIONS

The continuous intention-driven rehabilitation robot mainly could improve the voluntary motor function in muscle coordination during tracking tasks, and this improvement could be maintained after the training, as assessed by the 3-month follow up test. The voluntary motor improvement not only could be obtained at the training joint, e.g. the wrist joint in the robot-assisted wrist training, but also could be observed at the neighboring proximal joint, i.e., the elbow joint in the wrist training. Similar observations were also reported in a clinical trial study related to the continuous intention-driven robot-assisted elbow training study, i.e., the training improved the elbow function, as well as the shoulder function (Hu *et al.* 2007; Hu *et al.* 2008; Hu *et al.* 2009).

5.5 FUTURE STUDIES

One of the questions related to interactive rehabilitation robot development, which has not been well addressed by many studies, is that how the specific, or unique, design of a robot is related to the motor improvements achieved by this robot, in comparison with other similar interactive robots. Future works on randomized clinical trial studies are necessary for quantitatively understanding of the uniqueness of a rehabilitation robot with predictable training effects.

The success of a rehabilitation robot not only depends on the non-fatiguing motor, but also on the simulation of the interactive treatments conducted by a human physiotherapist. Most of current rehabilitation robots are very preliminary in treatment skill, or rehabilitation knowledge, when compared with a human physiotherapist. For example, the treatment of a robot usually is not adaptive with the recovery process of a subject. There is still a very large growing space for rehabilitation robot to be more intelligent.

5.6 ACKNOWLEDGEMENT

The Project was funded by Hong Kong Polytechnic University under Niche Areas Grant (1-BB50).

References

HUMAC NORM Testing & Rehabilitation System: User's Guide Model 770. Computer Sports Medicine, Inc., (2005).

Ashworth B., Preliminary trials of carisoprodol in multiple sclerosis. *Practitioner* **192**: 540–542, (1964).

Butefisch C, Hummelsheim H, Denzler P, Mauritz K. H., Repetitive training of isolated movements improves the outcome of motor rehabilitation of the centrally paretic hand. *J. Neurol. Sci.* **130**: 59–68, (1995).

Cauraugh J, Light K, Kim S, Thigpen M, Behrman A., Chronic motor dysfunciton after stroke: recovering wrist and finger extension by electromyography-triggered neuromuscular stimulation. *Stroke*, **31**: 1360–1364, (2000).

Cheng H. S., M. S. J, Lin C.C.K., Improving elbow torque output of stroke patients with assistive torque controlled by EMG signals. *J. Biomech. Eng.* **125**: 881–886, (2003).

Colombo R, Pisano F, Micera S, Mazzone A, Delconte C, Carrozza MC, Dario P, Minuco G., Robotic techniques for upper limb evaluation and rehabilitation of stroke patients. *IEEE T. Neur. Sys. Reh.* **13**: 311–323, (2005).

Dewald J. P. A, Sheshadri V, Dawson M. L, Beer R. F., Upper-limb discoordination in hemiparetic stroke: implications for neurorehabilitation. *Top Stroke Rehabil.* **8**: 1–12, (2001).

Dipietro L, Ferraro M, Palazzolo J. J, Krebs H. I, Volpe B. T, Hogan N., Customized interactive robotic treatment for stroke: EMG-triggered therapy. *IEEE Trans. Neural Syst. Rehabil.* **13**: 325–334, (2005).

Farmer J, Zhao X, van Praag H, Wodtke K, Gage F. H, Christie B. R., Effects of voluntary exercise on synaptic plasticity and gene expression in the dentate gyrus of adult mal Sprague-Dawley rats *in vivo*. *Neurosci.* **124**: 71–79, (2004).

Fasoli S. E, Krebs H. I, Stein J, Frontera W. R, Hogan N., Effects of robotic therapy on motor impairment and recovery in chronic stroke. *Arch. Phys. Med. Rehabil.* **84**: 477–481, (2003).

Ferraro M, Demaio J. H, Krol J, Trudell C, Rannekleiv K, Edelstein L, Christos P, Aisen M, England J, Fasoli SE, Krebs H, Hogan N, Volpe B. T, Assessing the motor status score: a scale for the evaluation of upper limb motor outcomes in patients after stroke. *Neurorehabilitation & Neural Repair* **16**: 283–289, (2002).

Flament D, Shapiro M. B, Kempf T, Corcos D. M., Time course and temporal order of changes in movement kinematics during learning of fast and accurate elbow flexions. *Exp. Brain Res.* **129**: 441–450, (1999).

Fugl-Meyer A. R, Jaasko L, Leyman I, Olsson S, Steglind S., The post-stroke hemiplegic patient. I: A method for evaluation of physical performance. *Scand. J. Rehabil. Med.* **7**: 13–31, (1975).

Georgopoulos A. P., On reaching. *Ann. Rev. Neurosci.* **9**: 147–170, (1986).

Gribble P. L, Mullin L. I, Cothros N, Mattar A., Role of cocontraction in arm movement accuracy. *J. Neurophysiol.* **89**: 2396–2405, (2003).

Hogan N, Krebs H. I, Charnnarong J, Srikrishna P, Sharon A., MIT-Manus: A workstation for manual therapy and training. In: *Proc. IEEE Workshop on Robot and Human Communication*, (1992).

Hu X, Tong K. Y, Song R, Tsang V. S, Leung P. O, Li L ., Variation of muscle coactivation patterns in chronic stroke during robot-assisted elbow training. *Arch. Phys. Med. Rehabil.* **88**: 1022–1029, (2007).

Hu X. L, Tong K. Y, Song R, Zheng X. J, Leung W. W. F., A comparison between electromyography-driven robot and passive motion device on wrist rehabilitation for chronic stroke. *Neurorehabilitation & Neural Repair* **23**: 837–846, (2009).

Hu X. L, Tong K. Y, Song R, Zheng X. J, Lui K. H, Leung W. W. F, Ng S, Au-Yeung S. S. Y., Quantitative evaluation of motor functional recovery process in chronic stroke patients during robot-assisted wrist training. *J. Electromyography Kinesiol* **18**, (2008).

Hummelsheim H, Maier-Loth M. L, Eickhof C., The functional value of electrical muscle stimulation for the rehabilitation of the hand in stroke patients. *Scand. J. Rehabil. Med.* **29**: 3–10, (1997).

Keith R. A, Granger C. V, Hamilton B. B, Sherwin F. S., The functional independence measure: a new tool for rehabilitation. *Advances in Clinical Rehabilitation* **1**: 6–18, (1987).

Krebs H. I, Hogan N, Aiesen M. L, Volpe B. T., Robot-aided neurorehabilitation. *IEEE Trans. Rehabil. Eng.* **6**: 75–87, (1998).

Lee S, Sankai Y., Power assist control for leg with HAL-3 based on virtual torque and impedance adjustment. In: *Proc. of IEEE SMC*, (2002).

Marchal-crespo L, Reinkensmeyer D. J., Review of control strategies for robotic movement training after neurologic injury. *Journal of NeuroEngineering and Rehabilitation* **6**: 1–15, (2009).

Ng M. F. W, Tong R. K. Y, Li L. S. W., A Pilot Study of Randomized Clinical Controlled Trial of Gait Training in Subacute Stroke Patients With Partial Body-Weight Support Electromechanical Gait Trainer and Functional Electrical Stimulation: Six-Month Follow-Up. *Stroke* **39**: 154–160, (2008).

Reinkensmeyer D. J, Dewald J. P. A, Rymer W. Z., Guidance-based quantification of arm impairment following brain injury: A pilot study. *IEEE Trans. Rehabil. Eng.* **7**: 1–11, (1999).

Reinkensmeyer D. J, Kahn L. E, Averbuch M, McKenna_Cole A. N, Schmit B. D, Rymer W. Z., Understanding and treating arm movement impairment after chronic brain injury: Progress with the ARM Guide. *J. Rehabil. Res. Dev.* **37**: 653–662, (2000).

Rosen J, Brand M, Fuchs M. B, Arcan M., A myosignal-based powered exoskeleton system. *IEEE Trans. cyb. Man. Cyb* **31**: 210–212, (2001).

Rosen J, M. B. F, Arcan M., Performances of hill-type and neural network muscle models: Towards a myosignal based exoskeleton. *Comput. Biomed. Res.* **32**: 415–439, (1999).

Schmit B. D, Dewald J. P. A, Rymer W. Z., Stretch reflex adaptation in elbow flexors during repeated passive movements in unilateral brain-injured patients. *Arch. Phys. Med. Rehabil.* **81**: 269–278, (2000).

Song R, Tong K. Y, Hu X. L, Li L., Assistive control system using continuous myoelectric signal in robot-aided arm training for patients after stroke. *IEEE T. Neur. Sys. Reh.* **16**, (2008).

Tong K. Y, Ng M. F, Li L. S., Effectiveness of gait training using an electromechanical gait trainer, with and without functional electric stimulation, in subacute stroke: A randomized controlled trial. *Arch. Phys. Med. Rehabil.* **87**: 1298–1304, (2006).

Volpe B. T, Ferraro M, Lynch D, Christos P, Krol J, Trudell C, Krebs H. I, Hogan N., Robotics and other devices in the treatment of patients recovering from stroke. *Current Atherosclerosis Reports* **6**: 314–319, (2004).

Volpe B. T, Krebs H. I, Hogan N, Edelstein O. L, Diels C, Aisen M., A novel approach to stroke rehabilitation: robot-aided sensorimotor stimulation. *Neurology* **54**: 1938–1944, (2000).

Chapter Six

Hand Rehabilitation Robot using Electromyography

Sze Kit Ho*, Raymond Kai-Yu Tong*, Mo Chen*, Hong Fu Zhou*, Peter Man Kit Pang*, Xiao Ling Hu* and Tai Wai Chan†

*Department of Health Technology and Informatics and The Hong Kong Polytechnic University, Hung Hom, Kowloon, Hong Kong SAR, China
†Industrial Centre, The Hong Kong Polytechnic University, Hung Hom, Kowloon, Hong Kong SAR, China

6.1 INTRODUCTION TO REHABILITATION ROBOTS

As technologies advance and better understanding of the stroke recovery, robots have caught the attention of the therapist and technologist that it can be used for rehabilitation because it can repetitively provide precise movements, collect good quantifiable measurements and never get tired from the long working hours. One of the first pioneers in robotic rehabilitation for upper extremities was the MIT Manus (Krebs *et al.* 1999). It supports the arm of the stroke patient on a horizontal plane and provides guided training of elbow and shoulder movements with visual, auditory and tactile feedbacks. A similar robotic training device is the Mirror-Image Motion Enabler (MIME) which uses the unimpaired arm to guide the shoulder and elbow movements of the impaired arm during bilateral training (Burgar *et al.* 2000). Another robotic device is the Bi-Manu-Track which trains the bilateral arm movement at the wrist joints (Hesse *et al.* 2003). As described in chapter 5, an upper and lower limbs rehabilitation robot named PolyJBot was developed to assist stroke subjects to actively train their wrist, elbow, ankle and knee joints using their own electromyography (EMG) as the intention driven signals (Tong and Hu 2008). Instead of passively trained by the robot, subjects are motivated to actively use their muscles during the training.

Biomechatronics in Medicine and Healthcare by Le Li and Raymond Kai-Yu Tong

www.panstanford.com
978-981-4241-61-8

6.1.1 Rehabilitation for Hand Functions

The loss of the hand functions are perceived by the stroke patients as a major problem and greatly affected their quality of life (QOL) (Broeks *et al.* 1999; Williams *et al.* 1999), and that the restoration of hand functions are important to the stroke subjects for their daily living. However, after went through the upper limb rehabilitation program, most stroke patients recovered some of the proximal motor functions at the shoulders and elbows but limited recovery for the distal motor functions at the wrists and hands (Chae *et al.* 2002; Chae and Hart 2003). As hand functions can do more complex tasks and require more muscle groups for fine control, the neural representation area at the motor cortex is larger. It will take longer time and more difficult for patient to retrain the hand functions. But the rehabilitation of hand functions is still achievable and under investigation. A few different groups around the world were already looking into hand rehabilitation using rehabilitation robot. For example, Masia *et al.* developed a hand module for the MIT-Manus which assists the grasping action (Masia *et al.* 2007). HWARD was a 3-degress of freedom (DOF) robotic device assists in grasping and releasing movements (Takahashi *et al.* 2005). The team of Lambercy *et al.* (chapter 4) developed the Haptic Knob and HandCARE to train the wrist pronation/supination and finger flexion/extension (Lambercy *et al.* 2007; Dovat *et al.* 2007). Kawasaki *et al.* built a 18-DOF hand motion assist robot (Kawasaki *et al.* 2007). A novel hand rehabilitation robot for hand functions training was developed as the extension of training for the upper extremities after the PolyJBot (Chapter 5).

6.2 DESIGN OF THE HAND REHABILITATION ROBOT

The hand rehabilitation robot is designed to train the hand functional tasks such as hand opening and hand grasp (i.e. palmar grasp and pinch). Each individual finger is powered by a separate actuator. This design requirement allows more complex pattern or task can be implemented. Hence a suitable actuator has to be found first. A few different actuators had been considered such as the voice coil motor, servo motor and linear actuator. However, the linear actuator was chosen because it can directly actuate the finger without the need to use gears or cable to transmit the power. And the micro linear actuator (ie. model L12) from the Firgelli, Canada meets our requirements with its small size, low cost and light weight characteristics.

According to Boissy *et al.*, the average grip force for the affected hand for stroke patient was about 130 N (Boissy *et al.* 1999). Comparing with other robot hand designs, maximum regulated output force for HWARD is 4-15 N (Cramer *et al.* 2007) while it was 16 N for Rutger Master Hand II (Bouzit *et al.* 2002) and 15 N for HandCare (Chapter 4.3.2). Therefore, the L12 linear actuator with 100 mm stroke length and 50:1 gear ratio would provide adequate speed (23 mm/s) and force (12 N) for assisting finger movement for stroke patient.

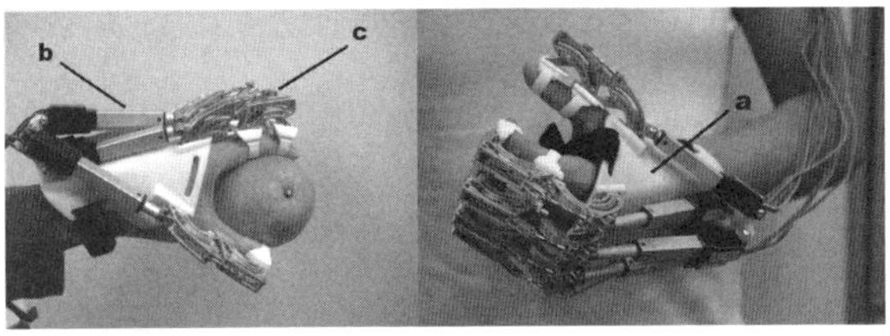

Figure 6.1 The task training hand system (a) actuators platform (b) linear actuator and (c) finger assembly. For color reference, see page 215.

6.2.1 Task Training Wearable Hand System

The first design is the task training wearable hand system which assists the user to practise the hand opening and palmar grasp functions with task oriented training (in Figure 6.1). It consists of a platform with five finger assemblies (one for each finger) and each finger assembly is actuated by one linear actuator. The linear actuator can move the metacarpal phalangeal (MCP) joint and interphalangeal (PIP) joint of the finger at the same time to generate finger extension and flexion. The range of motion for the MCP joint is 55° and the PIP joint is 65°. By adjusting the finger assembly to align the virtual centres to the MCP and PIP joint centres, the design can accommodate different palm size and finger length. It is a portable design where the total weight is approximately 500 grams. And the user can carry it around to practise hand function with their daily living activites.

6.2.2 Hand Function Training and Evaluation System

A hand function training and evaluation system is designed for training as well as evaluating hand functions such as the range of motion, finger forces and muscle control coordination of hand opening and hand grasp functions (in Figure 6.2). Position and force sensors have been integrated with motor system. It consists of two platforms that house the actuators and the arm. The poles of these two

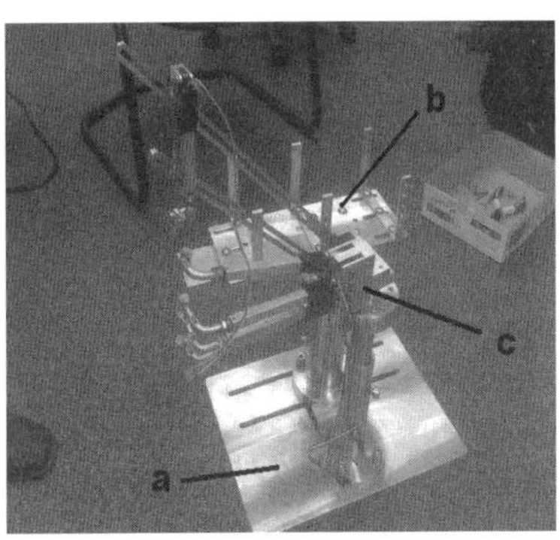

Figure 6.2 The hand function evaluation system (a) base support platform (b) hand support platform (c) actuators platform.

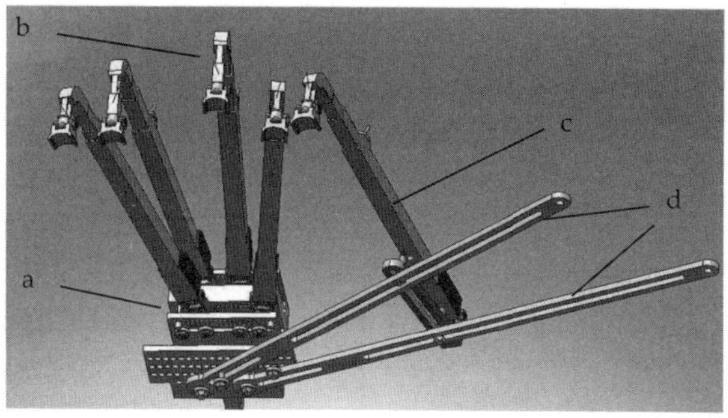

Figure 6.3 Platform to house the actuators (a) two levels actuator housing platform (b) finger actuators (c) thumb actuator (d) thumb actuator support bar.

platforms can be slided back and forward and sideway along the tracks on the base metal plate. Moreover, these poles can be rotated and elevated. The distance and the horizontal level can be adjusted for better alignment between the hand and the actuators. This flexible configuration of the hand function evaluation system also supports set up for right or left hand training.

6.2.2.1 Actuators Platform

Each finger is assisted by one linear actuator and the actuators need to be aligned with the finger movement path (Figure 6.3). A special platform was designed to house the actuators. It has two levels and the actuators can be freely placed at these levels. The advantage for this arrangement is that actuators can be placed closer together to fit for smaller hand size or palm width. Instead of four actuators placed side by side on the same level occupying wider space, two actuators for the middle and ring fingers can be placed on the first level while another two actuators for the index and last fingers can be placed on the second level. In addition, the angular direction of the actuator can be adjusted to align with the direction of the finger's flexion and extension to provide comfortable movement.

Two elongated rail bars are used to position the thumb actuator in two different settings to support the two hand functions ie. palmar grasp and pinch, as shown in Figure 6.4. The actuator platform is placed vertically so that all fingers are moving in horizontal level, reducing the gravity effects on the finger performance. And the arm of the patient can be comfortably placed on the arm holder.

6.2.2.2 Connecting Fingers

The finger is connected to the hand rehabilitation robot using a button connection (Figure 6.5). This is for easy attachment and detachment and act as a safety feature to avoid excessive force applied to the finger. Patient can unbuckle their fingers at anytime.

The 90 degree metal bars interconnect the fingers with the actuators. The metal bar screwed tightly with the stroke tip of the linear actuator. A mounting at the

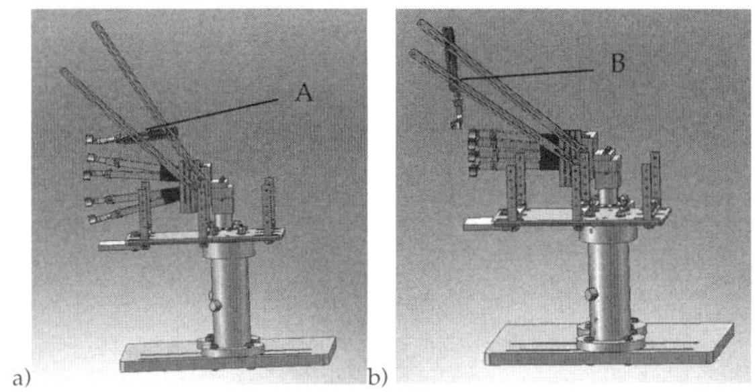

Figure 6.4 Thumb actuator configuration (a) palmar grasp (b) pinch.

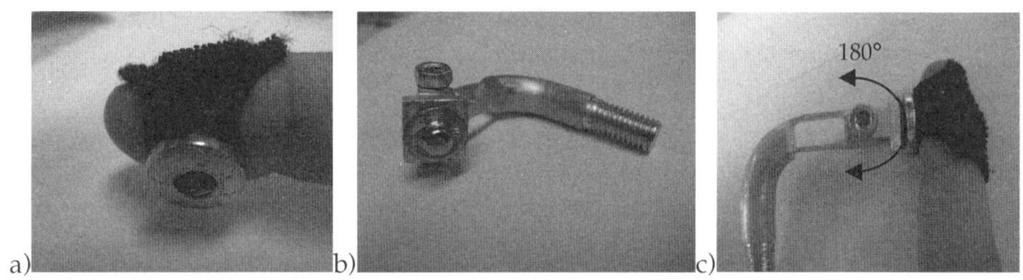

Figure 6.5 Connecting fingers using button connector (a) ring wrap around finger (b) metal bar with pivot mount (c) finger connect to metal bar.

front of the metal bar can rotate 180 degrees to allow finger to rotate along the tip of the bar when it is hand opening or hand grasp.

6.2.2.3 Position and Force Feedbacks

Each linear actuator is equipped with a linear slide potentiometer (ALPS model no. STRSA0N12S) which is used to measure the stroke extension of the actuator and hence this position feedback can be used to keep track of the finger position during training.

The metal bar of each actuator has a force transducer installed to measure the force applied by the finger. A pair of 5 mm foil strain gauges are installed in the cavity to measure the force during finger flexion and extension movements. Calibration is required to convert the feedback voltage into Newton (N). Multiple sand bags of 250 g are used to measure force up to 5 kg in both force directions (flexion and extension). Since the strain gauge has a good linearity, force beyond 5 kg or 49 N can still be measured.

6.3 EXPERIMENT PROCEDURE

When using the hand rehabilitation robot, subjects were asked to put their arms on the arm holder at a horizontal level. Wrist angle was fixed at zero degree to assure that gravity force would not interfere with the actual performance and hence the

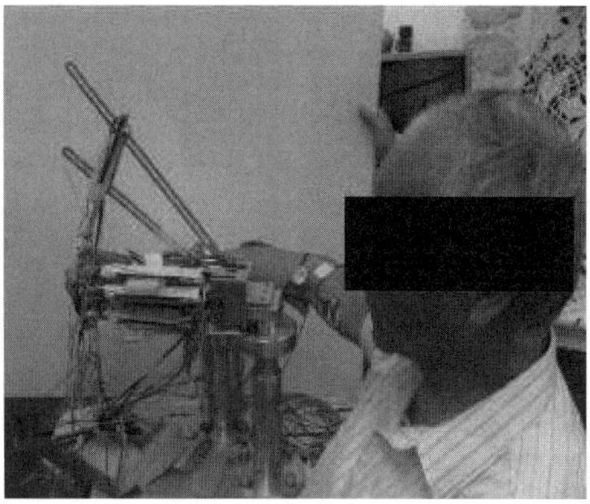

Figure 6.6 Experimental setup with an elderly subject.

measurement of the finger force would be generated from fingers only. Poles were adjusted to align the finger tips with the actuators. The actuator for the thumb was adjusted to provide the pinch movement. Figure. 6.6 shows the experimental setup for the right hand with one of the elderly subject.

6.3.1 Calibration of Range of Motion

Range of motion (ROM) measurements were required at the beginning of the evaluation, as individual's finger length and hand size was different. The travel range of each actuator needs to be adjusted to match the ROM of the corresponding finger. The range limit of each actuator was recorded and set for the hand opening and hand grasp during the training. As the travel distance of the finger tip varies according to the finger length, in order to align all the fingers for easier control, the ROM of each finger would be normalized to 100 percent according to the measured distance range (see Figure 6.7). After normalization, maximum flexion limit is mapped to 0%, and maximum extension limit is mapped to 100%.

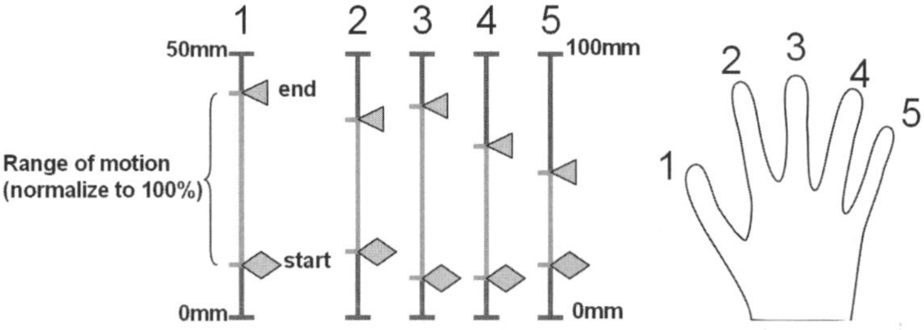

Figure 6.7 Calibration for the range of motion. The range of motion is represented by the space between the maximum flexion limit and the maximum extension limit.

6.3.2 EMG Electrode Placement

Two different muscle groups were selected for the detection of hand opening and hand grasp intention. As shown in the Figure 6.8, the EMG signals were collected from the extensor digitorum (ED) and the abductor pollicis brevis (APB). The ED signal was used for the control of hand opening while the APB signal was used for the control of hand grasp. Figure 6.9 displays the recorded EMG signals from the ED and APB muscles during a hand opening and hand grasp tasks.

6.3.3 Maximum Voluntary Contraction

Maximum voluntary contraction (MVC) can be used to evaluate the muscle strength of each subject every time at the beginning of the training. And the measured EMG signals of the MVC would be used for the normalization of the EMG signals for the control strategies. In order to measure the MVC more accurately, the hand rehabilitation robot would position the subject fingers randomly into 5 different hand positions according to the normalized ROM (ie. 0% means full palmar grasp or pinch while 100% means full hand opening) and the subject was asked to do two times MVC for hand grasp as well as two times MVC for hand opening.

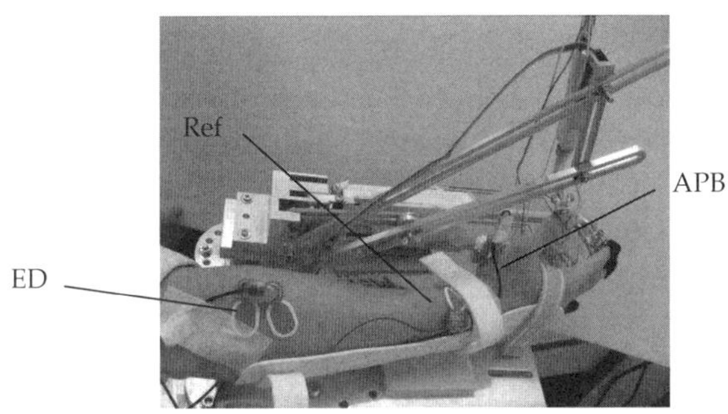

Figure 6.8 The setup showing the position of electrodes (APB, ED and reference).

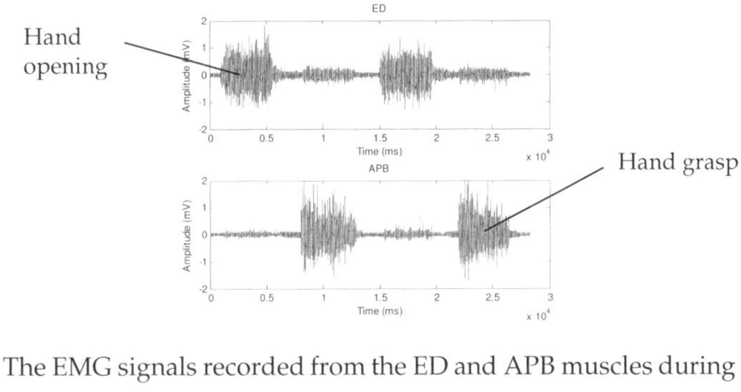

Figure 6.9 The EMG signals recorded from the ED and APB muscles during hand opening and hand grasp.

6.3.4 Control Strategies using Interactive EMG Signals

After the measurements of the MVC EMG signals and finger forces, three different training modes were provided to the subjects by the hand rehabilitation robot, namely the (1) continuous passive motion (CPM); (2) EMG-triggered motion (EMG-TRIG); and (3) continuous EMG-driven motion (cEMG). The first training mode provides passive motion to each finger for the hand opening and hand grasp tasks. In this mode, the subject was not required to provide any motor effort. The actuators would lead all the fingers according to the training task. In the EMG-triggered motion mode and the continuous EMG-driven motion mode, EMG signals are used to identify the intention of the hand opening and grasp from the subject during training. The EMG levels used in the EMG-TRIG mode and cEMG mode were normalized to the MVC value, which was defined as:

$$EMG = \frac{EMG_i - EMG_{i,rest}}{EMG_{i,IMVC} - EMG_{i,rest}} \tag{6.1}$$

where, EMG_i is the EMG of the agonist muscle i (ED during the extension, or APB during the flexion) after the processes of full wave rectification and moving average with 100ms window, $EMG_{i,rest}$ is the averaged EMG of muscle i during the resting state, and $EMG_{i,IMVC}$ is the EMG during maximum isometric contractions.

In the second mode (EMG-TRIG), the hand rehabilitation robot would wait for the EMG signals from ED or APB to reach above the threshold (commonly set at the 30% of the maximum voluntary contraction EMG signal strength) before initiating the motion of the training task. Once the EMG signal from the subject above the threshold, the robotic system would assist the subject to complete the training task.

The last training mode (cEMG) uses the EMG as the continuous driven signal for the training. Subject is required to continuously make voluntary muscle effort to complete the training task. The system actuates the hand opening or hand grasp task movements only when the real time EMG signal strength is higher than the threshold level and the system stops when the EMG signal strength is below threshold. Thus encourage the subject to continuous make effort to open or grasp their hands during training.

6.3.5 Hardware and Software Interfaces

All detected EMG signals, force and position feedbacks were sampled at a frequency of 1000 Hz with an USB NI data acquisition system (model: cDAQ-9172), and a LabView (version 8.5)-based application development platform for real-time control. The finger position inputs were used as a visual feedback for the subject, as shown in Figure 6.10.

The fingers' positions were displayed by the sliders during the finger tracking task. The target sliders move back and forward from 0% to 100% of the ROM of each finger in predefined t seconds. When the target sliders move, the subject' fingers (indicated by the control sliders) need to follow the movement of the target

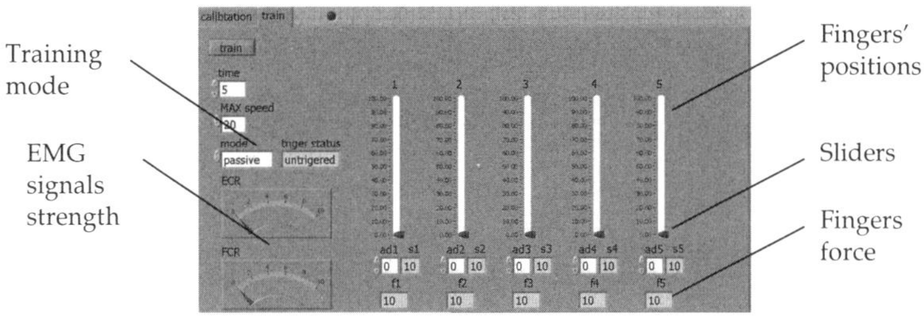

Figure 6.10 Graphical user interface of the hand rehabilitation robot.

as close as possible. Fingers force and EMG signals strength were displayed at the bottom as well.

6.4 PILOT CLINICAL EVALUATION OF HAND FUNCTIONS OF ELDERLY AND STROKE SUBJECTS

Five elderly subjects and five chronic stroke subjects were recruited in this pilot study. Both groups had 4 male and 1 female participants. The mean age of healthy elderly subjects was 67.2±3.6 years (range from 62 to 72 years old) while the mean age of chronic stroke subjects was 50.2±12.9 years (range from 35 to 64 years old). Table 6.1 summarizes the basic information of the elderly and stroke subjects and clinical assessment scores measured of the stroke subjects before the clinical trial. The assessments used were the Upper Extremities Fugl-Meyer Assessment (FMA-UE) for wrist and hand and the Action Research Arm Test (ARAT). The subject selection criteria are not having any cognitive, visual or attention deficits that would prevent them to follow the instructions or procedures. Both groups would use the right hand for training which implied the impaired hand for the stroke subject is on the same side too. There should be some residual active wrist and hand motion on the affected arm (see Table 6.1). Onset of stroke for the stroke subject should be at least 1 year and resulted from a single unilateral lesion only. This study was reviewed and approved by the human ethics committee of the local university and all subjects were informed with the experiment protocol and consents were requested.

Table 6.1 (a) Elderly subjects basic information (b) Stroke subjects and clinical assessment scores.

No (a)	Male/ Female	Age	No (b)	Male/ Female	Age	Lesion site	ARAT	FMA.W/H
E1	M	68	S1	M	39	L cerebral cortex	27	9
E2	F	62	S2	F	35	L basal ganglia	1	3
E3	M	72	S3	M	64	L basal ganglia	19	8
E4	M	67	S4	M	52	L cerebral cortex	28	14
E5	M	67	S5	M	61	L basal ganglia	7	8

The hand rehabilitation robot was set up for the right hand and adjusted for each subject's hand size. Calibrations of the range of motion were carried out and maximum voluntary contraction EMG signals and force for all subjects were recorded before training.

6.4.1 EMG Signal Analysis

Both stroke and elderly subjects were then requested to evaluate all 3 training modes. For each training mode, each subject was asked to perform two rounds of five cycles of hand opening (extension) and pinch (flexion). All EMG signals and the movement of all fingers were recorded for further analyses. Figure 6.11(a–f) shows the recorded EMG signals of ED and APB muscle groups as well as the position tracking movement of the index finger of the healthy elderly subject E4 and chronic stroke subject S4 for all 3 training modes.

For continuous passive motion, because it does not require any voluntary effort, both groups were able to complete the full range of hand opening and hand grasp under the assistance of the robotic system. Therefore, the EMG activation signals were very little. For EMG-triggered motion, both subject groups were able to trigger the movements of the robotic system. When comparing the EMG signal strength of the ED and APB between two groups, the elderly were stronger than the stroke group. In particularly, the stroke subject had difficulty in activating the APB muscle (ie. distal end). For the continuous EMG-driven motion training mode, as it required subject to continuously put effort to drive the movement, the duration of activated EMG signals were longer in both groups. The APB and ED EMG signals of stroke subject were not clearly distinguished from the

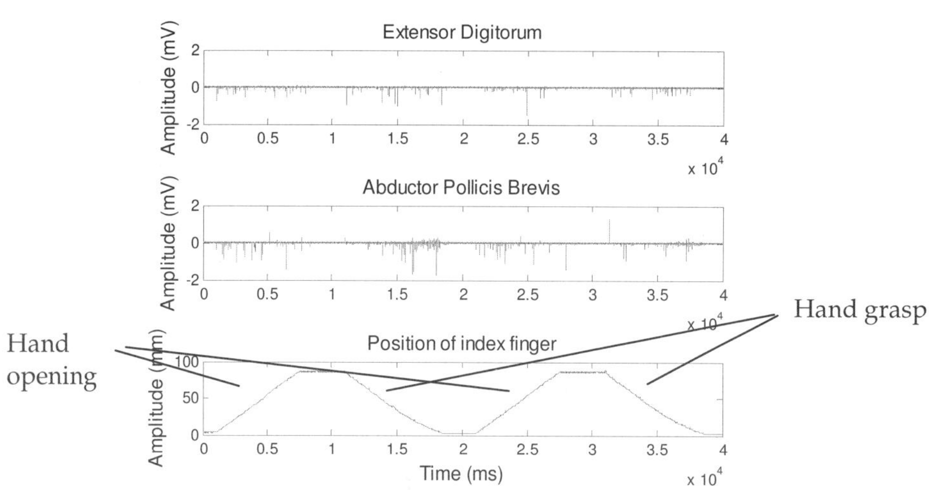

Figure 6.11a Continuous passive motion (CPM) for elderly subject E4. Top 2 rows are the EMG signals for ED and APB muscle groups. The bottom row is the position feedback of index finger movement.

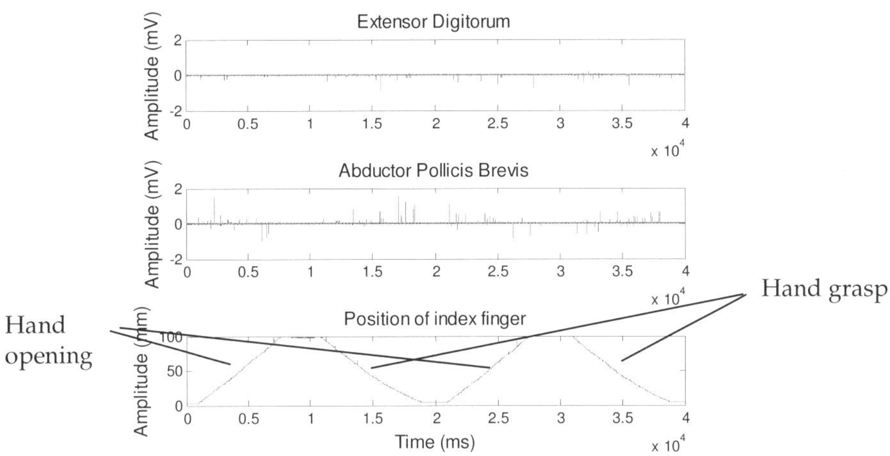

Figure 6.11b Continuous passive motion (CPM) for stroke subject S4. Top 2 rows are the EMG signals for ED and APB muscle groups. The bottom row is the position feedback of index finger movement.

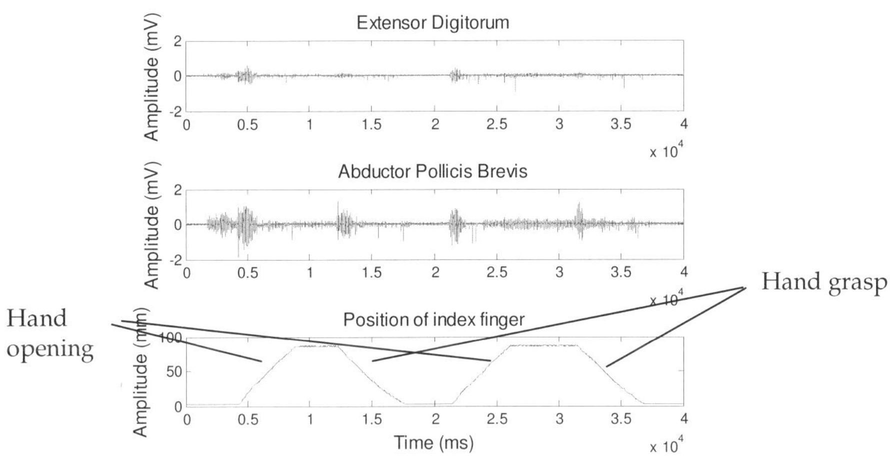

Figure 6.11c EMG-triggered motion for elderly subject E4. Top 2 rows are the EMG signals for ED and APB muscle groups. The bottom row is the position feedback of index finger movement.

hand opening or hand grasp tasks, showing that the stroke subject might have difficulty in muscle coordination when controlling these two muscle groups and cocontraction was observed.

6.4.2 Maximum Voluntary Force Analysis

Figure 6.12 shows the comparison charts of the maximum voluntary contraction forces of all fingers between the stroke and elderly groups. In both hand closing and hand opening tasks, stroke subjects had weaker finger forces than elderly

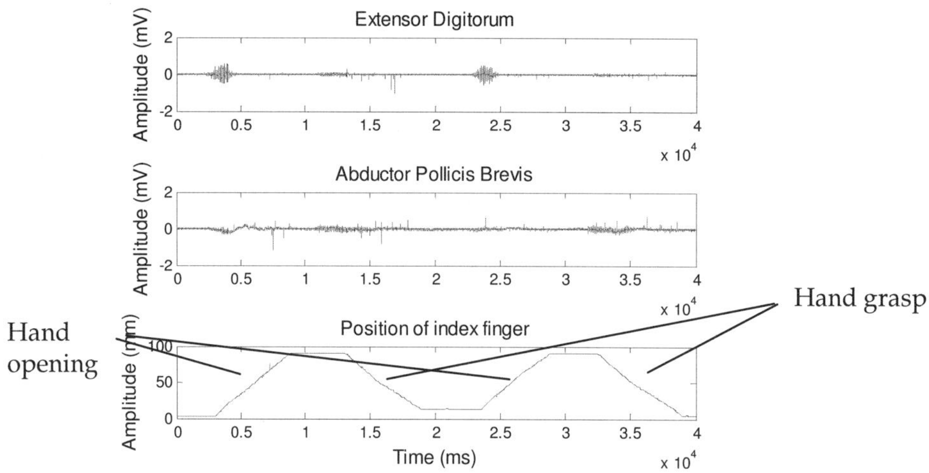

Figure 6.11d EMG-triggered motion for stroke subject S4. Top 2 rows are the EMG signals for ED and APB muscle groups. The bottom row is the position feedback of index finger movement.

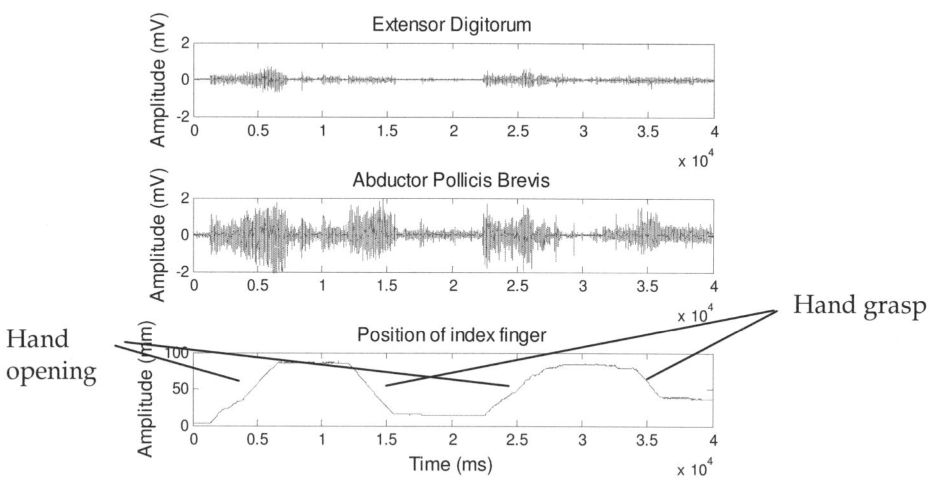

Figure 6.11e Continuous EMG-driven motion for elderly subject E4. Top 2 rows are the EMG signals for ED and APB muscle groups. The bottom row is the position feedback of index finger movement.

subjects. Because some stroke subjects had poor muscle co-ordination control, they could not open their hands, but rather flexed their fingers (opposite force) during extension motion. This could be the result of muscle co-contraction and spasticity where flexion muscles had stronger forces than extension muscles. Therefore, it is common that stroke subjects had more difficulty in hand opening than hand grasp. However, healthy elderly subjects did not encounter this problem.

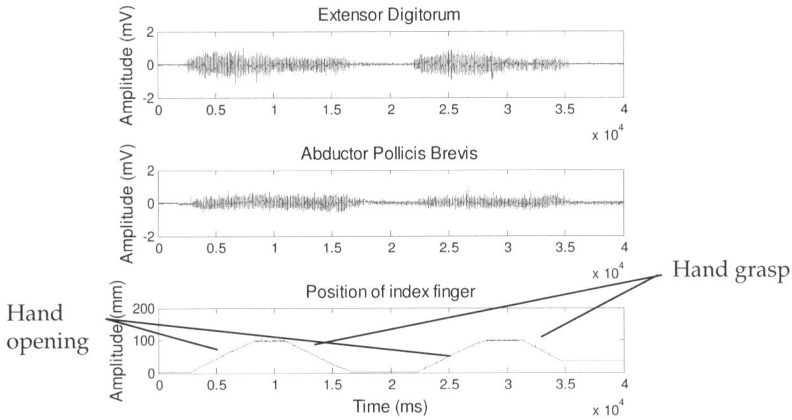

Figure 6.11f Continuous EMG-driven motion for stroke subject S4. Top 2 rows are the EMG signals for ED and APB muscle groups. The bottom row is the position feedback of index finger movement.

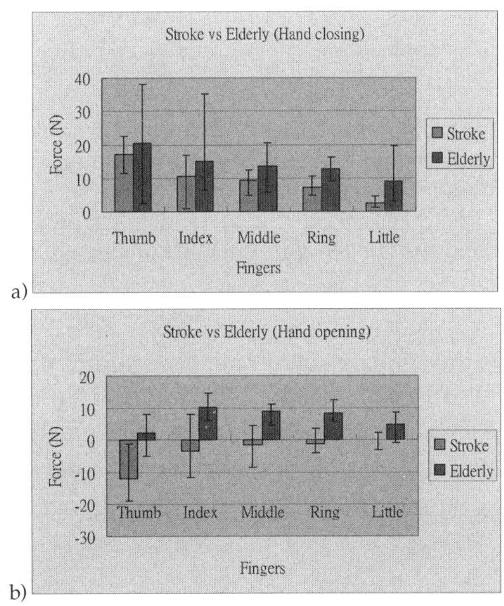

Figure 6.12 Maximum voluntary force between stroke and elderly groups during (a) hand grasp and (b) hand opening. The vertical bar is the maximum and minimum value within the group. The shaded bar is the mean value within the group. For color reference, see page 216.

6.4.3 Range of motion analysis

In the continuous EMG-driven mode, the movement is driven by the subjects' intention continuously. If the subject had difficulty in driving the system continuously, the range travelled would be less than 100%.

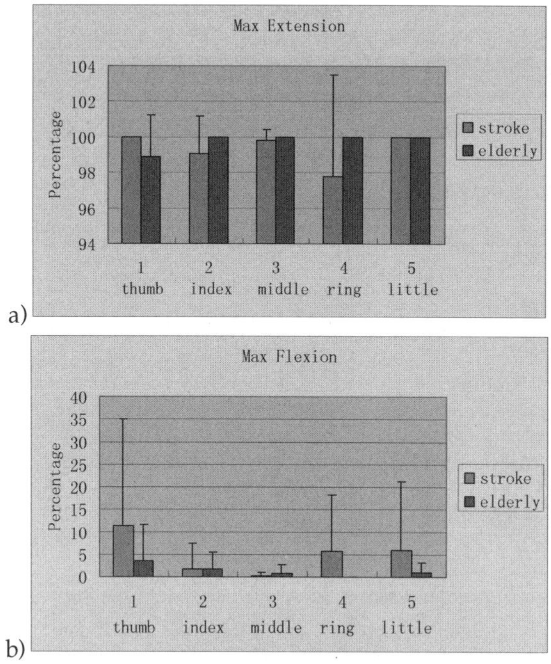

Figure 6.13 Comparison of the mean extension between 5 stroke and 5 elderly subjects during hand opening (extension). (a) Showing the maximum extension achieved in all cycles. Best result is 100% equals full extension. (b) Showing the maximum flexion achieved in all cycles. Best result is 0% equals complete hand grasp position. The vertical bar is the standard deviation and the shaded bar is the mean average. For color reference, see page 216.

Figure 6.13 shows the comparison of the maximum range between the elderly and stroke subjects. For hand opening task, the healthy elderly group covered almost the full range of extension whereas the stroke subjects had difficulty in extending their fingers. And for hand grasp task, the elderly had better muscle control than the stroke subjects to achieve more flexed position.

6.5 CONCLUSION

Rehabilitation of the distal motor functions of the upper extremity has been a challenge for the therapists for a long time and the recovery of hand functions is important to the stroke patients and elderly for their daily activities. With the new hand rehabilitation robot, stroke patients can actively train their hand opening and closing functions using their own EMG signals and learn. Learn to use their voluntary EMG signals to control the hand motion. Although stroke subjects had weak muscle strength and control, they demonstrated a better range of motion achieved during training with the assistance from the hand rehabilitation system. Further training with longer training period and greater intensity may be required for them to gain better muscle control. Using this new hand rehabilitation robot it demonstrated the feasibility for stroke subjects to train their hand functions with their own intention.

6.6 ACKNOWLEDGEMENT

The authors would like to thank for the financial support from the Innovative and Technology Council of the Hong Kong Special Administrative Region, China (grant no. GHP/003/07).

References

Boissy P., Bourbonnais D., Carlotti M. M., Gravel D. and Arsenault B. A., Maximal grip force in chronic stroke subjects and its relationship to global upper extremity function, Clin Rehabil, **13**, 354, (1999).

Bouzit M., Burdea G., Popescu G. and Boian R., The rutgers master II-new design force-feedback glove. In *IEEE/ASME Transactions on Mechatronics*, **7**(2), 256–263, (2002).

Broeks J. G., Lankhorst G. J., Rumping K. and Prevo A. J. H., The long-term outcome of arm function after stroke: Results of a follow-up study, *Disability & Rehabilitation*,**21**(8), 357–364, (1999).

Burgar C. G., Lum P. S., Shor P. C. and Machiel Van der Loos H. F., Development of robots for rehabilitation therapy: The Palo Alto VA/Stanford experience. *J. Rehabil. Res. Dev.*,**37**(6), 663–73, (2000).

Chae J. and Hart R., Intramuscular hand neuroprosthesis for chronic Non it survivors, *Neurorehabilitation & Neural Repair*, **17**, 109–117, (2003).

Chae J., Yang G., Park B. K. and Labatia I., Muscle weakness and cocontraction in upper limb hemiparesis: Relationship to motor impairment and physical disability, *Neurorehabilitation & Neural Repair*, **16**, 241–248, (2002).

Cramer S. C., Takahashi C. D., Der-Yeghiaian L, See J, Motiwala R. R. and Le V., Robot-Based Hand Motor Therapy after stroke, *Presented in the International Stroke Conference*, Feb. 2007, San Francisco, CA, (2007).

Dovat L., Lambercy O. and Johnson V., *et al.* A cable driven robotic system to train finger function after stroke. In: *IEEE 10th International Conference on Rehabilitation Robotics*, New York: IEEE;2007, 222–227, (2007)

Hesse S., Schulte-Tigges G., Konrad M., Bardeleben A. and Werner C., Robot-assisted arm trainer for the passive and active practice of bilateral forearm and wrist movements in hemiparetic subjects. *Arch. Phys. Med. Rehabil.*, **84**(6), 915–20, (2003).

Kawasaki H., Ito S. and Ishigure Y., *et al.* Development of a hand motion assist robot for rehabilitation therapy by patient self-motion control. In: *IEEE 10th International Conference on Rehabilitation Robotics*. New York: IEEE; 2007, 234–240, (2007).

Krebs H. I., Hogan N, Volpe B. T., Aisen M. L., Edelstein L. and Diels C., Overview of clinical trials with MIT-MANUS: a robot-aided neuro-rehabilitation facility. *Technol Health Care.* **7**(6), 419–23, (1999).

Lambercy O., Dovat L. and Johnson V., *et al.* Development of a robot-assisted rehabilitation therapy to train hand function for activities of daily living. In: *IEEE 10th International Conference on Rehabilitation Robotics*. New York: IEEE;2007, 678–682, (2007).

Masia L., Krebs H. I., Cappa P. and Hogan N., Design, characterization, and impedance limits of a hand robot. In: *IEEE 10th International Conference on Rehabilitation Robotics.* New York: IEEE; 2007, 1085–1089, (2007).

Song R., Tong K. Y., Hu X. L. and Li L., Assistive control system using continuous myoelectric signal in robot-aided arm training for patients after stroke, *IEEE T Neur Sys Reh*, 16, (2008).

Takahashi C., Der-Yeghiaian L., Le V.. and Cramer S. C., A robotic device for hand motor therapy after stroke. In: *Proceedings of IEEE 9th International Conference on Rehabilitation Robotics: Frontiers of the Human-Machine Interface. Chicago, Illinois*; 2005, 17–20,(2005).

Tong K. Y. and Hu X. L., "Service Robotics: Robot-Assisted Training for Stroke Rehabilitation," in *Service Robotics. Vienna, Austria: I-Tech Education and Publishing*, (2008).

Williams L. S., Weinberger M., Harris L. E., Clark D. O. and Biller J., Development of a Stroke-Specific Quality of Life Scale, *Stroke 30*, 1362–1369 (1999).

Chapter Seven

Functional Electrical Stimulation Leg Exercise: From Technology to Therapy

Nur Azah Hamzaid*,†, Che Fornusek* and Glen M Davis*
*Clinical Exercise and Rehabilitation Unit, University of Sydney, Lidcombe, NSW 2141, Australia
†Department of Biomedical Engineering, Faculty of Engineering, University Malaya, 50602, Kuala Lumpur, Malaysia

7.1 INTRODUCTION

Functional electrical stimulation (FES) is the application of external electrical currents to elicit muscle contractions using a neuromuscular stimulator, thereby bypassing the central nervous system (Holsheimer 1998). Muscle contractions via transcutaneous FES employs a control switch, a stimulator and a pair of electrodes deployed over the muscle belly (Sisto, 2009). When electrical stimulation is applied these muscles contract to produce motion, force and power.

Electrically stimulated contractions are employed to achieve 'functional' outcomes such as walking, standing or cycling, and to reverse foot-drop during gait in hemiplegic patients (Currier, 1992). In spinal cord injury (SCI) rehabilitation, FES is used to maintain or increase range of motion, ablate contractures, strengthen muscles, facilitate voluntary motor function, reduce spasticity, and prevent circulatory or orthostatic hypotension. In addition, FES is extensively used as a way of making possible exercise using the paralysed limbs (Sisto, 2009). Although not strictly "functional", FES-induced leg cycling has known benefits (Davis, 2008; Hamzaid, 2009) and it is broadly included because such benefits enhance functional outcomes.

7.2 EXERCISE FOR PEOPLE WITH NEUROLOGICAL DISABILITIES

Regular physical activity is beneficial not only for the able-bodied population, but also for people with neurological disabilities (Myslinski, 2005). Regular exercise

Biomechatronics in Medicine and Healthcare by Le Li and Raymond Kai-Yu Tong

www.panstanford.com
978-981-4241-61-8

induces numerous adaptations towards improved whole body fitness, particularly within the skeletal muscles. These adaptations have positive sequelae for the prevention and treatment of metabolic disorders (Hawley, 2009), especially amongst individuals with neurological pathophysiology.

Regular muscle strength and aerobic fitness training are normally prescribed to people with neurological disabilities to enhance their psychosocial and physical wellbeing (Skidmore, 2008). Individuals with stroke may perform exercise (Aziz, 2008) or task-oriented training (Rensink, 2009) to preserve and restore their fitness and functional capacity. People with traumatic brain injury (Bateman, 2001; Ross, 2009) may require regular exercise and physical training to improve their severely impaired wellbeing (Mayo Clinic, 2009).

7.2.1 Spinal Cord Injury and Exercise

SCI generally results from a traumatic lesion to the neural tracts within the spinal canal that results in sensory loss, motor deficit and bladder/bowel dysfunction (Anderson, 2002; Lifshutz, 2004). The most common causes of spinal cord injury are motor vehicle accidents (55%), followed by violence, falls, and recreational sports participation (Yeo, 1998).

Since the affected population is primarily young adults, and with improved medical treatment, the lifespan after SCI has significantly increased. However, as cervical or thoracic lesion SCI may lead to loss of lower limb movements, tetraplegia and paraplegia almost always result in significant physical deconditioning. Consequently, individuals with SCI often have significant reduction of their physical fitness due to limited movement capacity, which can lead to secondary degenerative disorders such as diabetes, hypertension and the early onset of cardiovascular disease (Jacobs, 2004). Effective rehabilitation, including aerobic fitness and muscular strength training can be useful preventive measures against secondary health problems.

Exercise is one possible strategy to reduce or reverse some of these post-injury complications (Jacobs, 2004). In individuals with SCI, voluntary exercise improves cardiovascular health, and increases the strength and endurance of the limbs that undergo training (Hicks, 2003). In contrast to voluntary exercise, FES-evoked training, which electrically stimulates the paralysed muscles to produce coordinated movements offers unique benefits to the paralysed limbs (Creasey, 2004). Theoretically, greater physical fitness can be achieved by including the lower limbs in the exercise as they make up the greater muscle mass of the body (Jacobs, 2004). Therefore FES leg exercise systems are now being integrated into their rehabilitation to optimize training (Sisto, 2009).

7.3 ELECTRICAL STIMULATION OF MUSCLES

Electrical stimulation-induced exercise applies trains of short, intense electrical pulses to generate muscle contractions and thereby elicit an exercise response (Dudley, 1999). Such artificially-evoked exercise usually involves the lower limbs, but may also involve the upper body via FES-assisted wrist exercise (Hartkopp, 2003) or arm cycling for tetraplegics (Gollee, 2002). The large muscle mass of the legs however implies that FES leg exercise has greater potential than voluntary arm exercise to train and improve cardiovascular fitness (Shephard, 1988; Haennel, 1992; Glaser 1994; Davis, 2008). The exercise performed during electrical stimulation can be as simple as isometric contractions through to more complex movements like leg raises (Hillegass, 1999), leg cycling (Fitzwater, 2002) or the lower-body component of rowing (Laskin, 1993).

The output of muscle stimulation using FES could be altered by modulating the current parameters, employing either monophasic or biphasic waveforms, current intensity, frequency, pulse duration and pulse train to elicit varied muscle contraction responses (Kralj, 1989).

7.3.1 Stimulation Waveforms

Trains of closely spaced stimulation pulses (Fig. 7.1, upper panel) are used to evoke muscle contractions. At a pulse frequency above 10–20 Hz in humans, the muscle fibre twitches (40–100 msec) begin to overlap and summate forming an extended muscle contraction (Baker, 2000). Increasing the pulse frequency further causes greater overlap and earlier force summation, until the individual twitches are completely fused into one smooth tetanic contraction. Tetanic summation depends upon the fibre characteristics of a particular muscle, but for de-efferented muscles it usually occurs at about 40 Hz pulse frequency (Shields, 1997; Gerrits, 2002). By adjusting the stimulation frequency (i.e. frequency modulation), between the fusion and the tetanus frequencies, the summation of fibre twitches and the resulting force can be modulated (Crago, 1980).

7.3.2 Pulse Frequency

During continuous stimulation, fatigue increases with higher stimulation frequency (Jones, 1979; Carroll, 1989; Hepple, 2003). There has been debate over whether the rate of fatigue is directly related to the frequency, the absolute number of pulses delivered (Marsden, 1983), both the frequency and the total number of

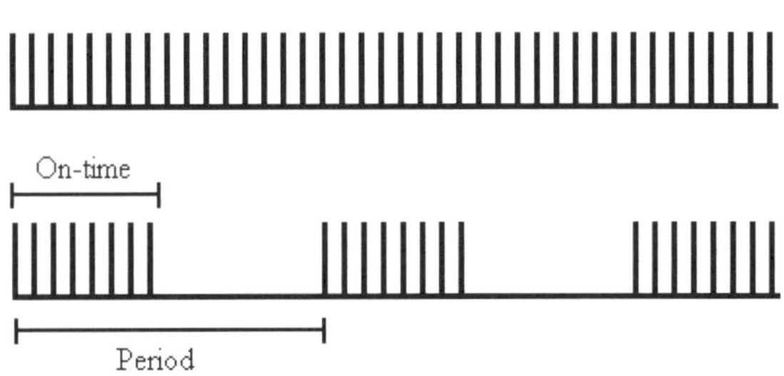

Figure 7.1 Continuous stimulation (top panel) and intermittent stimulation (bottom panel). For intermittent stimulation the duty cycle is equal to the on-time divided by the period.

pulses (Garland, 1992), or the increased forces produced at higher frequencies (Russ, 2002) by trying to understand what aspect of the stimulation frequency accelerates fatigue, researchers hope to develop new stimulation patterns such as variable frequency trains that will delay the occurrence of muscle fatigue (Bickel, 2003).

7.3.3 Intermittent Stimulation

Muscle stimulation during FES exercise can be continuous or intermittent. Intermittent stimulation (Figure 7.1, lower panel) involves repeated rhythmic trains of stimulation separated by periods without stimulation. During intermittent stimulation the "period" of repetition denotes the time between the start of consecutive stimulation bursts (Franken, 1993). The on-time is the length of a sequence of stimulation pulses during one cycle. The "duty cycle" is the on-time divided by the period. Both the duty cycle and the period of the intermittent stimulation have significant effect upon FES muscle fatigue.

Initially, a greater duty cycle produces a greater force time-integral (Lieber, 1993). However, fatigue rate increases with stimulation duty cycle (Baker, 1988), such that over an extended session a greater force-time-integral may not necessarily be produced (Lieber, 1993). This relationship is not surprising because increased contraction times require more energy and produce more metabolic byproducts, and because there is less recovery time between contractions. However, since a large proportion of the energy cost of a contraction is used to attain the initial muscle force (Russ, 2002) there must be an optimum duty cycle that represents the best trade-off between force output, fatigue, and the biomechanics of the task.

During intermittent stimulation for protocols with equivalent duty cycles, fatigue rate decreases as stimulation period is prolonged (Bergström, 1988; Hogan, 1998). Bergström *et al's* (1988) research, which investigated isometric muscle contractions, demonstrated that even though the total muscle contraction time and number of stimulation pulses were the same, fatigue developed faster in the protocols with shorter excitation periods. The metabolic cost of attaining a force is greater than maintaining the force. Hence, it is energetically 'expensive' and inefficient to produce short contractions (Bergström, 1988; Russ, 2002). However, if the length of the contraction is too long, then the amount of fatigue experienced will be greater (McTague, 1991). During long contractions ischemia may be induced by intramuscular pressure causing occlusion of blood circulation and an acceleration of fatigue (Petrofsky, 1975; Petrofsky, 2000). Higher contraction velocities also accelerate fatigue rate (Franken, 1993).

7.3.4 Electrode Types and Placements

A pair of electrodes is required to complete the circuit for current to flow through the muscles to evoke contractions. Spacing of the electrode pair effects the current

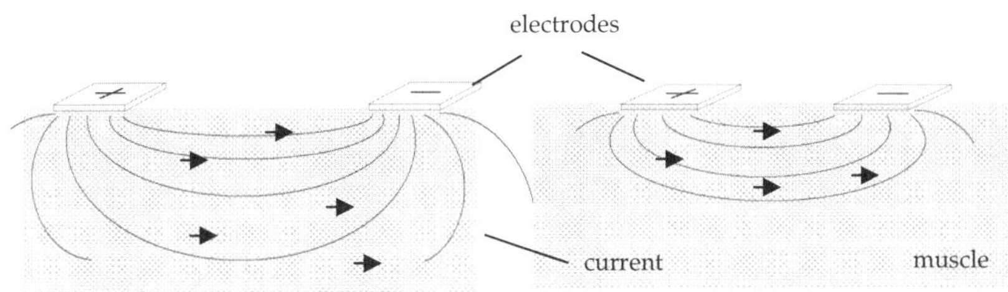

Figure 7.2 Current flowing through muscles with electrodes further apart gets deeper into muscle tissues compared to when the electrodes are closer together.

movement through muscle tissue (Sisto, 2009). Electrodes closer to each other allow the current to travel more superficially. Electrodes spaced further apart facilitate current travel deeper inside the muscle tissues (Fig. 7.2)

The electrode pairs could be surface electrodes which are the most commonly used for FES. Also, percutaneous electrodes (i.e. implanted in the muscle and exiting through the skin) or implanted electrodes, (i.e. completely implanted in the person's spinal roots) with radio frequency control outside the body could be used (Peckham 1987; Stein, 1992; Sisto, 2009). Implanted electrodes always provide greater precision of muscle movements; however the procedure is more invasive.

7.3.5 FES Muscle Fatigue and Muscle Fibre Recruitment

Onset of fatigue occurs faster during FES contractions than voluntary movements. During voluntary muscle contractions, individual motor units are activated independently at different times and rates leading to an asynchronous muscle fibre contraction pattern (Baker, 2000) and a reduction in fatigue. Additionally, motor fibre recruitment order via FES is the reverse of voluntary recruitment order, further accelerating fatigue. Motor units are recruited according to motor neurone position and geometry, with respect to the electrodes, as well as fibre size. During FES the large fast twitch fatigable units are recruited first and small slow twitch fatigue resistant units are recruited last (Hamada, 2004). This is because the electrical stimulation thresholds for the large neurons, which innervate the fast twitch fibres, are lower than for the small neurons which innervate the slow twitch motor units (Eccles, 1958).

As stimulation pulse intensity is increased, additional motor units are recruited. As more motor units are recruited and contribute to the contraction there is a non-linear increase in the force produced by the muscle (Kralj, 1989). If the stimulation intensity is high enough fibres from antagonist muscles may accidentally be recruited (Levin, 2000). At a given electrical muscle stimulation intensity there are no alterations in motor unit recruitment. Both the rapid fatigue during FES and the condition of paralysed muscle limit the functional outcomes or training benefits potentially delivered by any FES evoked systems (Sinclair, 1996).

7.4 FES-EVOKED EXERCISE

Originally FES was used as a technique to achieve standing and stepping amongst people with SCI (Vodovnik, 1965; Vodovnik, 1967). Individuals with SCI may be facilitated to perform upright ambulation with FES — sometimes with the assistance of orthoses. Nevertheless, the limitations in FES-evoked muscle contractions and the technology have to date made it impractical for extended walking outside of research laboratories (Kralj, 1989). However, more recently researchers have realized the potential of FES to produce exercise for peripheral and cardiorespiratory benefits in people with SCI (Phillips, 1984; Mutton, 1997). Even though the initial goal of FES for functional ambulation has yet to be achieved in a wider SCI population, the health benefits of FES evoked cycling exercise was discovered and has since been extensively acknowledged and investigated.

7.4.1 Benefits of FES-evoked Exercise

The health and fitness adaptation cycle continues as FES-evoked exercise is performed regularly. The regular muscle contractions accompanied by increased blood circulation can induce muscle hypertrophy which is also a well sought after cosmetic benefit amongst paraplegics and tetraplegics who normally have atrophied legs. An incomplete paraplegic may be able to perform better during training sessions if their muscular and cardiorespiratory capacities were enhanced, which might be a limiting factor before training (Postans, 2004). All these gains have the potential to increase ones psychological and social health and adaptation, which is important to reduce depression that is common amongst people with disabilities.

Increased muscle mass and size following electrical stimulation directly results in increased muscle strength and endurance (Kagaya, 1996), which further lead to increased functional exercise capacity (Petrofsky 1992a; Petrofsky, 1992b). With FES-evoked training, persons with SCI can perform exercise for longer training duration, at higher cadences, and increased resistance loads. Consequently, as FES-evoked functional capacity increases (i.e. evoked stepping distance, time or endurance), individuals who perform FES-evoked exercise will be able to exercise at higher cardiorespiratory intensity and eventually increase their aerobic fitness (Raymond, 2002). In short, carefully prescribed, FES-evoked exercise has demonstrated the ability to increase physical activity, life satisfaction, and well-being of people with SCI.

7.4.2 Performance Control

Research has been conducted to overcome the rapid muscle fatigue associated with FES that has limited the intensity of evoked exercise sessions. One way to overcome rapid muscle fatigue is to employ feedback control of the system. A user-controlled open-loop system is the most basic type of FES-system control, which is mostly employed during FES-evoked standing, stepping or short ambulation. In an open loop control the system does not change its stimulation properties regardless of the user's responses or performance, such as muscle fatigue when exercising or knee buckling during standing unless the user presses a switch (Kralj, 1989). Therefore, the only feedback the system has is the user's input which is based on the user's perception of their performance.

FES-evoked cycling exercise employs closed-loop control as it modifies the stimulation parameters based on training time, pedal or leg position, and in some modes based on the evoked forces. Position or motion sensors could be integrated as part of the closed loop system to detect critical body position or joint angles (Braz, 2006). Another example is the use of EMG to provide a signal that would indicate the initiation point during the start of an activity amongst people with incomplete SCI (Dutta, 2009). Surface EMG might also be utilized to detect early onset of muscle fatigue as a mode of fatigue compensation control (Winslow, 2003). The closed-loop systems allowed the stimulation parameters to be minimized and increased only as required to maintain a certain movement or position. This delayed the occurrence of muscle fatigue thus prolonged a training session (Winslow, 2003).

7.5 TECHNICAL DEVELOPMENT OF FES EXERCISE MACHINES

7.5.1 FES Cycling

FES-cycling elicits leg muscle contractions in appropriate sequence to produce cycling motion (Petrofsky, 1984; Wilder, 2002; Petrofsky, 2003). Generally the quadriceps, hamstrings, and gluteal muscle groups are used during FES-cycling (Glaser, 1994). Muscle contraction timing is controlled by a computer that stimulates each of the muscles at the correct crank angle to produce a pedalling movement (Petrofsky, 1984).

As the most popular mode of FES-evoked exercise, FES-evoked cycling may be the most economical way of training the leg muscles, and suitable for a wide range of persons with SCI. During FES cycling, the patient's body weight is always supported by seating and the training is highly repetitive. Furthermore a simple controller can automate the session. Therefore, only one person is required to monitor and run the system, making FES cycling a convenient and efficient mode of exercise for SCI individuals. A SCI person can begin FES-evoked cycling without much pre-training, in comparison to FES-evoked standing or walking which needs the leg muscles and bones to be strong enough to bear body mass in an upright posture.

In the past, FES cycling ergometer designs were dominated by devices that relied upon the electrically stimulated muscles to provide pedal drive and a mechanically or electrically braked flywheel to provide resistive loading. Over the years, advances have been made to the electronic braking and stimulation systems (Chen, 1997). However, controlling cycling cadence in this manner becomes more difficult when the desired target cadence is below 35 rev·min^{-1} and the resistive load is high.

7.5.2 Motorized FES Cycle Ergometers

An alternative to flywheel-braked cycling is to employ a motor to assist cycling (Eichhorn, 1984). For subjects with sufficient muscle power, the motor can be used to provide a pedalling resistance. The motor can also be used to calculate and correct for the energy required to passively move the legs and flywheel (Davis, 2001; Hunt, 2003). The motor has the advantage of enabling very weak subjects to perform FES cycling exercise, but a motorised system may pose an injury risk to the SCI subject's lower limbs. Safety precautions must be taken to limit the torque that the motor applies to the limbs of paralysed individuals. Recent technological advances have lead to the development of specialized low-power motorized cycle ergometers with safety features that prevent muscle injury (e.g. Motomed VIVA, Reck Medizentechnik GmβH, Germany) and can be integrated with FES.

7.5.3 Isokinetic FES Cycling Exercise

Recently, an isokinetic functional electrical stimulation leg cycle ergometer (iFES-LCE; Fig. 7.3) for people with spinal cord injury was developed (Fornusek, 2004). The iFES-LCE system was created from a motorized cycle ergometer, a computer, custom-designed software, and a laboratory-constructed six-channel transcutaneous neuromuscular stimulator.

It was designed to allow cycle training over a broad range of pedalling cadences (5-60 rev·min^{-1}), while providing accurate real-time feedback of muscle performance, to promote the development of both muscular strength and cardiorespiratory fitness. The inherent flexibility of the new system has made it very

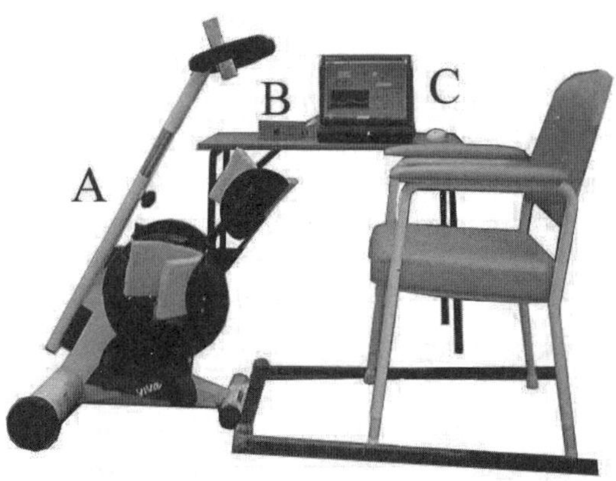

Figure 7.3 The iFES-LCE exercise system. Shown are a Motomed Viva® (A), the DS2000 neuromuscular stimulator (B), the control computer (C), and a chair for the subject. For color reference, see page 217.

useful as research and development tool. Examples of the iFES-LCE being used for research include the testing of biomechanical model for FES-evoked cycling (Sinclair 2001; Sinclair, 2004) and physiological response during FES-evoked cycling (Theisen, 2002).

Isokinetic exercise has long been recognised as a type of exercise whereby the muscle gains strength evenly throughout its range of movement, and is the fastest way to increase muscle strength. By definition, isokinetic exercise involves "an external means of holding the speed of body movements to a constant rate irrespective of the magnitude of forces generated by the participating muscles" (Hislop, 1967). Isokinetic exercise has been found to be an efficient, adaptable and reliable method of exercise (Grooten, 2002), thus most suitable in muscle strength building by individuals with SCI.

7.5.4 Isokinetic Cadence Control

Isokinetic motorized FES cycling systems have the advantage that cadence control is not reliant upon muscle stimulation. Non-motorized FES cycle ergometers rely upon the muscle stimulation to maintain the pedalling cadence. Relying on muscle stimulation to control pedalling cadence restricts the stimulation patterns that can be employed.

The mechanism of cadence control (i.e. motorized isokinetic vs. flywheel-braked isotonic FES-evoked cycling) at between 35–50 rev$\cdot$min^{-1} made no noticeable difference to the muscle powers generated or metabolic responses elicited (Fornusek, 2005).

Examples of stimulation intensity control schemes or modes that an isokinetic FES cycle can easily employ are manual control, a preset protocol, feedback control of power output, interval training, low cadence training, and eccentric training. Manual and preset protocol control of stimulation intensity is possible because the cycling motion does not rely on the muscle stimulation intensity; this is particularly useful for subjects who are very sensitive to muscle stimulation. Interval training has shown great potential to enhance the intensity of FES cycling (Janssen, 1996). Low cadence and eccentric training (Fornusek, 2009) may enhance the peripheral benefits of FES cycling.

The iFES-LCE is able to offer high-resistance low-cadence FES cycling. Muscle fatigue rates are less at lower pedal cadences (15 rev$\cdot$min^{-1}) during FES-evoked cycling and can produce higher muscle forces during FES-cycle training (Fornusek, 2004). Training with greater muscle forces has produced improved strength (Belanger, 2000; Hartkopp, 2003; Crameri, 2004) and hypertrophic gains (Dudley, 1999). Therefore, FES-LCE training at slow pedal cadences may confer improved strength and hypertrophic gains compared to higher pedal cadences (35-50 rev$\cdot$min^{-1}). Although the pedalling cadence affects the power output, it does not appear to influence the potency of cardiovascular stress (Fornusek, 2008). Therefore, low cadence training should be as effective as higher cadences for cardiovascular fitness training.

7.5.5 Isokinetic FES Leg Stepping Exercise

A more recent approach towards maximizing FES-evoked leg exercise dose potency has been to employ an elliptical stepping movement (Hamzaid, 2009). An isokinetic FES leg stepping trainer (iFES-LST) was developed to integrate the features of isokinetic exercise with evoked muscle contractions and elliptical stepping movements (Hamzaid, 2009). The stepping movement had less vertical displacement than normal cycling would have and had greater ratio of horizontal:vertical displacement (Hamzaid, 2007). The authors hypothesised that the evoked muscle contractions would facilitate longer muscle activation times to produce the elliptical movement (Hamzaid, 2006), facilitated by a 'slider-crank' mechanism (Shigley, 1995) as illustrated in Fig. 7.4. Thus, leg training might approximate the known movements of walking, but in a seated posture, with potential benefits to the patient.

The primary leg muscles were stimulated in repetitive sequence based on the position of the legs. A continuous potentiometer was utilized to deduce the accurate crank angular position from which the leg position was derived. Evoked leg muscle contractions translated into the legs producing stepping power onto the pedals, which could be quantified given the muscles were conditioned enough and the stimulation current is sufficiently high.

The elliptical stepping trainer elicited greater metabolic cost and higher mechanical efficiency compared to traditional FES-evoked cycling (Hamzaid, 2009). The gain in power production by changing the mechanical foundation (i.e. cycling to stepping) was greater than the power production increase when optimizing the stimulation pattern during FES-evoked stepping (Hamzaid, 2008).

Another feature of the iFES-LST was the released ankle joint in plantar-dorsiflexion facilitated by a custom-made ankle foot orthoses (AFO). The AFO

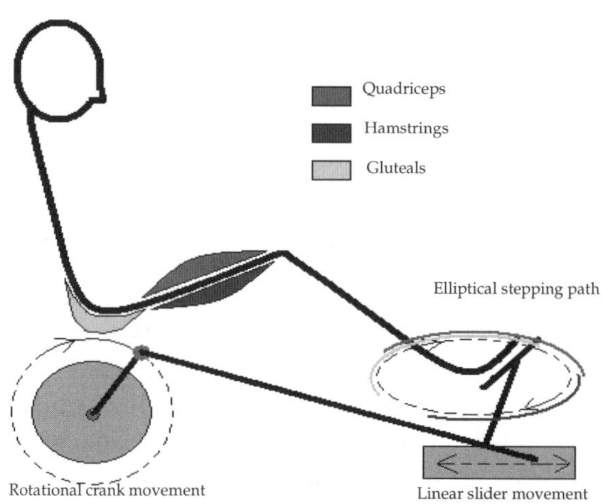

Figure 7.4 Joint and linkages of an elliptical stepper. Primary muscles and the muscle stimulation path is illustrated. For color reference, see page 217.

supported the weight of the legs from the pedal while pivoting around the heel area (Kim, 2007). The main function of the AFO was as a cavity for the SCI users' leg to control the involuntary lateral knee movements due to gravity and movement while they were seated on the exercise machine. However, the released ankle joint allowed constrained FES-induced leg movements to the sagittal plane.

The AFO produced greater ankle joint power than released-ankle cycling (Hamzaid, 2009). This feature may assist ankle joint restrengthening in which FES-evoked seated stepping is more relevant to walking as compared to cycling. Nevertheless, the current state of research does not support the use of released ankle joint during FES-evoked cycling. For example, ankle power was found to be 10% less when released than during fixed ankle cycling (van Soest, 2005). Further research has to be conducted to design the optimal of ankle foot orthoses during FES (Trumbower, 2005). A well designed constrained-ankle orthoses combined with FES would be able to achieve the best physio-therapeutical effects. In short, by optimizing the mechanical foundation of the system, a more dose-potent mode of exercise could be attained.

7.6 CONCLUSIONS

FES-evoked exercise systems can enhance the aerobic fitness, muscle strength and endurance, and improve physiological outlook in individuals with SCI. Future uses of these devices will play a role in "activity-based therapies", both during acute rehabilitation and to provide benefits to those with long-standing SCI.

References

Anderson A. J., "Mechanisms and pathways of inflammatory responses in CNS trauma: spinal cord injury." *J. Spinal Cord. Med.* **25**(2), 70–9; discussion 80, (2002).

Aziz N. A., J. Leonardi-Bee., *et al.* "Therapy-based rehabilitation services for patients living at home more than one year after stroke." *Cochrane Database of Systematic Reviews* (2) (2008).

Baker L. L., K. Cole., *et al.* "Effects of duty cycle and frequency on muscle fatgiue during isometric electrically stimulated quadriceps contractions." *Phys. Ther.* **68**, 835 (1988).

Baker L. L., C. L. Wederich., *et al.* Neuromuscular Electrical Stimulation: A Practical Guide. CA, (2000).

Bateman A., F. J. Culpan., *et al.* "The effect of aerobic training on rehabilitation outcomes after recent severe brain injury: A randomized controlled evaluation." *Archives of Physical Medicine and Rehabilitation* **82**(2), 174–82 (2001).

Belanger M., R. B. Stein., *et al.* "Electrical stimulation: can it increase muscle strength and reverse osteopenia in spinal cord injured individuals?" *Arch. Phys. Med. Rehabil* **81**(8), 1090–8 (2000).

Bergström M., and E. Hultman., "Energy cost and fatigue during intermittent electrical stimulation of human skeletal muscle." *J. Appl. Physiol.* **65**(4), 1500–5 (1988).

Bickel C. S., J. M. Slade., *et al.* "Fatigability and variable-frequency train stimulation of human skeletal muscles." *Phys. Ther.* **83**(4), 366–73 (2003).

Braz G. P., M. Russold., *et al.* Motion Sensors Feedback in FES Gait: *A Novel Control Strategy. World Congress on Medical Physics and Biomedical Engineering*, Seoul, South Korea, (2006).

Carroll S. G., R. J. Triolo., *et al.* "Tetanic responses of electrically stimulated paralyzed muscle at varying interpulse intervals." *IEEE Trans. Biomed. Eng.* **36**(7), 644–53 (1989).

Chen J. J., N. Y. Yu., *et al.* "Applying fuzzy logic to control cycling movement induced by functional electrica stimulation." *IEEE Trans. Neural Syst. Rehabil. Eng.* **5**(2), 158–69 (1997).

Crago P. E., P. H. Peckham., *et al.* "Modulation of muscle force by recruitment during intramuscular stimulation." *IEEE Trans. Biomed. Eng.* **27**(12), 679–84 (1980).

Crameri R. M., P. Cooper., *et al.* "Effect of load during electrical stimulation training in spinal cord injury." *Muscle Nerve.* **29**(1), 104–11 (2004).

Creasey G. H., C. H. Ho., *et al.* "Clinical applications of electrical stimulation after spinal cord injury." *J. Spinal. Cord. Med.* **27**(4): 365–75,(2004).

Currier D. P. and R. M. Nelson, Eds. Dynamics of Human Biologic Tissues. Philadelphia, F. A. Davis Company, (1992).

Davis G. M., N. A. Hamzaid and C. Fornuset. "Cardiorespirotory, metobolic, and Biomechanical Responses during Functional Electrical Simulation Leg Exereise: Heolth and Fitness Bemefits." Artificial organs. **32**, 625–659 (2008).

Davis G. M., P. Sinclair., *et al.* Improvements Relating to Muscle Stimulation Systems. Australia, The University of Sydney, (2001).

Dudley G. A., M. J. Castro., *et al.* "A simple means of increasing muscle size after spinal cord injury, a pilot study." Eur *J. Appl. Physiol. Occup Physiol.* **80**(4), 394–6 (1999).

Dutta A., R. Kobetic., *et al.* "Gait Initiation With Electromyographically Triggered Electrical Stimulation in People With Partial Paralysis." *Journal of Biomechanical Engineering-Transactions of the Asme* **31**(8) (2009).

Eccles J. C., R. M. Eccles., *et al.* "The action potentials of the alpha motoneurones supplying fast and slow muscles." *J. Physiol* **142**(2), 275–91 (1958).

Eichhorn K. F., W. Schubert., *et al.* "Maintenance, training and functional use of denervated muscles." *J. Biomed. Eng.* **6**(3), 205–11 (1984).

Fitzwater R., "A personal user's view of functional electrical stimulation cycling." *Artif. Organs.* **26**(3), 284–6 (2002).

Fornusek C., An Isokinetic Functional Electrical Stimulation Leg Cycle Ergometer for Indviduals with Spinal Cord Injury. Sydney, The University of Sydney, Australia. PhD, 318 (2005).

Fornusek C., S. Ahmadi., *et al.* Eccentric Functional Electrical Stimulation Cycling. 14th Annual International Functional Electrical Stimulation Society Conference. Seoul, Korea 83–4 (2009).

Fornusek C. and G. M. Davis., "Maximizing muscle force via low-cadence functional electrical stimulation cycling. *Journal of Rehabilitation Medicine* **36**(5), 232–7 (2004).

Fornusek C. and G. M. Davis., "Cardiovascular and metabolic responses during functional electric stimulation cycling at different cadences." *Archives of Physical Medicine and Rehabilitation* **89**(4), 719–25 (2008).

Franken H. M., P. H. Veltink., *et al.* "Fatigue of Intermittently Stimulated Paralyzed Human Quadriceps During Imposed Cyclical Lower Leg Movements." *J. Electromyogr Kinesiol* **3**(1), 3–12 (1993).

Garland D. E., C. A. Stewart., *et al.* "Osteoporosis after spinal cord injury." *J. Orthop Res.* **10**(3), 371–8 (1992).

Gerrits H. L., M. T. Hopman., *et al.* "Effects of training on contractile properties of paralyzed quadriceps muscle." *Muscle Nerve* **25**(4), 559–67 (2002).

Glaser R. M., "Functional neuromuscular stimulation. Exercise conditioning of spinal cord injured patients." *Int J. Sports Med.* **15**(3), 142–8 (1994).

Gollee H., K. J. Hunt., *et al.* An Apparatus for FES-assisted Arm-Cranking Exercise in Tetraplegia. *The 7th Annual Conference of the IFESS*, Ljubljana, Slovenia (2002).

Grooten W. J., A. V Puttemans., *et al.* "Reliability of isokinetic supine bench press in healthy women using Ariel Computerized Exercise System." Scandinavian *Journal of Medicine & Science in Sports* **12**(4), 218–22 (2002).

Haennel R. G., G. D. Snydmiller., *et al.* "Changes in blood pressure and cardiac output during maximal isokinetic exercise." *Arch. Phys. Med. Rehabil* **73**(2), 150–5 (1992).

Hamada T., T. Kimura., *et al.* "Selective fatigue of fast motor units after electrically elicited muscle contractions." *J. Electromyogr Kinesiol* **14**(5), 531–8 (2004).

Hamzaid N., G. M. Davis., *et al.* Isokinetic Cycling versus Elliptical Stepping, A Kinematic and Electromyography Analysis. *15th International Conference on Mechanics in Medicine and Biology*. Singapore. **15**,514–5 (2006).

Hamzaid N. A. and G. M. Davis., "Health and Fitness Benefits of Functional Electrical Stimulation-Evoked Leg Exercise for Spinal Cord–Injured Individuals, A Position Review." *Topics in Spinal Cord Injury Rehabilitation* **14**(4), 88–121 (2009).

Hamzaid N. A., C. Fornusek., *et al.* "Mechanical design and driving mechanism of an isokinetic functional electrical stimulation-based leg stepping trainer." *Australasian Physical Engineering Science in Medicine* **30**(4), 323–6 (2007).

Hamzaid N. A., C. Fornusek., *et al.* Development of an Isokinetic FES Leg Stepping Trainer (iFES-LST) for Individuals with Neurological Disability. *IEEE 11th International Conference on Rehabilitation Robotics*, Kyoto, Japan (2009).

Hamzaid N. A., C. Fornusek., *et al.* Stimulation Angle Variation in Isokinetic Stepping. *International Functional Electrical Stimulation Society* Conference, Freiburg, Germany (2008).

Hamzaid N. A., K. Pithon., *et al.* Metabolic Cost and Mechanical Efficiency of FES-Evoked Leg Cycling and Elliptical Stepping. *14th Annual International Functional Electrical Stimulation Society Conference*. Seoul, Korea, 79–81 (2009).

Hartkopp A., S. D. Harridge., *et al.* "Effect of training on contractile and metabolic properties of wrist extensors in spinal cord-injured individuals." *Muscle Nerve* **27**(1), 72–80 (2003).

Hawley J. A and J. O. Holloszy., "Exercise, it's the real thing!"*Nutrition Reviews* **67**(3), 172–8 (2009).

Hepple R. T., D. J. Krause., *et al.* "V(O2) max is unaffected by altering the temporal pattern of stimulation frequency in rat hindlimb in situ." *J. Appl. Physiol* **95**(2), 705–11 (2003).

Hicks A. L., K. A. Martin., *et al.* "Long-term exercise training in persons with spinal cord injury, effects on strength, arm ergometry performance and psychological well-being." *Spinal Cord.* **41**(1), 34–43 (2003).

Hillegass E. A. and G. A. Dudley., "Surface electrical stimulation of skeletal muscle after spinal cord injury." *Spinal Cord.* **37**(4), 251–7 (1999).

Hislop H. J. and J. J. Perrine., "The isokinetic concept of exercise." *Phys. Ther.* **47**(2), 114–7 (1967).

Hogan M. C., E. Ingham., *et al.* "Contraction duration affects metabolic energy cost and fatigue in skeletal muscle." Am *J. Physiol.* **274**(3 Pt 1), E397–402 (1998).

Holsheimer J., "Concepts and Methods in Neuromodulation and Functional Electrical Stimulation, An Introduction." *Neuromodulation* **1**(2), 57–61 (1998).

Hunt K. J., A. J. Cathcart., *et al.* Workrate and cadence control for exercise testing in FES cycling. *IFESS From Technology to Marlet Bridging the Gap*, Maroochydore, Sunshine Coast, Queensland, Australia (2003).

Jacobs P. L. and M. S. Nash., "Exercise recommendations for individuals with spinal cord injury." *Sports Medicine* **34**(11), 727–51 (2004).

Janssen T., R. Glaser., *et al.* Improving FES-Leg Cycle Ergometer Performance in Individuals who have Plateaued During Long-term Training. *RESNA '96 Proceedings*, Salt Lake City, Utah (1996).

Jones D. A., B. Bigland-Ritchie., *et al.* "Excitation frequency and muscle fatigue, mechanical responses during voluntary and stimulated contractions." *Exp. Neurol.* **64**(2), 401–13 (1979).

Kagaya H., Y. Shimada., *et al.* "Changes in muscle force following therapeutic electrical stimulation in patients with complete paraplegia." *Paraplegia* **34**(1), 24–9 (1996).

Kim I., N. A. Hamzaid., *et al.* Design Considerations of Lower Limb Support for Elliptical Stepping Exercise by Spinal Cord Injured Individuals. *5th Australasian Congress on Applied Mechanics*, Brisbane, Australia, Engineers Australia (2007).

Kralj A. and T. Bajd, Eds., Functional Electrical Stimulation, Standing and Walking after Spinal Cord Injury. Florida, CRC Press (1989).

Laskin J. J., E. A. Ashley., *el al.* "Electrical stimulation-assisted rowing exercise in spinal cord injured people. A pilot study." *Paraplegia.* **31**(8), 534–41 (1993).

Levin O., J. Mizrahi., *et al.* "Transcutaneous FES of the paralyzed quadriceps, is knee torque affected by unintended activation of the hamstrings?" *J. Electromyogr Kinesiol* **10**(1), 47–58 (2000).

Lieber R. L. and M. J. Kelly., "Torque history of electrically stimulated human quadriceps, implications for stimulation therapy." *J. Orthop Res.* **11**(1), 131–41 (1993).

Lifshutz J. and A. Colohan., "A brief history of therapy for traumatic spinal cord injury." *Neurosurg Focus* **16**(1), E5 (2004).

Marsden C. D., J. C. Meadows., *et al.* ""Muscular wisdom" that minimizes fatigue during prolonged effort in man, peak rates of motoneuron discharge and slowing of discharge during fatigue." *Adv. Neurol* **39**, 169–211 (1983).

Mayo Clinic Ed., Mayo Clinic Guide to Living with a Spinal Cord Injury. New York, Demos Health (2009).

McTague M. and S. Lynch., The effect of ON OFF times on fatigue during electrical stimulation of the quadriceps muscle, *Dept. Phys. Ther.*, Univ So Calif (1991).

Mutton D. L., A. M. Scremin., *et al.* "Physiologic responses during functional electrical stimulation leg cycling and hybrid exercise in spinal cord injured subjects." *Arch. Phys. Med. Rehabil* **78**(7), 712–8 (1997).

Myslinski M. J., "Evidence-based Exercise Prescription for Individuals with Spinal Cord Injury." *Journal of Neurologic Physical Therapy* **Jun**(2005) 104–016.

Peckham P. H., "Functional electrical stimulation, current status and future prospects of applications to the neuromuscular system in spinal cord injury." *Paraplegia* **25**(3), 279–88 (1987).

Petrofsky J. S., "Functional Electrical-Stimulation, a 2-Year Study." *Journal of Rehabilitation* **58**(3), 29–34 (1992a).

Petrofsky J. S. and M. Laymon., "The effect of previous weight training and concurrent weight training on endurance for functional electrical stimulation cycle ergometry." Eur *J. Appl. Physiol* (2003).

Petrofsky J. S., C. A. Phillips., *et al.* "Bicycle Ergometer For Paralyzed Muscle." *Journal of Clinical Engineering* **9**(1), 13–9 (1984).

Petrofsky J. S., R. R. Rochelle., *et al.* "The assessment of the static component in rhythmic exercise." Eur *J. Appl. Physiol Occup Physiol* **34**(1), 55–63 (1975).

Petrofsky J. S. and R. Stacy., "The effect of training on endurance and the cardiovascular responses of individuals with paraplegia during dynamic exercise induced by functional electrical stimulation." Eur *J. Appl. Physiol Occup Physiol* **64**(6), 487–92 (1992b).

Petrofsky J. S., R. Stacy., *et al.* "The relationship between exercise work intervals and duration of exercise on lower extremity training induced by electrical stimulation in humans with spinal cord injuries." Eur *J. Appl. Physiol* **82**(5–6), 504–9 (2000).

Phillips C. A., J. S. Petrofsky., *et al.* "Functional Electrical Exercise - a Comprehensive Approach for Physical Conditioning of the Spinal Cord Injured Patient." *Orthopedics* 7, 1112 (1984).

Postans N. J., J. P. Hasler., *et al.* "Functional electric stimulation to augment partial weight-bearing supported treadmill training for patients with acute incomplete spinal cord injury, A pilot study." *Archives of Physical Medicine and Rehabilitation* **85**(4), 604–10 (2004).

Raymond J., G. M. Davis., *et al.* "Cardiovascular responses during submaximal electrical stimulation-induced leg cycling in individuals with paraplegia." *Clin. Physiol Funct Imaging* **22**(2), 92–8 (2002).

Rensink M., M. Schuurmans., *et al.* "Task-oriented training in rehabilitation after stroke, systematic review." *J. Adv. Nurs.* **65**(4), 737–54 (2009).

Ross L. F., L. A. Harvey., *et al.* "Do people with acquired brain impairment benefit from additional therapy specifically directed at the hand? A randomized controlled trial." *Clin. Rehabil.* **23**(6), 492–503 (2009).

Russ D. W., M. A. Elliott., *et al.* "Metabolic costs of isometric force generation and maintenance of human skeletal muscle." Am *J. Physiol Endocrinol Metab.* **282**(2), E448–57 (2002).

Russ D. W., K. Vandenborne., *et al.* "Effects of muscle activation on fatigue and metabolism in human skeletal muscle." *J. Appl. Physiol* **92**(5), 1978–86 (2002).

Shephard R. J., E. Bouhlel., *et al.* "Muscle mass as a factor limiting physical work." *J. Appl. Physiol* **64**(4), 1472–9 (1988).

Shields R. and Y. Chang., "The Effects of Fatigue on the Torque-frequency Curve of the Human Paralysed Soleus Muscle." *J. Electromyogr Kinesiol* **7**(1), 3–13 (1997).

Shigley J. E. and J. J. J. Uicker., Theory of Machines and Mechanisms, McGraw-Hill, Inc (1995).

Sinclair P. J., G. M. Davis., *et al.* "Pedal forces produced during neuromuscular electrical stimulation cycling in paraplegics." *Clinical Biomechanics* **11**(1), 51–7 (1996).

Sisto S. A., E. Druin., *et al.*, Eds. Spinal Cord Injuries, *Management and Rehabilitation.* Missouri, Mosby Elsevier (2009).

Skidmore F. M., S. L. Patterson., *et al.* "Pilot safety and feasibility study of treadmill aerobic exercise in Parkinson disease with gait impairment." *Journal of Rehabilitation Research and Development* **45**(1), 117–24 (2008).

Stein R. B., P. H. Peckham., *et al.*, Eds. Neural Prostheses, Replacing Motor Function after Disease or Disability. New York, Oxford University Press (1992).

Trumbower R. D. and P. D. Faghri. "Kinematic analyses of semireclined leg cycling in able-bodied and spinal cord injured individuals." *Spinal. Cord.* **43**(9), 543–9 (2005).

van Soest A. J., M. Gfohler., *et al.* "Consequences of ankle joint fixation on FES cycling power output, a simulation study."*Med. Sci. Sports Exerc* **37**(5), 797–806 (2005).

Vodovnik L., W. J. Crochetiere., *et al.* "Control of Skeletal Joint by Electrical Stimulation of Antagonists." *Med. Biol. Eng.* **5**,97–109 (1967).

Vodovnik L. and W. D. McLeod., "Electronic detours of broken nerve paths." *Med. Electr.* **20**, 110–6 (1965).

Wilder R. P., E. V. Jones., *et al.* "Functional electrical stimulation cycle ergometer exercise for spinal cord injured patients." *J. Long. Term. Eff. Med. Implants.* **12**(3), 161–74 (2002).

Winslow J., P. L. Jacobs., *et al.* "Fatigue compensation during FES using surface EMG." *Journal of Electromyography and Kinesiology* **13**(6), 555–68 (2003).

Yeo J. D., J. Walsh., *et al.* "Mortality following spinal cord injury."*Spinal Cord* **36**(5), 329–36 (1998).

Chapter Eight

Combined Functional Electrical Stimulation (FES) and Robotic System Driven by User Intention for Post-Stroke Wrist Rehabilitation

Xiaoling Hu, Raymond Kai-Yu Tong, Rui Li, Jingjing Xue, Szekit Ho and Pengnan Chen

Department of Health Technology and Informatics, The Hong Kong Polytechnic University, Hung Hom, Kowloon, Hong Kong SAR, China

8.1 INTRODUCTION

The extent of the restoration of limb functions after stroke is highly associated with the intensive practice of the affected limbs by their own neuromuscular efforts (Broeks *et al.* 1999; Farmer *et al.* 2004). Functional electrical stimulation (FES) can stimulate the muscles through electrical current, which generates limb movement by activating a person's own muscles to restore motor functions and also evoke sensory feedback during muscle contraction to the brain to promote motor relearning (Chae and Yu 1999; Chae *et al.* 2000; Chan *et al.* 2008). On the other hand, rehabilitation robotic system can provide external assistive support to body parts (e.g. limbs), which help persons to experience limb movements at the paretic side to improve related sensory-motor functions during limb movements (Volpe *et al.* 2004; Riener *et al.* 2005). Both FES systems and rehabilitation robots have been used for rehabilitation applications on disabled persons(Volpe *et al.* 2000; Tong and Hu 2008). However, most FES and robot devices are applied to a paralyzed limb in a passive way, i.e. the supports from an FES or a robot are not related to the voluntary residual motor activities of a person (Popovic *et al.* 2002; Sinkjaer *et al.* 2003). Some FES or robotic systems involve voluntary motor inputs, e.g. electromyography (EMG) or torque (Hesse *et al.* 2003; Hara 2008). While, these systems only use the voluntary inputs as a triggering signal to initiate a start signal

Biomechatronics in Medicine and Healthcare by Le Li and Raymond Kai-Yu Tong

www.panstanford.com
978-981-4241-61-8

of a motion, and the remained motion are pre-programmed by FES or robot in a passive pattern.

Currently, FES and rehabilitation robot are still separate systems. In comparison with FES, robot system uses the motor to provide external assistive force; it does not have the effect as in FES, which directly activates a person's own motor power from the paretic muscles to generate the assistive force. However, difficulties also could be encountered when using FES to activate groups of muscles with dynamic limb movements, since electrode size and the number of FES channels would be challenges of whether the paretic muscle groups could achieve movements with desired kinematic qualities, such as speeds and trajectories. FES can cause muscle contractions, and this contraction could activate feedback from natural sensors in the body through the afferent nerves back to the central nervous system, which may help in motor relearning during training (Chae and Yu 1999; Bhakta 2000). It is possible that a combined rehabilitation system with both FES and robotic supports may enhance the training effects by either pure robot or FES training.

Upper limb functions are highly related to the daily activities of a person. However, in rehabilitation training, many stroke survivors experienced reasonable motor recovery of their proximal upper limb (shoulder and elbow) but limited wrist recovery at the distal (Chae and Yu 1999; Bhakta 2000). Improvement of the wrist functions can directly increase the usage of the affected hand of persons after stroke (Broeks*et al.* 1999). In this chapter we introduced a combined FES-robot system, which may assist wrist rehabilitation training for persons after stroke interactively to their voluntary residual motor intentions.

8.2 THE COMBINED FES-ROBOT SYSTEM

The FES-robot system could assist wrist training for persons after stroke continuously and interactively according to their voluntary residual motor intentions detected by electromyography (EMG) during training. The system was developed based on the robotic prototype of the continuous interactive rehabilitation robot as introduced in Chapter 5. Figure 8.1(a) shows the experimental setup of the FES-robot system when doing the wrist training, with EMG and FES electrodes attached on the antagonist muscle pairs of flexor carpi radialis (FCR) and extensor carpi radialis (ECR). The EMG and FES electrode configuration on a muscle is shown in Figure 8.1(b). A subject would be asked to conduct the wrist flexion and extension in a horizontal plane from -45° (the negative sign represented extended positions) to 60° (the positive sign represented flexed positions) with a selected velocity by tracking with a target cursor. During a wrist tracking task, both the robot and the FES parts would provide assistance to the subject, and the detailed structure of the FES-robot system is illustrated in Figure 8.2(a).

The system mainly consisted of an FES part, a robot part, and a personal computer (PC) based control platform. The interface between the PC and the

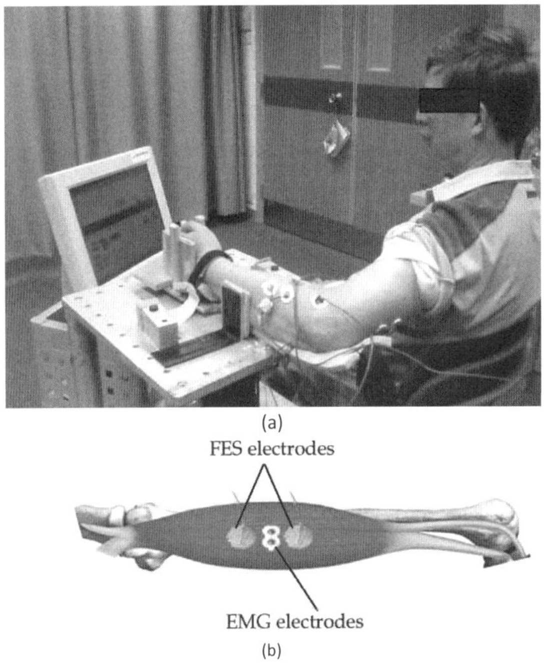

Figure 8.1 The FES-robot training experimental setup (a). The configuration of the FES electrodes and EMG electrodes on a muscle (b). For color reference, see page 218.

FES/robot parts was an analog-digital card. The PC-based control platform had three functions:

(1) to provide a programmed tracking task and guide a subject through visual feedback;
(2) to control the FES and robot parts providing assistance during tracking; and
(3) to save data during training.

The FES part was a two-channel programmable voltage stimulator. In this study, the outputs of a channel of the stimulator were square pulses with constant amplitude of 100 V, inter-pulse interval at 25 ms (i.e., stimulation frequency of 40 Hz), and varied pulse width from 0–200μs. The robotic part of the FES-Robot system had one-degree of freedom, i.e. wrist flexion and extension on the horizontal plane, was designed and fabricated for assisting the wrist movements, as illustrated in Figure 8.2(b). A two-layer of aluminum plates were connected by four aluminum pillars inside of a motor and torque sensor tower. The lower plate was fixed to the base of the tower. The direct drive brushless AC servo motor was fixed to the lower plate. The motor was connected to a torque sensor. The other end of the torque sensor was connected to a manipulandum with an orthosis to fix the palm. During the training, the palm of the paretic side of a subject was placed into the orthosis on the manipulandum which could rotate with the motor; and the wrist angle signals were measured via readings of the positions of the

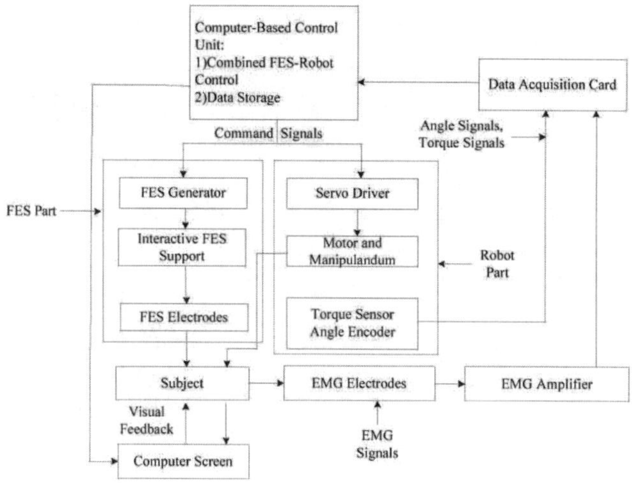

(a)

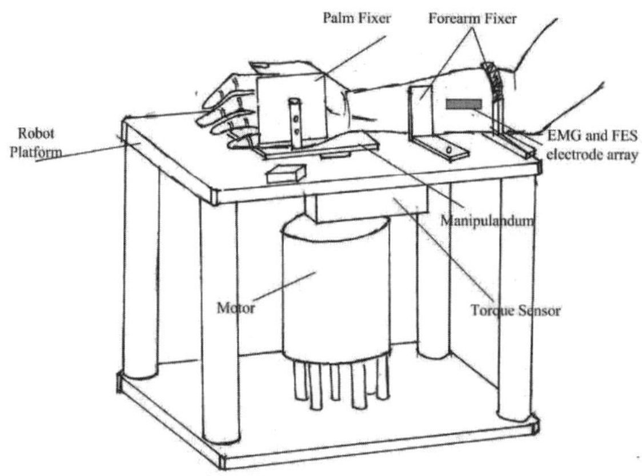

(b)

Figure 8.2 The system diagram of the FES-Robot system (a), and an illustration of the structure for the motor part (b).

manipulandum. A belt was used to fasten the wrist joint in order to keep the joint position still during palm movement.

The control algorithm for the assistive FES and torque could be described as follows:

$$\text{Assistance}_{\text{FES}-\text{robot}} = \text{Assistance}_{\text{Robot}} + \text{Assistance}_{\text{FES}} \tag{8.1}$$

where, $\text{Assistance}_{\text{FES}-\text{robot}}$ represented the ultimate support of the FES-robot system, $\text{Assistance}_{\text{Robot}}$ was the support from the robot part applied to the manipulandum, $\text{Assistance}_{\text{FES}}$ was the support from the FES part applied to the FES electrodes. The robotic assistance for the FES-robot system was same as the algorithm for the continuous intention-driven wrist robot introduced in Chapter 5.

The assistance from the FES part was defined as

$$\text{Assistance}_{\text{FES}} = \begin{cases} \text{K} \cdot \text{W}_{\text{max,FCR}} \cdot \text{M}_{\text{Flexion}}, & \text{During the flexion tracking phase} \\ \text{K} \cdot \text{W}_{\text{max,ECR}} \cdot \text{M}_{\text{Extension}}, & \text{During the extension tracking phase} \end{cases}, \tag{8.2}$$

where, K was a constant gain factor set before experiment, ranging from 0 to 1, $W_{\text{max,FCR/ECR}}$ was the maximum stimulation impulse width applied on the FCR or ECR muscles, which were the threshold values to evoke maximal wrist flexion and extension when the forearm was put horizontally on a table with the wrist joint started at its neutral position. $M_{\text{Flexion/Extension}}$ in Eq. 8.1 was defined as

$$\text{M}_{\text{Flexion/Extension}} \doteq \frac{\text{EMG}_{\text{m,Flexion/Extension}} - \text{EMG}_{\text{mREST}}}{\text{EMG}_{\text{mIMV}} - \text{EMG}_{\text{mREST}}}, \tag{8.3}$$

where $\text{EMG}_{\text{m,Flexion/Extension}}$ was the EMG of the agonist muscle, m, in its contraction phase during the tracking (e.g. the EMG of FCR during the wrist flexion phase, or the EMG of ECR during the wrist extension phase); EMG_{mREST} was the averaged EMG of the muscle, m, during its resting state; and EMG_{mIMV} was the maximal EMG value of the muscle, m, during its isometric voluntary contractions (IMVC). All EMG signals were first processed by the full wave rectification and moving average with 100 ms window before input into Eq. 8.3. It was understood that during the electrical stimulation, stimulation artifacts would contaminate EMG signals. Sample-and-hold software (S/H, by LABVIEW) was applied for reducing the stimulation artifacts after the EMG signals were digitized. The S/H program had the functions first to detect the onset of a stimulation artifact (usually

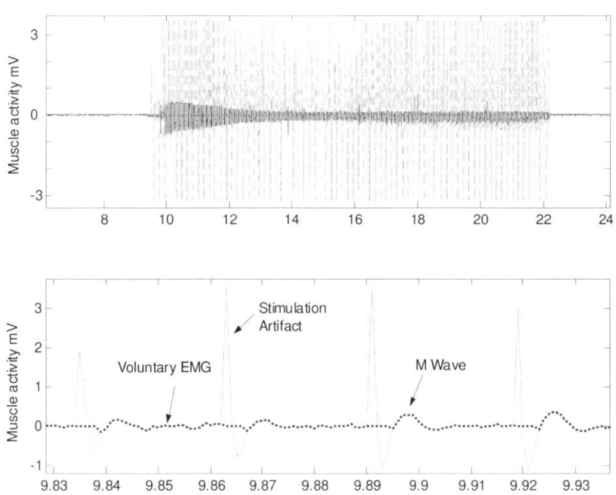

Figure 8.3 The captured EMG signals after the process of sample-and-hold. The upper panel shows the EMG signal before (dotted line) and after (solid line) the process of sample-and-hold. The lower panel shows the enlarged signals in the upper panel. For color reference, see page 218.

followed with a very sharp rising phase as shown in Figure 8.3), then to set the output signal to be zero during a preset blocking period (3–5 ms in this study), which was obtained though observation on the stimulation artifact duration on a subject before experiment. It was noticed that besides the EMG generated from voluntary muscle contractions, M-waves evoked by electrical stimulation also could be captured during tracking tasks assisted with FES (see Figure 8.3). EMG signals used in Eq. 8.3 were the signals after the sample-and-hold process, the rectification, and then the moving average. The FES-robot system also could generate interactive resistive torques as the interactive robot system introduced in Chapter 5.

8.3 SYSTEM PERFORMANCE EVALUATION

The developed FES-robot system was first evaluated on its assistive function on wrist tracking tasks by persons after stroke. In the evaluation, two different wrist tracking speeds, i.e., 10°/s and 20°/s, were used. For each tracking trial, there were 5 cycles of wrist flexion and extension from -45° to 60°. In our previous continuous intention-driven robot-assisted wrist training only 10°/s was selected (Hu *et al.* 2007; Hu *et al.* 2008; Song *et al.* 2008; Hu *et al.* 2009). It was an empirical speed that the subjects would not feel too easy or too difficult to follow during the training process. In the FES-robot evaluation, five subjects with chronic stroke (at lease 1 year after onset of stroke, male, aged from 36 to 56 with mean±SD=48±7) were recruited after obtaining approval from the Human Subjects Ethics Sub-Committee of the Hong Kong Polytechnic University. All of the subjects were hemiplegia due to single cerebral unilateral ischemic event, whose spasticity of wrist flexion/extension at the paretic side was measured by the Modified Ashworth Scale (MAS, equal to 1.8±0.7 at the wrist joint) (Ashworth 1964). The voluntary motor function of the paretic upper limb for the subjects was scored by the Fugl-Meyer Assessment (FMA, 19.8±5 shoulder/elbow, and 11.2±4.2 wrist/hand) (Fugl-Meyer *et al.* 1975). Each subject was required to conduct wrist tracking tasks supported by the FES-robot system with five different assistive combinations as shown in Table 8.1, and two different tracking speeds

Table 8.1 Combination of assistances from the FES and robot parts.

System Assitance	FES Gain	Robot Gain
M5f5	50%	50%
M1f1	100%	100%
M0f1	100%	0%
M0f0	0%	0%
M1f0	0%	100%

The FES ain and robot gain are in accordance with the definition in Eq. 5.2 and in Eq. 5.3 of Chapter 5.

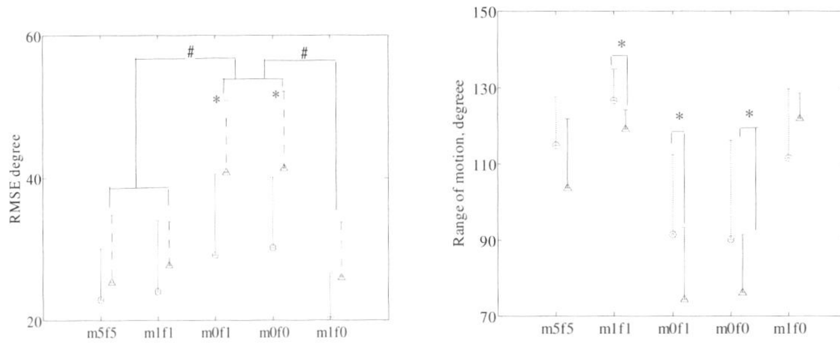

Figure 8.4 The RMSE and the maximal ROM achieved by the subjects with different FES and robot assistive combinations and with different tracking speeds (circles are for 10°/s, deltas are for 20°/s). Differences with statistical statistical significance ($P<0.05$) were denoted by "#" with respect to the FES and robot combinations (ANOVA tests) and "*" to the tracking speed (t-tests).

(i.e., 10°/s and 20°/s). In the tracking tasks, EMG signals were collected from the muscles of FCR, ECR, biceps brachii (BIC), and triceps brachii (TRI). The tracking performance was evaluated by EMG parameters (i.e., EMG co-contraction and EMG activation level), root mean squared error (RMSE) between the target and the actual tracking positions, the maximal range of motion (ROM) during tracking. The detailed calculation methods for the EMG parameters could be found in Chapter 5. Each tracking task was repeated twice, and the mean value of an evaluation parameter was taken as an experimental reading for statistical analysis. During the evaluation, a rest of 2 minutes was taken by a subject to avoid fatigue; and the sequence of the evaluation trials with different combinations of assistance was randomly assigned.

After collected the data from the subjects, the evaluation parameters during the FES-robot assisted tracking were summarized. Figure 8.4 shows the RMSE and the maximal ROM of the subjects during the wrist tracking tasks with different FES and robot assistive combinations and with the two different tracking speeds, i.e., 10°/s and 20°/s. The RMSE reflected the wrist tracking accuracy of the tested limb. It was found that with a faster tracking speed (20°/s), the tracking performance was lowered when no assistance was provided from the FES-robot system (in case of m0f0). With pure support from the FES part, the tracking RMSE had the largest mean values for both tracking speeds. The RMSE had the relatively low values in the assistive patterns of m5f5, m1f1, and m1f0. It suggested that with the support from the robot part, or the combined supports from both the FES and robot parts the tracking performance was improved. Different tracking speeds affected the maximal ROM greatly (Figure 8.4). It was observed that in the tracking trials with 10°/s the maximal ROMs were significantly higher than those with 20°/s in assistive patterns of m1f1, m0f1, and m0f0. The mean values of the maximal ROM for m5f5, m1f1, and m1f0 were higher than those for m0f1 and m0f0, in which the assistive pattern of m1f1 had the highest mean values for both tracking speeds. The data in RMSE and the maximal ROM implied that with the supports

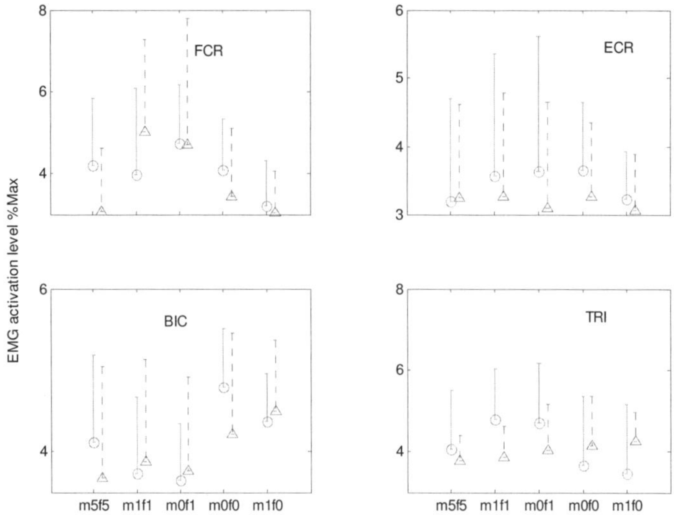

Figure 8.5 The EMG activation levels of the muscles of FCR, ECR, BIC, and TRI during the tracking tasks with different FES and robot assistive combinations and different tracking speeds (circles are for 10°/s, deltas are for 20°/s).

from the FES and robot parts the overall tracking performance could be improved, in comparison with those no system support at all or the pattern with only FES assistance.

Figure 8.5 shows the EMG activation levels of the antagonist muscle pairs related to the wrist and the elbow joints. It was found that the EMG activation levels of the FCR muscle in tracking tasks with FES assistance were higher than those without FES. It was because that during electrical stimulation on the FCR, evoked muscular potentials, i.e., M waves, besides the voluntary EMG would be detected. However, higher ECR EMG activation levels during assistive patterns with FES (m5f5, m1f1, m0f1) were not observed in this study, especially in the cases with the tracking speed of 20°/s. In the experiment, most of the subjects had more difficulties in following the tracking target moving with 20°/s than with 10°/s. The subjects always paused in tracking when they felt hard to follow the target cursor in trials with 20°/s. It could be a reason for the lowered EMG activation level in tracking with 20°/s even with FES assistance. This was also associated with the worse tracking performance measured with the RMSE and the maximal ROM. The EMG activation levels for the BIC muscle were lowered in the assistive patterns with FES (m5f5, m1f1, m0f1) compared to the patterns of m1f0 and m0f0, which implied that the elbow flexor was relaxed in the wrist tracking, whereas the pure robot-assisted tracking could not lower down the activity in the elbow flexor.

The reduced BIC activations when introducing FES assistance also resulted in a decrease in co-contraction indexes in the muscle pairs of FCR&BIC and ECR&BIC during the tracking (Figure 8.6). A reduction in co-contraction index of a muscle pair mainly reflected the decrease of overlap in the contracting phase for the two

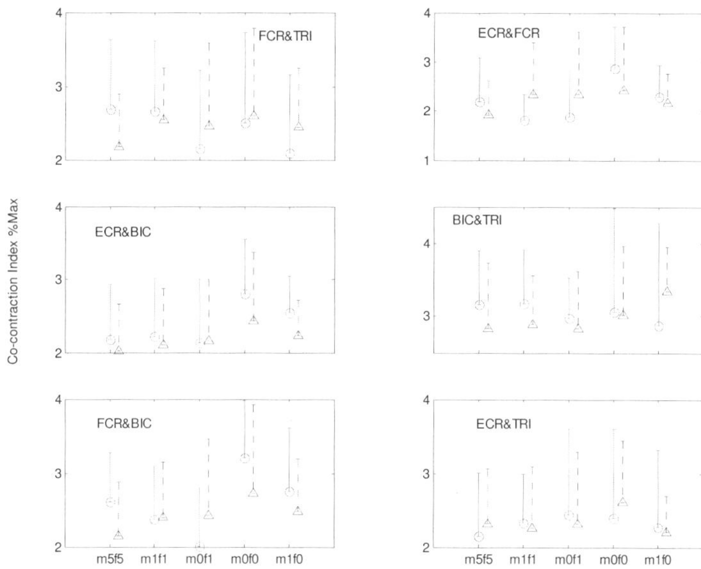

Figure 8.6 The Muscle co-contraction indexes of the muscle pairs during the tracking tasks with different FES and robot assistive combinations and with different tracking speeds (circles are for 10°/s, deltas are for 20°/s).

muscles (Hu *et al.* 2007; Hu *et al.* 2008; Hu *et al.* 2009). For an unimpaired subject, it is expected that the muscles related to the elbow joint should be quite when doing the wrist tracking. However, for persons after stroke, compensatory muscle activities related to the proximal joints, such as the elbow and shoulder, are commonly observed when they are required to conduct wrist movements (Dewald *et al.* 1995; Dewald *et al.* 2001). The results in the system evaluation suggested that introducing FES could reduce the correlated elbow movements during the wrist flexion and extension. Chae, J. *et al.* indicated in their study on neuromuscular stimulation for motor relearning in hemiplegia that electrical stimulation not only evoked contractions in the paretic muscle, but also stimulate the sensory feedback in the affected muscle (Chae and Yu 1999; Chae *et al.* 2000), which could increase the awareness from the subject to use the target muscles, rather than using compensatory motions from other body parts. The co-contraction between the ECR&FCR during the tracking could reflect the coordination of the two muscles in the simple wrist extension and flexion movements. When the tracking speed was 20°/s, there was almost no difference in the ECR&FCR co-contraction index among different system assistive patterns. It might be that the target tracking speed was too fast for the subjects to follow even with the FES-robot assistances. However, for the 10°/s tracking speed, the ECR&FCR co-contraction index had its maximal mean value when there was no assistance from the FES-robot (i.e., m0f0); and the minimal mean value was observed when both FES and robot part give 100% assistance (i.e., m1f1). It suggested that with the assistance of the FES-robot, the muscle co-ordination for the wrist joint could be improved in the un-trained persons after stroke with 10°/s during the wrist tracking. This speed was then used in a FES-robot assisted wrist training for chronic stroke.

8.4 FES-ROBOT ASSISTED WRIST TRAINING

After the FES-robot system evaluation, we also conducted a preliminary study on the training effectiveness of the system on persons with chronic stroke. The five subjects attended the system evaluation, were recruited for a 20-session FES-robot assisted wrist training one month later. Before the training, clinical assessments of FMA (shoulder/elbow and wrist/hand), MAS (elbow and wrist), the action research arm test (ARAT)(Carroll 1965), and the FIM instrument (Keith *et al.* 1987) were measured. The training intensity was assigned as 3 to 5 sessions per week, and the whole training program was finished within 7 consecutive weeks. In each training session, there were 14 wrist tracking trials, and each trial had five wrist extension/flexion cycles. The experimental setup for the training was same as that for the evaluation (Figure 8.1). The assistive combination from the FES-robot system was 1:1 for the FES and robot parts (i.e., m1f1, m5f5, m0f0 described in Table 1), since the performance in muscle coordination capabilities were better when both the FES and robot gave support during the tracking. For the 14 tracking trials in a training session, alternative FES-robot assistance were applied with the scheme as described in Figure 8.7. Robotic resistances with different resistive coefficient values (0%, 10%, and 20% of the maximal wrist torque values during IMVC, with the detailed definition in Eq 5.3, Chapter 5) There were totally 7 types of assistive and resistive combinations, and each of them was repeated twice in the training with the first and the last wrist tracking trials had the gain combination of 0% assistive and 0% resistive. The reason for applying different gain values in the training was that the subjects could sense some changes in the training, which motivated them to concentrate on the tracking tasks; meanwhile, verbal encouragement was also used during the training.

The FES-robot training effects were assessed by the pre- and post- evaluation of clinical scores, i.e., FMA, MAS, ARAT, and FIM. The FMA mainly measures

Table 8.2 The clinical scores measured before and after the FES-robot assisted wrist training.

	FMA (Shoulder/ Elbow)	FMA * (Wrist/ Hand)	MAS (Elbow)	MAS * (Wrist)	ARAT *	FIM
Pre-Training	19.8 ± 5.1	11.2 ± 4.2	1.4 ± 0.7	1.8 ± 0.7	20.1 ± 5.1	65.4 ± 1.4
Post-Training	22.2 ± 4.7	19.7 ± 3.7	0.8 ± 0.5	0.5 ± 0.4	29.3 ± 6.5	65.4 ± 1.4

The items marked with "*" showed significant difference after a paired-t-test with $P < 0.05$.

the voluntary functions of the upper limb, which could be roughly divided into the shoulder/elbow part and the wrist/hand part. Increases in the FMA scores suggest an improvement in the related motor functions. The MAS measures the involuntary muscle spasticity when doing passive joint movements (such as extension/flexion to test the flexors and the extensors). A decrease in the MAS reflexes released muscle spasticity in the associated muscles. The ARAT also measures the upper limb voluntary functions, while more focuses on hand/finger functions. Most of the ARAT tasks require voluntary motions of fingers, such as pinch, grip, and grasp. Increased ARAT score suggested improved upper limb motor functions, especially in the hand and fingers. Increased scores in the FIM instrument may reflect improved independency in general tasks related to daily activities. Besides the clinical scores, the motor recovery process was also monitored by the parameters of RMSE, EMG activation levels of ECR, FCR, BIC, and TRI muscles, and co-contraction indexes of the different muscle pairs in tracking trials when there was neither FES and robot supports, nor resistive torque (i.e., 0% assistance and 0% resistance). Table 8.2 shows the comparison between the clinical scores before and after the training. Improvements with statistical significance ($P<0.05$, paired-t-test) were found in the FMA (Wrist/Hand), MAS (Wrist), and ARAT in the post-training tests. The increased FMA (Wrist/Hand) suggested an improvement in the voluntary motor function in the wrist joint; and the improved ARAT score also suggested a better voluntary performance in finger functions, which was absent in our previous pure interactive robot-assisted wrist training (Hu *et al.* 2009). It was interesting that when doing the post-training ARAT assessments, the main improvement in almost all subjects was in the finger pinch function, e.g. picking up a marble with different sizes. A release in muscle spasticity related to the wrist joint was found after the training as assessed by the MAS (wrist). However, the release of muscle tone in the elbow joint was not significant at present. There was no change in the daily independency after the training either, as assessed by the FIM instrument.

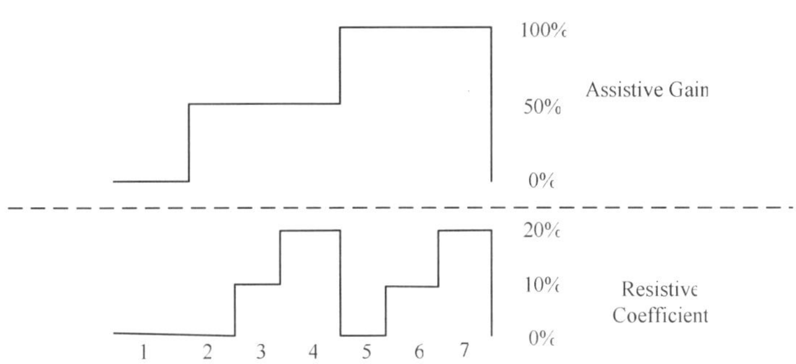

Figure 8.7 The assistive and resistive scheme used in a training session. The assistive gains are the gain values of both the FES and robot parts in the interactive control. The resistive coefficient is a percentage value applied to the constant resistance during the wrist flexion and extension phases.

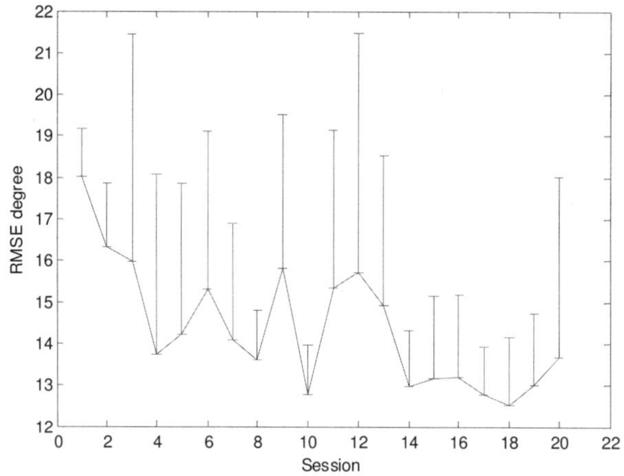

Figure 8.8 The RMSE variation across the training session for the tracking trials without assistance or resistance from the FES-robot system.

Figure 8.8 shows the variation of the RMSE for the tracking trials. The RMSE decreased throughout the whole training process, which implied the improved tracking skill of the affected limbs. The decreasing trend of the RMSE ended in the later part of the training (after session 14), which suggested a relative stable performance achieved by the subjects. Figure 8.9 shows the variation of the EMG activation levels of the different muscles across the training sessions. Decreases in the EMG activation levels were found in the muscles of FCR, ECR, and BIC. The decrease of the FCR and ECR EMG levels could be related to the release of the muscle spasticity, in accordance with the MAS wrist score. It was found the

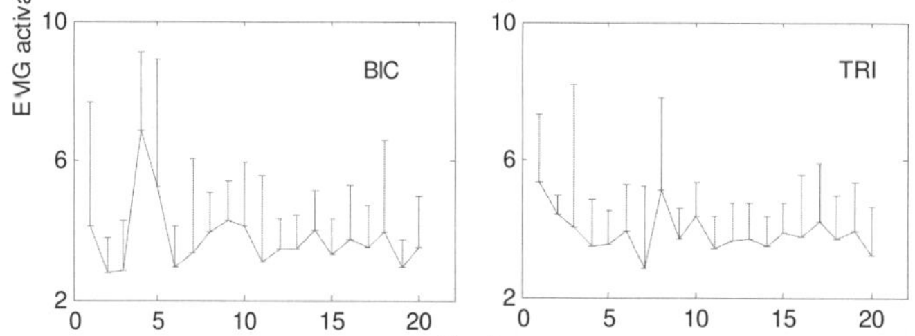

Figure 8.9 The EMG activation levels for the ECR, FCR, BIC, and TRI muscles during the training for the tracking trials without assistance or resistance from the FES-robot system.

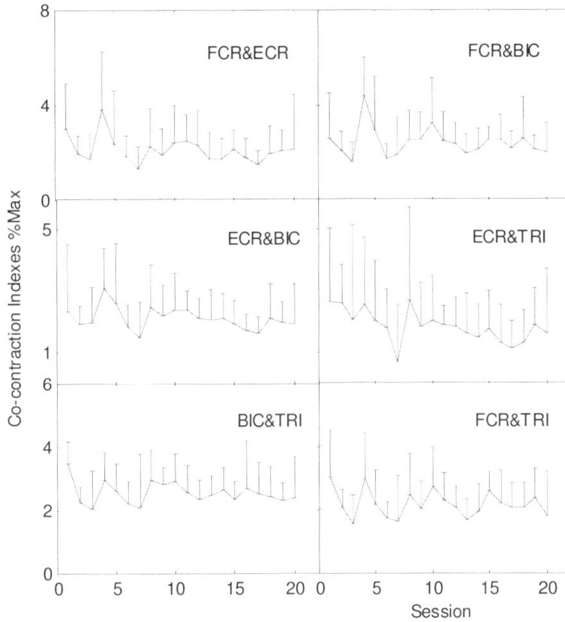

Figure 8.10 The co-contraction indexes of the muscle pairs during the training for the tracking trials without assistance or resistance from the FES-robot system.

EMG activation levels for the flexors (i.e., FCR and BIC) had a quick decrease in the first several training sessions; and after that, the EMG levels of the two flexors were stable. It possibly implied that the FES-robot treatment might lead to a fast spasticity reduction. In our previous studies on pure-robot assisted wrist or elbow training, there was no steady state ever reached by the decreasing trend of muscle activation levels within 20 training sessions (Hu *et al.* 2007; Hu *et al.* 2009).

The variations in the muscle co-contraction indexes during the FES-robot assisted training were shown in Figure 8.10. Decreasing trends were observed in the muscle pairs of FCR&ECR, FCR&BIC, and ECR&TRI. The decrease of FCR&ECR and FCR&BIC co-contraction indexes reached to their steady state in the first half training sessions; and these decreases indicated a better co-ordination of the muscles when doing the tracking even without the assistance from the FES-robot system. The decrease of the ECR&TRI throughout the training sessions was in accordance with the trend for the ECR activation level. It also implied that the variation in the co-contraction of this pair of muscles was mainly caused by the ECR. The results in the muscle co-contractions suggested that the individual muscle activities had become more independent, and the elbow movements were gradually isolated from those for the wrist. The FES-robot assisted wrist training also showed a faster improvement in the muscle co-ordinations, measured by the co-contraction indexes, in comparison with the previous pure robot assisted training (Hu *et al.* 2007; Hu *et al.* 2009). It possibly implied that with the involvement of FES, robot-assisted training could speed up the recovery process.

8.5 CONCLUSIONS

In this chapter, a novel FES-robot system for post-stroke rehabilitation on the wrist joint was introduced. The FES-robot could continuously interactive to the voluntary intention of a person after stroke, by detecting the residual EMG signals from the paretic limb. The FES-robot assisted wrist tracking could immediately reduce excessive muscle activities in the elbow flexor, and also could improve the tracking performance measured by the maximal ROM and tracking RMSE. In the FES-robot assisted wrist training, it was also observed faster recoveries in muscle co-ordination and release in wrist muscle spasticity compared with those in the pure robot-assisted trainings (Hu*et al.* 2007; Hu *et al.* 2009). In future studies, large scale randomized clinical trials will be conducted to provide more solid and conclusive training effects of the FES-robot system.

8.6 ACKNOWLEDGEMENT

The project was funded by the Research Grants Council of the Hong Kong Special Administrative Region, China (grant no. PolyU 5318/09E).

References

Ashworth B (1964) Preliminary trials of carisoprodol in multiple sclerosis. *Practitioner* 192:540–542.

Bhakta BB (2000) Management of spasticity in stroke. *British Medical Bulletin* 56:476–485.

Broeks JG, Lankhorst GJ, Rumping K, Prevo AJ (1999) The long-term outcome of arm function after stroke: results of a follow-up study. *Disability & Rehabilitation* 21:357–354.

Carroll D (1965) A quantitative test of upper extremity function. *J Chronic Dis.* 18:479–491.

Chae J, Kilgore K, Triolo R, Yu D (2000) Neuromuscular stimulation for motor neuroprosthesis in hemiplegia. *Crit. Rev. Phys. Rehabil. Med.* 12:1–23.

Chae J, Yu D (1999) Neuromuscular stimulation for motor relearning in hemiplegia. *Crit. Revs. Phy. Rehab. Med.* 11:279–297.

Chan MK, Tong KY, Chung K (2008) Bilateral upper limb training with functional electric stimulation in patients with chronic stroke. Neurorehabilitation and Neural Repair In press.

Dewald JPA, Pope PS, Given JD, Buchanan TS, Rymer WZ (1995) Abnormal muscle coactivation patterns during isometric torque generation at the elbow and shoulder in hemiparetic subjects. Brain 118.

Dewald JPA, Sheshadri V, Dawson ML, Beer RF (2001) Upper-limb discoordination in hemiparetic stroke: implications for neurorehabilitation. *Top Stroke Rehabil.* 8:1–12.

Farmer J, Zhao X, van Praag H, Wodtke K, Gage FH, Christie BR (2004) Effects of voluntary exercise on synaptic plasticity and gene expression in the dentate gyrus of adult mal Sprague-Dawley rats in vivo. *Neurosci.* 124:71–79.

Fugl-Meyer AR, Jaasko L, Leyman I, Olsson S, Steglind S (1975) The post-stroke hemiplegic patient. I: A method for evaluation of physical performance. *Scand J. Rehabil. Med.* 7:13–31.

Hara Y (2008) Neurorehabilitation with new functional electrical stimulation for hemiparetic upper extremity in stroke patients. *J. Nippon Med. Sch.* 75.

Hesse S, Schulte-Tigges G, Konrad M, Bardeleben A, Werner C (2003) Robot-assisted arm trainer for the passive and active practice of bilateral forearm and wrist movements in hemiparetic subjects. *Arch. Phys. Med. Rehabil.* 84:915–920.

Hu XL, Song R, Tong KY, Tsang SF, Leung PO, Li L (2007) Variation of Muscle Coactivation Patterns in Chronic Stroke During Robot-Assisted Elbow Training. *Arch. Phys. Med. Rehabil.* 88:1022–1029.

Hu XL, Tong KY, Song R, Zheng XJ, Leung WFW (2009) A comparison between electromyography-driven robot and passisve motion device on wrist rehabilitation for chronic stroke. *Neurorehabil. Neural Repair* 23:837–846.

Hu XL *et al.* (2009) Quantitative Evaluation of Motor Functional Recovery Process in Chronic Stroke Patients during Robot-Assisted Wrist Training,. Journal of Electromyography and Kinesiology. **19**: 639–650.

Keith RA, Granger CV, Hamilton BB, Sherwin FS (1987) The functional independence measure: a new tool for rehabilitation. *Advances in Clinical Rehabilitation* 1:6–18.

Popovic MR, Popovic DB, Keller T (2002) Neuroprostheses for grasping. *Neurol. Res.* 24:443–452.

Riener R, Nef T, Colombo G (2005) Robot-aided neurorehabilitation for the upper extremities. *Med. Biol. Eng. Comp.* 43:2–10.

Sinkjaer T, Haugland M, Inmann A, Hansen M, Nielsen KD (2003) Biopotentials as command and feedback signals in functional electrical stimulation systems. *Medical Engineering & Physics* 25:29–40.

Song R, Tong KY, Hu XL, Li L (2008) Assistive control system using continuous myoelectric signal in robot-aided arm training for patients after stroke. *IEEE Transactions on Neural Systems and Rehabilitation Engineering* 16:371–379.

Tong KY, Hu XL (2008) Robot-Assisted Training for Stroke Rehabilitation. In: Takahashi Y (ed) Service Robotics, Austria.

Volpe BT *et al.* (2004) Robotics and other devices in the treatment of patients recovering from stroke. *Current Atherosclerosis Reports* 6:314–319.

Volpe BT, Krebs HI, Hogan N, Edelstein OL, Diels C, Aisen M (2000) A novel approach to stroke rehabilitation: robot-aided sensorimotor stimulation. *Neurology* 54:1938–1944.

Chapter Nine

Development of Robots for Active Rehabilitation of the upper Limbs on the Transverse Plan for Stroke Patients

Chou-Ching K. Lin*, Ming-Shaung Ju†, Pin-Cheng Kung† and Shu-Min Chen‡

* *Department of Neurology, National Cheng Kung University Hospital, Taiwan*
† *Department of Mechanical Engineering, National Cheng Kung University, Taiwan*
‡ *Department of Physical Medicine and Rehabilitation, National Cheng Kung University, Taiwan*

9.1 INTRODUCTION

Rehabilitation program is the main stay of treatment for patients suffering from trauma, stroke or spinal cord injury. Conventionally, these programs rely heavily on the experience and manual manipulation of the therapists. The rehabilitation movements can be roughly divided into passive and active types. In the passive movements, the affected limbs are passively moved by the external forces, while in the active movements, the patients actively move their limbs under a designed external assistance or resistance. Since the number of patients is large and the treatment is time-consuming, it is a big advance if robots can assist in performing treatment. In addition, it is possible to construct new treatment maneuvers with the robots. Many robotic systems have been developed for assisting rehabilitation of the upper limbs. One of the major difficulties in realizing rehabilitation with robots is the controller design. In the rehabilitation robots that are designed for free active movement, mostly single-level not hierarchical controller is implemented. Usually one form of admittance controllers is utilized. Although the benefits of imposing assistant or resistant force have not being fully established (Kahn *et al.*, 2006), most robotic systems give guidance about the path and impose forces during the movements. In the rehabilitation robots that are designed for passive movements or active movements with external assistance or resistance, the controller is usually divided into the high and low levels. The low-level controller

Biomechatronics in Medicine and Healthcare by Le Li and Raymond Kai-Yu Tong

www.panstanford.com
978-981-4241-61-8

achieves the position control, force control, or novel controls of pneumatic and cable-wired actuators on each degree of freedom. Usually one form of impedance controllers is utilized. Impedance control and admittance control are duality but may not be mutually convertible in non-linear systems (Marchal-Crespo and Reinkensmeyer, 2009). The high-level controller schedules the trajectories or paths that potentially achieve the purpose of rehabilitation. Simple linear movement with simple velocity profile is relatively easy to design. Yet, manual treatments usually involve complex maneuvers with resistive or assistive force imposed at specific times of the movement. Circular or more complex movements with predefined imposing force are more difficult to design. In the following, the existing robotic systems for the rehabilitation of the upper limbs with an emphasis on controller implementation are reviewed.

Hogan *et al* (Krebs *et al.*, (1998). designed a planar robot (MIT-Manus) with impedance control for guiding patients to do movements along the specified planar trajectories. A five-bar-link drive mechanism with decoupled joint dynamics (Asada and Youcef-Toumi, 1984), which facilitated the controller design, was adopted for constructing the robot. Noritsugu *et al.*, (1997). for treating patients with trauma, designed an arm-like robot with 2 degree-of-freedom (DoF) and developed four modes of planar linear motion. Each actuator comprises two rubber artificial muscles (Rubbertuator RUB-835S (link 1), RUB-825S (link 2) from Bridgestone Company, Japan) to strengthen the generated torque. Impedance control for position was implemented. Hybrid position/force controllers (Raibert, Craig and Hybrid, 1981; Suh *et al.*, 1991), controlling position in one direction and force in the orthogonal direction, have the advantage of simultaneously maintaining the desired movement trajectory and force for the planar movements. Lum and co-workers (Burgar *et al.*, 2000) developed the mirror-image motion enabler (MIME) robot that enabled 3 dimensional (3D) rehabilitation movements of the affected side guided by the intact side according to the master-slave principle. The robot and its controller were based on a commercially available model (Staubli PUMA-560). The robot provided a viscous resistance in the direction of desired movement and spring-like forces in all other directions. Thus, the system had position control in one direction and velocity-dependent force control in the other direction. Cozens (1999), using a single-axis robot and torque control mode, applied resistive or assistive torque to the elbow for rehabilitation of patients with spasticity and weakness. Colombo *et al.*, (2005). designed a planar robot based on three linear motion guides and implemented admittance control. Reinkensmeyer *et al.*, (1999) developed ARM-guide that had a passive linear constraint to limit the movement of the upper limb to a linear path and a single motor to assist arm movement. The robot, in a general sense, also implemented position control in one direction and force control in the other direction. Yet, the position control was provided by the hardware constraint. Similar to an admittance controller, a counterpoise assistive controller that compensated for gravity and elbow passive properties was implemented for force control. Bi-Manu-Track (Hense *et al.*, 2003) was developed for rehabilitation of the distal parts of the upper limb and allowed wrist flexion/extension and forearm pronation/supination. PLEMO-P1 (Kikuchi *et al.*, 2009), having 2-DoF force-feedback function in its working plane and 1 uncontrollable DoF to adjust the inclination angle of the working plane, used electrorheological fluid brakes to generate resistive forces during active movements. Exercise Machine for Upper Limb (EMUL) (Koyanagi *et al.*, 2003), using electrohrheological fluid actuators and having a similar mechanism as PLEMO-P1, supported active 3D movements. The robot was said to be safer because of its specific actuators. ACtive REhabilitation robotic device (ACRE 2) (Doornebosch *et al.*, 2007) had 5 DoF and supported 4 modes of 3D movements with impedance control. GENTLE/S (Coote *et al.*, 2003), combing a commercial robot (HapticMASTER robot, Moog-FCS B.V., The Netherlands) and virtual reality technology, implemented admittance control and was able to assist free active 3D movements. ACT^{3D} (Sukal *et al.*, 2005) was based on the same HapticMASTER robot and had similar functions. REHAROB (Toth *et al.*, 2005) combined 2 6-DoF industrial robots and was implemented with 3D passive movements. As the technology has advanced, more complicated robots with multiple degrees of freedom were designed. NeRebot (Fanin *et al.*, 2003) was a 3 DoF wire-based robot for 3D passive movements and its successor MeriBot (Rosati *et al.*, 2005) was a 5 DoF wire-based robot that was augmented with 2 more mechanical DoF and had a larger working space. Some of the more recent robots are in the category of the so-called exoskeleton. ARMin (Nef *et al.*, 2007), possessing a haptic display and semi-exoskeleton kinematics with 4 active DoF and 2 passive DoF, could deliver patient-cooperative arm therapy. Rehabilitation modes with both active and passive movements in 3D space were implemented and the controller was basically a PD controller for torque control. Robot assisted UPper Extremity Repetitive Therapy (RUPER T^{TM}) (He *et al.*, 2008), using "McKibben" type pneumatic actuators, was a light-weighted and portable exoskeleton robot. It provided 5 DoF movements (shoulder elevation (flexion), elbow extension, humeral external rotation, forearm supination, and wrist/hand extension). The controller consisted of a modified PID feedback controller with a nonlinear filter. Additionally, three of the joint controllers had a feedforward controller built upon iterative learning algorithm in parallel. It is noted that most of these robots, irrespective of their DoF, are aimed at rehabilitation of proximal joints, i.e., shoulder and elbow joints.

Additional problems in designing controllers for rehabilitation robots are the uncertainty about the biomechanical properties of subjects' upper limb, the non-linear dynamics of robots such as the Coulomb friction in the mechanism and the interaction with another unresolved controller (the human control). In a classical design process, the control parameters are determined according to the system model and its parameters. For a robot-assisted rehabilitation program, the subject is also part of the dynamic system and the dynamic model of the subject is not as clear and invariable as the mechanical system. Fuzzy control(Wang, 1994; Rugh, 1991; Lee *et al.*, 1998) is known for coping with nonlinear systems and systems that have uncertainty in its parameters. Yet, a main problem associated with fuzzy control is how to guarantee the global stability (Tanaka and Wang, 2001). Many researchers have tried to maintain the stability by fine tuning a stable linear PID controller and the function of the fuzzy logic was the tuner (Ibrahim, 2002; Moon and Lee, 2003; Deskur *et al.*, 1998).

In the above review, there are 17 rehabilitation robots for upper limbs and only five robots have dimension of movements less than 3. Yet, we decided to develop a planar robot based on the following reasons, (1) the design of controller and therapeutic trajectories becomes more difficult as the DoF and movement dimension increase and (2) the knowledge about how to design the beneficial movement trajectories, especially in 3D, is currently lacking.

9.2 OUR PLANAR REHAB ROBOT FOR UPPER LIMBS

We have devoted ourselves to develop a 2-DoF robot specialized for rehabilitation of the upper limbs in the horizontal plane in the past 10 years (Ju *et al.*, 2001; Wu *et al.*, 2002; Ju *et al.*, 2005) (Fig. 9.1a). Our robot system consists of a robot mechanism, motion controller, position and force/torque sensors, and a personal computer (Fig. 9.1b). During the rehabilitation, the subject's hand grasps a clamp that allows free pronation/supination. The commands calculated by the personal computer are sent to drivers of two AC motors of the robot. The inputs to the controller, consisting of end-point force and position information, are used both for closed-loop control and for later off-line analyses. We adopt the five-bar-link drive mechanism (Asada *et al.*, 1984) for constructing the robot (Fig. 9.1c). The motors are located at the base (origin of X-Y coordinate system), in order to minimize the inertial loading of the whole robot system. The main advantage of the design is that when the physical configuration of the 4 links satisfies the relation of Eq. (1), the dynamic equation of the robot can be theoretically decoupled as Eq. (2),

$$\frac{m_4}{m_3}\frac{l_{g4}}{l_{g3}} = \frac{l_2}{l_1}, \tag{9.1}$$

$$\begin{bmatrix}\tau_1\\ \tau_2\end{bmatrix} = \begin{bmatrix}h_{11} & 0\\ 0 & h_{22}\end{bmatrix}; \begin{bmatrix}\ddot{\theta}_1\\ \ddot{\theta}_2\end{bmatrix} \tag{9.2}$$

where m_3, m_4, l_{g3} and l_{g4} are the masses and lengths to the centers of mass of third and fourth links respectively, l_1 and l_2 are lengths of first and second links respectively, τ_1 and τ_2 are the input torques of the robot joints respectively, h_{11} and h_{22} are constants, and θ_1 and θ_2 are the angles of first and second links relative to the horizontal axis (X), respectively. Eq. (2) means that the two axes are independent and it makes the controller design process simpler. During the design process, we find that friction has significant effects on the robot performance and the friction torque can be added to Eq. (2), as

$$\begin{bmatrix}\tau_1\\ \tau_2\end{bmatrix} = \begin{bmatrix}h_{11} & 0\\ 0 & h_{22}\end{bmatrix}\begin{bmatrix}\ddot{\theta}_1\\ \ddot{\theta}_2\end{bmatrix} + \begin{bmatrix}\tau_{f1}\\ \tau_{f2}\end{bmatrix} \tag{9.3}$$

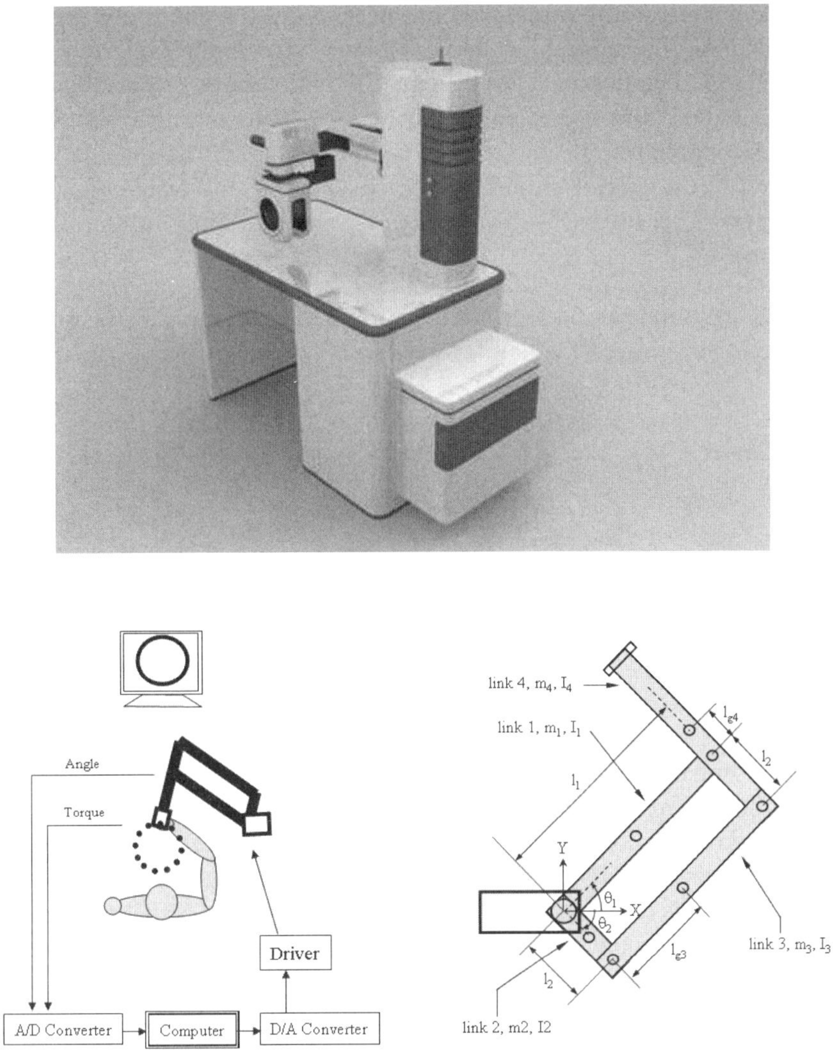

Figure 9.1 Upper: a photo of our planar robot for rehabilitation of the upper limbs, lower left: the components of the robot and lower right: the five-bar-link drive mechanism.

$$\tau_{fk} = \begin{cases} b_f \cdot \dot{\theta}_k + \tau_c & when\ \dot{\theta}_k > 0 \\ b_f \cdot \dot{\theta}_k - \tau_c & when\ \dot{\theta}_k < 0 \end{cases} \quad k = 1,2 \tag{9.4}$$

where τ_{f1} and τ_{f2} are torques to be compensated, b_f is a constant for viscous friction term and τ_c is a static Coulomb friction torque (Phillips and Ballou, 1993). b_f and τ_c are determined empirically (Lu *et al.*, 1993). For the overall control scheme, we adopt the hybrid position/force control,[6] i.e., controlling force in the tangential direction of the movement and controlling position in the orthogonal direction. The main goal of control is to keep the hand of the subject in a predefined track and to impose an assistant or resistant force along the moving direction.

Since force is the control variable along the moving direction, position can not be controlled and the subject can move with an individually preferred speed. In the scheme, the direction of force control (S_T) is determined first by a selection matrix ($\mathbf{S}_S$) and the direction of position control (S_N) is determined accordingly by another selection matrix (**I** - $\mathbf{S}_S$), where **I** is the identity matrix.

The end position error along S_N is calculated first and transformed into the equivalent end force error (F_N) by a predefined stiffness constant(K_s), i.e.,

$$\Delta F_N = Ks \cdot \Delta X_N \tag{9.5}$$

where ΔX_N is the end position error along S_N in one time step. ΔF_N is transformed to the needed torque acting on joints by the Jacobian matrix (J),

$$\tau_N = J^T \cdot \Delta F_N = J^T \cdot Ks \cdot \Delta X_N \tag{9.6}$$

where

$$J = \begin{bmatrix} -l_1 \cdot \sin(\theta_1) & -l_4 \cdot \sin(\theta_2 + \pi) \\ l_1 \cdot \cos(\theta_1) & l_4 \cdot \cos(\theta_2 + \pi) \end{bmatrix}. \tag{9.7}$$

τ_N and $\Delta\tau_N$ are the inputs to the fuzzy logic and are regarded as error and error change in the logic, respectively. In the fuzzification process, inputs (τ_N and $\Delta\tau_N$) are scaled and mapped to the five triangle-shaped membership functions. One membership degree is obtained for each scaled input and membership function combination. Then, each combination of mapped inputs activates one control action according to the inference rule table. The control rule table was determined based on the step response of a presumed second-order system. The final output of the position fuzzy controller is obtained in the defuzzification process by using the center-of-gravity method.

Force control is implemented in the tangent direction of actual movement. By this convention, the robot is able to provide a desired resistive or assistive force to the subjects (Chou, 1997). Since the properties of the subject are unknown a priori, it is impossible to determine the optimal control parameters exactly. Therefore we combine a conventional linear PI (proportional-integral) controller and a fuzzy PI tuner as the force controller. The purpose of the fuzzy PI tuner is to compensate for the nonlinear dynamics (joint friction) of the robot and the unknown disturbing force from the subject. The force error along S_T direction (ΔF_T) is transformed into joint torque error (τ_T) by J^T. τ_T and change of it ($\Delta\tau_T$) are fed to the fuzzy PI tuner. The fuzzy PI tuner has separate fuzzy logics for P and I parts, and each operates in a similar way as in the position controller. The outputs from the fuzzy logic (K_{Pc} for P part and K_{Ic} for I part) are linearly combined with the conventional PI controller,

$$\tau_F = \tau_T \cdot (K_P + K_{Pc}) + \int \tau_T \cdot (K_I + K_{Ic})\, dt, \tag{9.8}$$

where K_P and K_I are the parameters for the conventional PI controller respectively and τ_F is the final output of the force control. The maximal values of K_{Pc} and K_{Ic} are set to be equal to K_P and K_I, respectively.

As mentioned in the Introduction, stability is one of the main concern for fuzzy controllers. The stability of our robot system is investigated by the conventional describing function analyses. According to Aracil and Gordillo, (Aracil and Gordillo, 2004) the describing function of the fuzzy force PI-controller can be defined as

$$[C_F(a, \omega p + C_L(a, \omega p] \cdot e(a, \omega p, \tag{9.9}$$

where e (a, ω pgs assumed to a simple sinusoidal function a·sin(ωt), both a and ω are constants, and

$$C_L(a, \omega pg K_P + K_I/(a \cdot \omega p, \tag{9.10}$$

$$C_F(a, \omega pg = \mathrm{g1} \cdot sp(a) + k2 \cdot si(a/\omega)/s, \tag{9.11}$$

$$sp(a) = \min\left[1, \frac{2}{\pi}\left(\sin^{-1}\frac{K_P}{a} + \frac{K_P}{a}\sqrt{1-(\frac{K_P}{a})^2}\right)\right], \tag{9.12}$$

$$si(a) = \min\left[1, \frac{2}{\pi}\left(\sin^{-1}\frac{K_I}{a} + \frac{K_P}{a}\sqrt{1-(\frac{K_P}{a})^2}\right)\right], \tag{9.13}$$

K_I and K_P are the saturation limits of fuzzy logic for integration and proportional parts, respectively. The condition for the first harmonic balance is 1 + [C_F(a, ωp) + C_L(a, ωp)]·G = 0. The stability of the fuzzy controller is then visualized by drawing a series of curves of [C_F(a, ωp + C_L(a, ωp)] against -G^{-1}. The analyses shows that, with the implemented fuzzy controller, the robot arm is stable in face of disturbance of frequencies from 10 to 0.01 Hz and magnitudes from 0.1 to 100 N (Fig. 9.2). In other words, the robot arm will be stable in the expected therapeutic maneuver ranges.

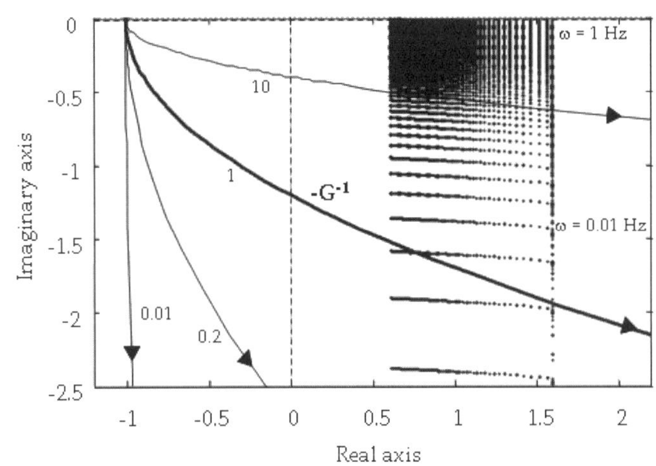

Figure 9.2 Results of describing function analyses.

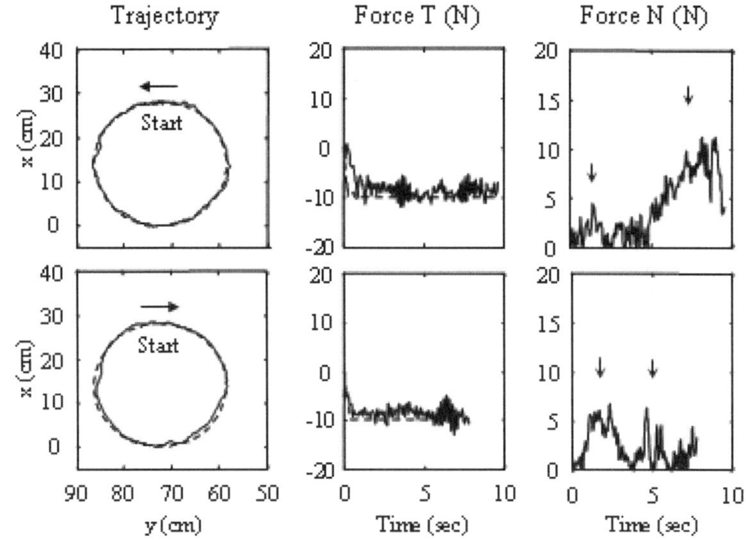

Figure 9.3 Circular active movements against a load of 10 Newtons.

We design three types of movement trajectories, namely, linear, circular and figure eight. The normal linear movement trajectory is an outward movement from the chest of 28 cm in length and the oblique linear movement trajectory is an oblique (45°) outward movement from the chest of 21.2 cm in length. The circular movement trajectory is a circular movement with a diameter of 28 cm. The figure-8 movement trajectory consists of two ellipses (14×28 cm) with their short axes in alignment in radial direction and with opposite moving directions. Since the movement velocity is not controlled, in the design process a trajectory is partitioned into 4000 segments by length along the trajectory instead of the lapsed time (Yoshikawa, 1990). We also used a randomly timed perturbation force to test the control capability of the subject to maintain the trajectory.

Fig. 9.3 shows example results of circular active movements of a normal subject against a load of ten Newtons. The trajectory was well maintained with the position error less than 1.25 cm during the whole trajectory. The control system kept a resistive load of 10 Newtons. In the third column, the force along the direction normal to the movement shows that the subject could follow the trajectory well, except when the subject needed to change direction in the left-right axis (arrows).

Fig. 9.4 shows examples of applying randomly timed perturbation torques to test the control capability in a normal subject and a stroke patient. The perturbation imposed a constant force of 7.5 Newtons along the direction normal to the movement for a fixed interval, as indicated by the dotted wedge. It is clear that the perturbation caused a larger deviation from the desired trajectory in the stroke patient.

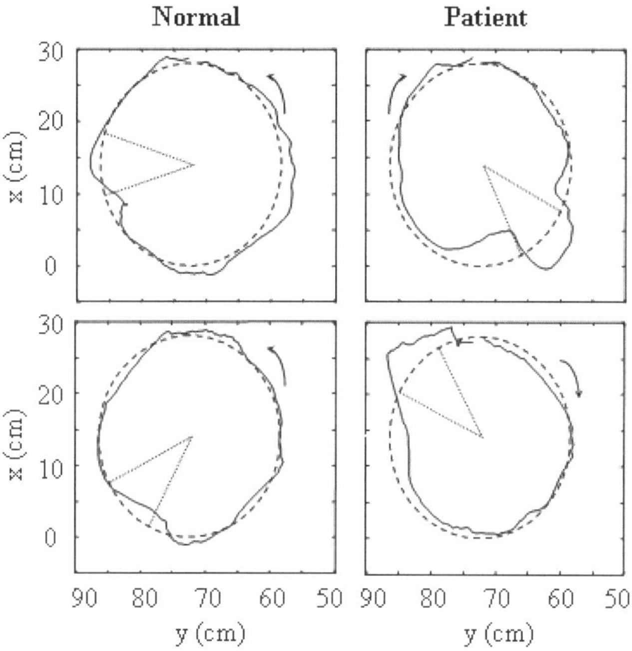

Figure 9.4 Random perturbation as a test of control capability in a normal subject and a stroke patient.

9.3 EVALUATION OF BENEFITS FOR REHABILITATION WITH ROBOTS

The main manifestations of motor deficits in stroke patients include weakness, loss of dexterity, spasticity and abnormal synergy. In clinical practice, MRC scale (Bates, 1995), Brunnstrom's Stage (BrS) (Brunnstrom, 1970), the FuglMeyer assessment (FM) (Fugl-Meyer *et al.*, 1975), the Functional Independence Measure (FIM) (Tinetti, 1986), and the Modified Ashworth Scale (MAS)(Bohannon and Smith, 1987) are used to semi-quantify motor deficits and functional capability. Although these clinical indices reflect motor deficits they are ordinal and heavily depend on the judgment of raters.

Many robotic systems have relevant parameters for quantification of treatment efficacy Gerachshenko *et al.*, 2008; Schwerin *et al.*, 2008; Sakatani *et al.*, 2007). These parameters may originate form kinematics, kinetics and electromyogram (EMG). Usually, the efficacy of robot system in rehabilitation is reported with results from scale evaluation and quantitative parameters. FM and FIM are by far the most used scale parameters. The pioneering MIT-Manus (Kwakkel *et al.*, 2008; Wolbrecht *et al.*, 2008) showed a beneficial effect of robot-assisted upper limb treatment of severely affected stroke patients. MIME system (Rosati *et al.*, 2007; Hesse *et al.*, 2005) has been validated for chronic patients that could provide the affected limb to perform a mirror movement of the movement defined by the intact limb. Arm reaching therapy for chronic patients has been verified with Arm Guide (Colombo *et al.*, 2008). Kwakkel *et al* (Kwakkel *et al.*, 2008). did a systematic review and meta-analyses on the effects of robot-assisted therapy on upper limb recovery after stroke. Only randomized clinical trials were included in the review and ten studies, involving 218 patients, were included in the synthesis. Meta-analysis, using upper limb part of FM score as the parameter, showed a non-significant heterogeneous summary effect size (SES) in terms of motor recovery. Sensitivity analysis of studies involving only shoulder-elbow robotics demonstrated a significant homogeneous SES for motor recovery. No significant SES was observed for functional ability (ADL), using FIM score as the parameter. The authors attribute the failure to observe improvement in ADL to the improper choice of ADL scales. Another review article by Prange *et al* (2006). reached very similar conclusions.

While the effects of rehabilitation with robots are mostly reported on motor recovery and improvement in ADL in the past, we focused more on the abnormal synergy. In the upper limbs, the abnormal synergies include the flexor synergy (characterized by simultaneous shoulder abduction, elbow flexion, and forearm supination) and the extensor synergy (characterized by simultaneous shoulder adduction, elbow extension, and forearm pronation). At the initial stage of stroke recovery, abnormal synergies of the affected limbs are facilitated in a reflex level. After a period of treatment, abnormal synergies are broken down and voluntary normal movements are facilitated. Quantification of abnormal synergies can be used as an objective indicator of recovery. In recent studies, quantitative assessment indices of abnormal synergies have been developed based on kinematics, (Dipietro *et al.*, 2007; Micera *et al.*, 2005; Sukal *et al.*, 2007; Ellis *et al.*, 2008) kinetics (Dewald *et al.*, Beer *et al.*, 2004; Ellis *et al.*, 2005), EMG (Gerachshenko *et al.*, 2008; Dewald *et al.*, 1995; Lum *et al.*, 2003), transcranial magnetic stimulation(Schwerin *et al.*, 2008) and functional magnetic resonance images during voluntary movements of stroke patients. Abnormal coactivation of the elbow flexors with the shoulder abductors, extensors, external rotators, elevators and retractors has been found in the affected limbs of stroke patients (Dewald *et al.*, 2001; Ellis *et al.*, 2005; Dewald *et al.*, 1995; Lum *et al.*, 2003). Prior to pronator contraction, corticomotor excitability of the antagonist biceps brachii was increased post-stroke (Gerachshenko *et al.*, 2008). These studies focused on observing the patient's abnormal synergies under static conditions. However, most movements in daily activities are dynamic. Researchers have determined that abnormal shoulder abductor/elbow flexor coupling limited stroke patients from reaching out in the work area (Sukal *et al.*, 2007; Ellis *et al.*, 2008; Beer *et al.*, 2004). In addition, stroke patients exhibited high correlation between shoulder and elbow angles during a circle-drawing task (Dipietro *et al.*, 2007) These studies have demonstrated that abnormal synergies occurred during voluntary movements. In addition, most of the studies have focused on the analysis of abnormal synergies in proximal joints such as the shoulder and elbow rather than in distal joints. We considered both the proximal and distal parts of the upper extremity at the same time. In summary, the synthesized results concluded that the robots showed

Table 9.1 Quantitative and clinical indices in the initial and fourth month evaluations

Index	Initial[$1]	4th month[$1]	p[$2]
r	-0.25	-0.02	<0.05
I	82.9	56.9	<0.05
C	-7.0	-36.9	0.09
BrS	3	4	0.13
MAS	2	1	0.25
FM	20	32	<0.05

[$1] Values are medians
[$2] Wilcoxon signed-rank test

benefits for the motor recovery, especially in the proximal joints, but no influence on functional ability.

We performed, in addition to the conventional rehabilitation for 0.5 hours, rehabilitation with the robot for another 0.5 hours, 3 times per week for 4 months. Seven stroke patients in the chronic stage were recruited. Rectilinear movements in 4 directions (right-left, forward-backward and two 45° oblique directions) were chosen as the rehabilitation movements. In addition to the traditional scales (BrS, MAS and FM), we developed three indicators to quantify the abnormal synergy. r was the correlation coefficient between the elbow joint angle and the supination/pronation angle of the forearm, I (Integration of Absolute Deviation of Torque) was used to quantify the total variation of forearm pronation-supination torque and C was a parameter derived from principle component analyses of 8 surface EMG of upper limbs during movements. The whole results are summarized in Table 9.1.

Two of three quantitative indicators (r and I) showed significant improvement after 4 months of rehabilitation with the robot, while one of three semi-quantitative scales, FM showed significant improvement. The reason that there was no difference in BrS, and MAS scores might be that BrS was invented for the global status and MAS was specific for hypertonia, i.e., they were not indicators for abnormal synergies. In addition, these scales are rather coarse and might not be able to differentiate subtle difference. In summary, our preliminary results indicated that rehabilitation with robots may help to break the abnormal synergies.

9.4 FUTURE DEVELOPMENT

One logical extension of the planar robots is to 3D robots. However, as mentioned in the Introduction, many problems and challenges need to be solved before the 3D robots can be practically useful. There are other modifications and augmentations, including rehabilitation of the hand and wrist, self-control by EEG, custom-tailored treatment protocol, developing evidence-based evaluation parameters and designing more efficient movements, that can make the robot systems more powerful.

The main function of our planar robot is for rehabilitating the elbow and shoulder joints. However, in stroke patients, motor impairments of the wrist and hand usually accompany those of elbow and shoulder joints. For the upper limbs, the function of hands is the main focus, and the function of the proximal parts is supportive. After completing the planar robot for elbow-shoulder rehabilitation, we modify the wrist fixation part so that the pronation-supination movement of the forearm can also be controlled and rehabilitated (Kung *et al.*, 2005). Two types of movements are designed, i.e., passive and active movements. The passive movement means that the subject is asked to relax his forearm and the robot guides the forearm to complete the movement. The main function of the passive movements is to reduce the muscle tone of the forearm and to increase the ROM. In the active mode, subjects have to move actively along a planned trajectory and the robot applies either a resistant or an assistant torque. Active movements are designed to help patients to increase muscle power. Two treatment trajectories, i.e., seesaw-like and ramp-and-hold trajectories, are designed to mimic the facilitation techniques of the physical therapists. In the seesaw-like trajectory the robot can cyclically stretch the forearm of the subject. Hogan's group also has developed a wrist rehabilitation robot, which can be combined with the original MIT-MANUS (Krebs *et al.*, 2007).

The next step is for rehabilitation of the hand. In terms of the joint number, hand is the most complicated part of the upper limb and the design of robots for hand rehabilitation is the most difficult part. Hogan's group developed two generations of robots for hand rehabilitation (Masia *et al.*, 2006) and is still on the way of improving the system. We also developed several prototypes, but none is satisfactory (Hong *et al.*, 2006; Shih *et al.*, 2007). More studies to gain insight into what is essential for hand rehabilitation may be needed before a practical rehabilitation robot for hands can be designed.

Currently, the rehabilitation robots are controlled by pre-written programs and subjects interact with the robots through parameters, such as force, position and compliance. The subjects can not control the behavior of the robots. Allowing subjects to have control over the robots may have the benefits of tailoring the treatment individually. EEG is a commonly used control source for brain-computer interface (BCI) (Wolpaw *et al.*, 2000) , which is defined as an artificially reconstructed connection between a subject's brain and the environment. BCI is developed to help subjects with motor impairments to regain environmental control or communication with others. Using the subjects' own EEG as the control source may have the benefits of training the brain and promoting plasticity of the cortex. If the required imagery attempts correspond to the natural control for the rehabilitating movements, it is also possible that the setup may promote the repair of the corrupted efferent connection. We implemented the idea in a rehabilitation device of fingers. The results (Chen *et al.*, 2009) indicate that the idea is plausible. Yet, the benefits for fingers and for the brain need to be validated.

The individual difference among subjects are huge, because variation in the pre-morbid capability, the size and the location of stroke lesions and the intensity of rehabilitation. It is more logical to design and implement a custom-tailored

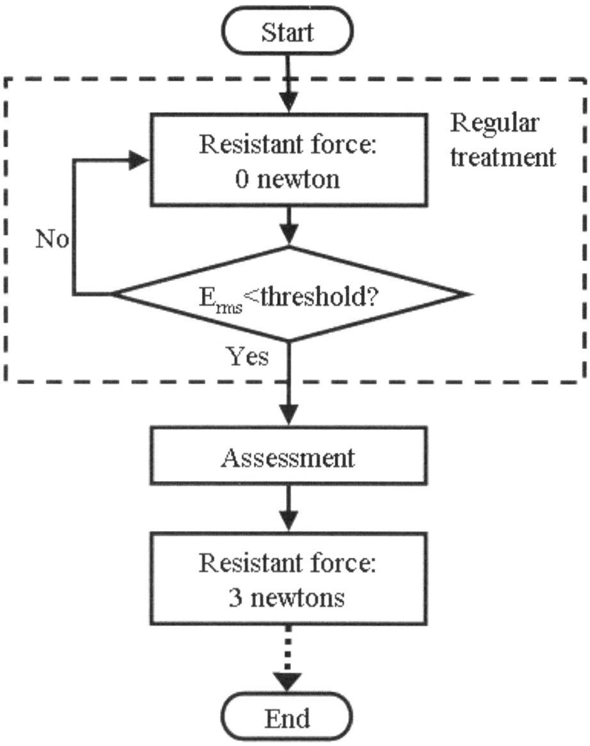

Figure 9.5 Flow chart for customized rehabilitation program.

rehabilitation program. In manual rehabilitation, therapists have a feeling of the subject's status and perform rehabilitation individually. However the feeling or the measure is qualitatively or even elusive. In the robotic rehabilitation, the rehabilitation program is uniform or is adjustable but there is no definite rule for adjustment. Hogan's group tried several modes of performance-based treatments with robots (Krebs *et al.*, 2003). The results were promising but needed to be verified. We did a study on a custom-made flow chart for patients rehabilitating with the robot (Wu *et al.*, 2002). The basic idea is to change the resistant load periodically based on the quantitative performance parameters (Fig. 9.5). The study is preliminary, in the sense that many parameters in the rehabilitation program can also be changed during the progress. It requires more extensive studies to determine what is the optimal combination and temporal relation of changes.

9.5 CONCLUSIONS

In this chapter, we reviewed the existing robot systems and their controllers for the purpose of upper limb rehabilitation. Robot systems were shown to improve motor recovery, more significant in proximal part, but not in functional ability.

We presented our approach with a planar robot. Our results indicated robot rehabilitation may also assist to break abnormal synergy. Future trends for the rehabilitation with the planar robot are outlined in the last part.

References

Kahn, L. E., Zygman, M. L., Rymer, W. Z. and Reinkensmeyer, D. J., Robot-assisted reaching exercise promotes arm movement recovery in chronic hemiparetic stroke: a randomized controlled pilot study, *J. Neruoeng. Rehabil.*, **3**, 12 (2006).

Marchal-Crespo, L. and Reinkensmeyer, D. J., Review of control strategies for robotic movement training after neurologic injury, *J. Neuroeng. Rehabil.*, **6**, 20 (2009).

Krebs, H. I., Hogan, N., Aisen, M. L. and Volpe, B. T., Robot-aided neurorehabilitation, *IEEE Trans. Rehab. Eng.*, **6**, 75–87 (1998).

Asada, H. and Youcef-Toumi, K., Analysis and design of a direct-drive arm with a five- bar-link parallel drive mechanism, *Tran. ASME J. Dyn. Syst. Meas. Contr.*,**106**, pp. 255–230 (1984).

Noritsugu, T. and Tanaka, T., Application of rubber artificial muscle manipulator as a rehabilitation robot," *IEEE/ASME Trans. Mechatron.*, **2**, 259–267 (1997).

Raibert, M. H. and Craig, J. J. Hybrid, position/force control of manipulators, *Trans. ASME J. Dyn. Syst. Meas. Contr.*, **102**, 126–133 (1981).

Suh, H., Hong, J. H., Oh, S.-R. and Kim, K. B., Fuzzy rule based position/force control of industrial manipulators, *IEEE/RSJ Intl. Workshop Intelligent Robots Syst.*, **3**, 1617–1622 (1991).

Burgar, C. G., Lum, P. S., Shor, P. and van der Loos, H. F., Development of robots for rehabilitation therapy: The Palo Alto VA/Stanford experience. *J. Rehabil. Res. Dev.*, **37**, 663–673 (2000).

Cozens, J. A., Robotic assistance of an active upper limb exercise in neurologically impaired patients, *IEEE Trans. Rehab. Eng.*, **7**, 254–256 (1999).

Colombo, R., Pisano, F., Micera, S., Mazzone, A., Delconte, C., Carrozza, M. C., Dario, P. and Minuco, G., Robotic Techniques for upper limb evaluation and rehabilitation of stroke patients, *IEEE Trans. Neural Sys. Rehab. Eng.*, **13**(3), 311–324 (2005).

Reinkensmeyer D., Takahashi C. and Timoszyk W., Evaluation of an assistive controller for reaching following brain injury, *Proc. 1st Joint BMES/EMBS Conf.*, p. 631 (1999).

Hesse S, Schulte-Tigges G, Konrad M., Bardeleben A. and Wermer C Robot-assisted arm trainer for the passive and active practice of bilateral forearm and wrist movements in hemiparetic subjects, *Arch. Phys. Med. Rehabil.*, **84**, 915–920 (2003).

Kikuchi T, Fukushima K, Furusho J and Ozawa T., Development of quasi-3DOF upper limb rehabilitation system using ER brake: PLEMO-P1, *J. Phys. Conf. Series.* **149**, 1–4 (2009).

Koyanagi K, Imada Y, Furusho J, Ryu U, Inoue A. and Takenaka K., 3-D Rehabilitation robot system for upper limbs and its force display techniques, *ICAT*, (2003).

Doornebosch A. J, Cools H. J. M, Slee-Turkenburg M. E. C, van Elk M. G. and Schoone-Harmsen M., Robot-mediated ACtive Rehabilitation (ACRE2) for the hemiplegic upper limb after a stroke: A pilot study *Technology and Disability*, **19**, 199–203 (2007).

Coote S, Stokes E, Murphy B. and Harwin W., The effect of GENTLE robot mediated therapy on upper extremity dysfunction post stroke, *Proc 8th ICORR*, pp. 59–62 (2003).

Sukal T. M, Ellis M. D, and Dewald J. P. A., Dynamic characterization of upper limb discoordination following hemiparetic stroke, *Proc 9th ICORR*,pp.519–521 (2005).

Toth A., Fazekas, G. Arz, G., Jurak, M. and Horvath, M., Passive robotic movement therapy of the spastic hemiparetic arm with REHAROB: report of the first clinical test and the follow-up system improvement, *Proc 9th ICORR*, (2005).

Fanin C., Gallina P., Rossi A., *et al.* NeRebot: a wire-based robot for neurorehabilitation. *Proc 8th ICORR*, (2003).

Rosati, G, Gallina, P, Masiero, S. and Rossi, A., Design of a new 5 d.o.f. wire-based robot for rehabilitation, *Proc 9th ICORR*, pp.431–433 (2005).

Nef, T, Mihelj, M. and Riener R., ARMin: a robot for patient-cooperative arm therapy, *Med. Bio. Eng. Comput.*, **45**, 887–900 (2007).

He, J., Balasubramanian, S. and Wei, R., Designing interactive and intelligent control for rehabilitation robots, eds. Xiong, *et al.*, *ICIRA 2008, Part II, LNAI 5315, pp. 7–16*, (2008).

Wang L-X., *Adaptive Fuzzy Systems and Control: Design and Stability Analysis* (Prentice Hall, Englewood Cliffs NJ, USA), (1994).

Rugh W. J., Analytical framework for gain scheduling, *IEEE Contr. Syst Magazine*, **11**(1), 79–84, (1991).

Lee S. H, Kim S. G. and Lim J. T., Fuzzy-logic-based fast gain-scheduling control for nonlinear suspension systems, *IEEE Trans. Industrial Electronics*, **45(6)** 953–955 (1998).

Tanaka K. and Wang H. O., *Fuzzy Control Systems Design and Analysis* (John Wiley & sons, Inc., New York, USA), (2001).

Ibrahim A.-A. S., Nonlinear PID controller design using fuzzy logic, *IEEE MELECON 2002* pp. 595–599 (2002).

Moon U.-C. and Lee K. Y., Hybrid algorithm with fuzzy system and conventional PI control for the temperature control of TV glass furnace, *IEEE Trans. Contr Syst Tech*, **11**(4), 548–554 (2003).

Deskur J, Muszynski R. and Sarnowski D., Tuning and investigation of combined fuzzy controller, *7th Intl Conf. Power Electronics and Variable Speed Drives*, pp.21–23 (1998).

Ju M. S, Lin D. H, Lin C. C. K, Hwang I. S. and Chen S. M. Application of fuzzy theory in development of a robot for neuro-rehabilitation of elbow, *ASME Summer Bioeng. Conf.*, (2001).

Wu S. Y., Ju, M. S., Lin C. C. K., Hwang I. S. and Chen S. M., Treatment trial of using robot for neuro-rehabilitation of upper extremities, *Proc. 2002 Conf. BME Tech.*, (2002).

Ju, M. S, Lin, C. C. K, Lin, D. H, Hwang, I. S. and Chen, S. M. Torque-angle hybrid fuzzy control for a rehabilitation robot. *IEEE Trans. Neural Syst. Rehab. Eng.* **13**(3), 349–358 (2005).

Phillips S. M. and Ballou K. R., Friction modeling and compensation for an industrial robot, *J. Robot. Syst.*, **10**, 947–971 (1993).

Lu Z., Shimoga K. B. and Goldenberg A. A., Experimental determination of dynamic parameters of robotic arms, *J. Robot. Syst.*, **10**, 1009–1029 (1993).

Chou Z. Y., *Contact force control in soft boundary condition*, M.S. thesis, Department of Mechanical Engineering and Technology, National Yung-Lin Technology College, Taiwan (in Chinese), (1997).

Aracil, J. and Gordillo, F., Describing function method for stability analysis of PD and PI fuzzy controllers, *Fuzzy Sets and Systems*, **143**, 233–249 (2004).

Yoshikawa T., *Foundations of Robotics: Analysis and Control* (MIT Press, Cambridge, USA), (1990).

Bates B., *A Guide to Physical Examination and History Taking* (Lippincott philadelphia, USA, p. 513), (1995).

Brunnstrom S., *Movement Therapy in Hemiplegia* (Harper & Row New York, USA), (1970).

Fugl-Meyer A. R, Jaasko L and Leyman I., The post-stroke hemiplegic patient. 1. A method for evaluation of physical performance *Scand. J. Rehabil. Med..*, **7**, 13–31 (1975).

Tinetti M. E., Performance-oriented assessment of mobility problems in elderly patients. *J. Am. Geriatr. Soc.*, **34**, 119–26 (1986).

Bohannon R. W. and Smith M. B., Interrater reliability of a modified ashworth scale of muscle spasticity *Phys. Ther.*, **67**, 206–7 (1987).

Gerachshenko T, Rymer W. Z. and Stinear J. W., Abnormal corticomotor excitability assessed in biceps brachii preceding pronator contraction post-stroke. *Clin. Neurophysiol.*, **119**, 683–92 (2008).

Schwerin S, Dewald J. P. A., Haztl M., Jovanovich S., Nickeas M. and MacKinnon C., Ipsilateral versus contralateral cortical motor projections to a shoulder adductor in chronic hemiparetic stroke: Implications for the expression of arm synergies *Exp. Brain Res.*, **185**, pp. 509–19 (2008).

Sakatani K., Murata Y., Fujiwara N., Hoshino T., Nakamura S., Kano T. and Katayama Y., Comparison of blood-oxygen-level-dependent functional magnetic resonance imaging and near-infrared spectroscopy recording during functional brain activation in patients with stroke and brain tumors. *J. Biomed. Opt.* 12, (2007).

Kwakkel G, Kollen B. J. and Krebs H. I., Effects of robot-assisted therapy on upper limb recovery after stroke: A systematic review, *Neurorehabil. Neural Repair*, **22**, 111–21 (2008).

Wolbrecht E. T., Chan V, Reinkensmeyer D. J. and Bobrow J. E., Optimizing compliant, model-based robotic assistance to promote neurorehabilitation, *IEEE Trans. Neural. Syst. Rehabil. Eng.*, **16**, 286–97 (2008).

Rosati G., Gallina P. and Masiero S., Design, implementation and clinical tests of a wire-based robot for neurorehabilitation, *IEEE Trans. Neural. Syst. Rehabil. Eng.*, **15**, 560–569 (2007).

Hesse S, Werner C, Pohl M, Rueckriem S, Mehrholz J and Lingnau M. L., Computerized arm training improves the motor control of the severely affected arm after stroke — A single-blinded randomized trial in two centers, *Stroke*, **36**, pp. 1960–1966 (2005).

Colombo R, Pisano F, Micera S, Mazzone A, Delconte C, Carrozza M. C., Dario, p. and Minuco G. Assessing mechanisms of recovery during robot-aided neurorehabilitation of the upper limb, *Neurorehabil. Neural Repair.*, **22**, 50–63 (2008).

Kwakkel G, Kollen B. J. and Krebs H. I., Effects of robot-assisted therapy on upper limb recovery after stroke: A systematic review, *Neurorehabil. Neural Repair*, **22(2)**, 111–121 (2008).

Prange G. B., Jannink M. J. A., Groothuis-Oudshoorn C. G. M., Hermens H. J. and Ijzerman M. J., Systematic review of the effect of robot-aided therapy on recovery of the hemiparetic arm after stroke. *J. Rehabil. Res. & Dev.*, **43**(2), pp.171–184 (2006).

Dipietro L, Krebs H. I., Fasoli S. E., Volpe B. T., Stein J, Bever C., and Hogan N., Changing motor synergies in chronic stroke *J. Neurophysiol.*, **98**, 757–768 (2007).

Micera S, Carpaneto J, Posteraro F, Cenciotti L, Popovic M. and Dario P., Characterization of upper arm synergies during reaching tasks in able-bodied and hemiparetic subjects *Clin. Biomech.*, **20**, 939–946 (2005).

Sukal T. M., Ellis M. D. and Dewald J. P. A., Shoulder abduction-induced reductions in reaching work area following hemiparetic stroke: neuroscientific implications, *Exp. Brain. Res.*, **183** 215–223 (2007).

Ellis M. D., Sukal T, DeMott T. and Dewald J. P. A., Augmenting clinical evaluation of hemiparetic arm movement with a laboratory-based quantitative measurement of kinematics as a function of limb loading, *Neurorehabil. Neural Repair*, **22**, 321–329 (2008).

Dewald J. P. A. and Beer R. F. Abnormal joint torque patterns in the paretic upper limb of subjects with hemiparesis, *Muscle Nerve* **24**, 273–83 (2001).

Beer R. F., Dewald J. P. A., Dawson M. L. and Rymer W. Z., Target-dependent differences between free and constrained arm movements in chronic hemiparesis, *Exp Brain Res*, **156**, 458–470 (2004).

Ellis M. D., Holubar B. G., Acosta A. M., Beer R. F. and Dewald J. P. A. Modifiability of abnormal isometric elbow and shoulder joint torque coupling after stroke, *Muscle Nerve* **32**, 170–178 (2005).

Dewald J. P. A., Pope P. S., Given J. D., Buchanan T. S. and Rymer W. Z., Abnormal muscle coactivation patterns during isometric torque generation at the elbow and shoulder in hemiparetic subjects, *Brain*, **118**, 495–510 (1995).

Lum P. S., Burgar C. G. and Shor P. C. Evidence for strength imbalances as a significant contributor to abnormal synergies in hemiparetic subjects, *Muscle Nerve*, **27**, 211–21 (2003).

Schwerin S, Dewald J. P. A., Haztl M, Jovanovich S, Nickeas M. and MacKinnon C., Ipsilateral versus contralateral cortical motor projections to a shoulder adductor in chronic hemiparetic stroke: implications for the expression of arm synergies, *Exp Brain Res.*, **185**, 509–19 (2008).

Sakatani, K, Murata, Y, Fujiwara, N, Hoshino, T, Nakamura, S, Kano, T., *et al.* Comparison of blood-oxygen-level-dependent functional magnetic resonance imaging and near-infrared spectroscopy recording during functional brain activation in patients with stroke and brain tumors, *J. Biomed. Opt*, (2007).

Kung B. C, Ju M. S, Lin C. C. K and Chen S. M. Clinical assessment of forearm pronation/supination torque in stroke patients, *J. Med. Biol. Eng.*, **25(1)**, 39–43 (2005).

Krebs H. I., Volpe B. T., Williams D, Celestino J, Charles S. K., Lynch D. and Hogan N. Robot-aided neurorehabilitation: A Robot for wrist rehabilitation, *IEEE Trans Neural Syst Rehabil Eng*, **15**(3), 327–335 (2007).

Masia, L., Krebs, H. I., Cappa, P. and Hogan, N. Whole-arm rehabilitation following stroke: Hand module, *Biomed. Robot. & Biomechatron.*, pp. 1085–1089 (2006).

Hong, C. S., Ju, M. S. and Lin, C. C. K.(2006) Development of a robot for neruo-rehabilitation of hand, *Intl. Symposium BME*, Taipei, Taiwan, p.180.

Shih M. C., Lin C. C. K. and Ju, M. S. A study of brain-computer interface (BCI) controlled prosthetic hand, *XXI Congr. Intl. Soc. Biomech.*, Taipei, Taiwan, (2007).

Wolpaw J. R., Birbaumer N, Heetderks W. J., McFarland D. J., Peckham P. H., Shalk G, Donchin E, Quatrano L. A., Robinson C. J. and Vaugham TM. Brain–computer interface technology: A review of the first international meeting *IEEE Trans Rehab Eng.*, **8**, 164–173 (2000).

Chen, C. W., Lin, C. C. K. and Ju, M. S. Hand orthosis controlled by using brain-computer interface, *J. Med. Biol. Eng.*, **29**(5), 234–241,(2009).

Krebs H. I., Palazzolo J. J., Dipietro L, Ferraro M, Krol J, Rannekleiv K, Volpe B. T. and Hogan N. Rehabilitation robotics: Performance-based progressive robot-assisted therapy, *Auton. Robot.*, **15**(1), 7–20 (2003).

Chapter Ten

Upper Extremity Rehabilitation Systems and Augmented Feedback

Birgit I. Molier*, Gerdienke B. Prange*, Thijs Krabben*,
Michiel J. A. Jannink*,†, Jaap H. Buurke*,‡ and Hermie J. Hermens*,§

*Roessingh Research and Development, 7500AH Enschede, The Netherlands
†University of Twente, Department of Biomedical Engineering, 7500AE Enschede, The Netherlands
‡Rehabilitation Centre 'the Roessingh', 7500AH Enschede, The Netherlands
§University of Twente, Department of Biomedical Signals and Systems, 7500AE Enschede, The Netherlands

10.1 INTRODUCTION

With ageing, the incidence of neurological diseases, such as stroke, increases strongly. This induces a substantial increase of the strain on health care. By using innovative technologies, such as robotics and augmented feedback, intensive practice with reduced amount of health care professionals can be accomplished.

In this chapter an overview is given of the problems and possible solutions concerning arm rehabilitation for stroke survivors, based on current research.

10.2 STROKE

A stroke, or cerebrovascular accident (CVA), is a major cause of mortality and permanent disability in the world. In Europe the estimated amount of people experiencing a first stroke varies between 460 thousand and 1.1 million people every year (Ijzerman 2005). In the US every year around 780 thousand people experience a first or recurrent stroke (Rosamond 2008).

10.2.1 Definition

Stroke can be defined as a neurological deficit due to damage to the blood supply of the brain. This can be ischemic or hemorrhagic. An ischemic stroke is due

Biomechatronics in Medicine and Healthcare by Le Li and Raymond Kai-Yu Tong

www.panstanford.com
978-981-4241-61-8

to an obstruction of a blood vessel, occurring in approximately 85 percent of the cases. A hemorrhagic stroke is due to a rupture of a blood vessel, which occurs in approximately 15 percent of the cases (Rosamond 2008).

10.2.2 Impairments

Due to blood deficiency, as a direct consequence of the stroke, brain tissue is destructed. This can result in a variety of sensory, motor, cognitive and psychological impairments. This includes sensory loss, hemispatial neglect, aphasia, muscle weakness, spasticity, limited movement coordination, attention and memory deficits, depression and behavioral changes (Speach 1995).

Concerning the motor domain, a stroke often leads to damage of descending nerve pathways from the brain to the spinal cord, and of neural communication between brain areas. A reduction in integration of sensory and motor information combined with altered nerve signals, limits the selective activation of muscles. Coupled activation of muscles is often observed, such as shoulder abduction and elbow flexion, called muscle synergies. Without selective and voluntary control of muscles, arm and hand functionality is impaired, causing serious limitations in activities of daily living (Dewald 1995, Beer 1999).

Weakness is a common impairment of the upper extremity in 77 percent of the patients with a first-ever stroke (Lawrence 2001). Even after six months, 60 percent of stroke survivors have a hemiparetic arm which remains without function, due to for example weakness, synergistic coupling or spasticity in the arm (Kwakkel 2003).

10.2.3 Recovery

Spontaneous neurological recovery occurs after stroke. This involves short-term and long-term (from six months onward) physiological mechanisms in the brain (Kwakkel 2004). The extent of the neurological recovery varies among patients. Though, the recovery of motor functions follows a stereotypical sequence (Kreisel 2006).

When damage in the brain is detected, enhancement of active brain tissue surrounding the damaged area (infarct) occurs. Within days the swelling from excessive accumulation of plasma fluid in the tissue surrounding the infarct is reduced. Therefore reperfusion of the blood deprived brain area around the infarcted area can occur and the ischemic penumbra is resolved. Also the diaschisis, which is a malfunction of remote brain areas due to lack of neural input, is diminished. Due to these short-term mechanisms related brain areas can regain their neural communication (Speach 1995, Krakauer 2005).

A longer-term mechanism involved in natural neurological recovery is neural plasticity: cortical representations of, for example motor actions change during recovery. Cortical reorganization can occur in areas adjacent to and remote from the infarcted area, both in the infarcted (ipsilesional) and opposite (contralesional) hemisphere. Processes enabling cortical reorganization are:

— activation of previously inactive neurons: unmasking of latent synapses;
— facilitation of alternative networks;
— and collateral sprouting: growth of new axons.

These processes allow development of new paths for neural communication, to sidestep those neural paths that were damaged due to the infarct. To induce cortical reorganization these processes need to be stimulated, which can be induced by rehabilitation therapy (Speach 1995, Krakauer 2005, Kwakkel 2004).

10.3 REHABILITATION THERAPY

Spontaneous neurological recovery can be stimulated by rehabilitation therapy. Stimulation of sensory and motor areas induces reorganization of brain tissue through which motor skills can be relearned. This process of motor relearning can improve arm function. Several key elements of motor relearning for rehabilitation therapy have been identified (Schaechter 2004).

10.3.1 Key Elements

Several studies into principles of motor relearning and processes of cortical reorganization are performed. They provide a neurophysiological basis for key elements that have the potential for stimulation of restoration of arm and hand function after stroke (Krakauer 2005).

10.3.1.1 Intensity

Intensity of training is defined as the number of repetitions (frequency) of a particular movement in a certain period of time. Several studies have indicated that training with a higher frequency or longer duration stimulates functional recovery of the arm (Kwakkel 1999, 2006). From brain studies it is known that repetition of movements strengthens the representation of the trained movements in the brain (Fischer 2001).

10.3.1.2 Task-specificity

Functional exercises are exercises which focus on activities of daily living that are relevant for the patient's independence. Several studies have shown that functional training results in a more normalized brain activity pattern (Schaechter 2004). Such normalization of brain a activity is related to improvements in motor control and functional abilities. (Nelles 2001) Therefore, task-specific exercises of activities of daily living are important to stimulate motor recovery after stroke (Fischer 2001).

10.3.1.3 Active-initiation

It is shown in brain studies that cortical activity during active execution of movements is larger than during passive movements. Also, motor cortex excitability is higher after active movement training. Therefore exercise therapy focusing on active initiation and execution of movements is associated with improved arm function, and is essential to implement in rehabilitation therapy (Kaelin-Lang 2005, Feys 1998).

10.3.1.4 Motivation and Feedback

Motivation and feedback are also important elements for rehabilitation therapy. Addition of augmented feedback to exercises can stimulate the learning process by making patients more aware of their performance. In several review studies the additional motivational effect of virtual environments has been shown to be positive (Holden 2005, van Vliet 2006, Henderson 2007).

10.3.2 Current Therapies

A number of current therapy strategies incorporate several of these key elements (intensity, task-specificity, active-initiation, motivation and feedback).

10.3.2.1 CIMT

Constrained-induced movement therapy (CIMT) combines three key elements of motor learning in therapy; intensity, task-specificity, and active-initiation. The unaffected arm is restricted from being used, by means of wearing a sling, and therefore the patient is forced to use the affected arm and hand. This therapy has shown positive effects on arm and hand function in stroke survivors. A drawback of CIMT is that only patients with a considerable level of hand function, at least 20 degrees wrist and 10 degrees finger extension, are eligible for treatment (Wolf 2002).

10.3.2.2 Mirror-therapy

During a mirror therapy, patients place a mirror beside the unaffected arm. In this way the view of the affected arm is blocked, thereby creating the illusion that the affected arm is moving as well as the unaffected arm. This therapy uses two key elements: intensity and active-initiation. Studies on mirror therapy show beneficial effects on the treatment for the hemiparetic arm (Ezendam 2009). A drawback of mirror-therapy is the potential reliance of the patient on the image of the apparently functional arm. If the reliance is too large, the intention of using the affected arm decreases.

10.3.2.3 TNMES

Therapeutic neuromuscular electrical stimulation (TNMES) of the wrist and finger extensors is a therapy in which muscles are stimulated without voluntary muscle contraction. TNMES makes use of the key element intensity in therapy. An increase of muscle force of the stimulated muscles is mentioned in some studies as a beneficial effect of TNMES. However, it is not known whether improvements on arm and hand function are clinically relevant or whether functional improvements can be achieved (De Kroon 2002).

10.4 ROBOTIC DEVICES

To enhance motor relearning during rehabilitation therapy, integration of the previously mentioned key elements is essential. Unfortunately in current clinical practice this is labor-intensive and requires one-to-one manual interactions with therapists, which poses a high strain on therapists (Volpe 2002). With the upcoming technologies of robotic devices and augmented feedback it is possible to provide a combination of intense, task-specific, and interactive therapy in a motivating environment. With robotic devices, patients may therefore achieve increased gains from rehabilitation treatment (Feys 1998, Kwakkel 1999).

10.4.1 Passive and Active Movement

Robotic devices can be used in rehabilitation therapy for passive, active-assisted and active-resisted movement training. The training modality depends on the amount of assisting force provided by the robot; total assistance for passive movements, no assistance for active movements, and force against the movement direction for active-resisted.

Studies reporting the design and development of robotic devices have been reported extensively. However, only a few studies examine the effect of robotic devices on stroke rehabilitation in a clinical setting. Overall, robot-aided therapy on the upper extremity in stroke survivors seems to improve both short and long-term motor functions, but functional improvements are rarely seen. These studies mainly focused on the proximal arm, while proper control of both arm and hand are pre-requisites for many activities of daily living (Prange 2006, Kwakkel 2008).

10.4.2 Gravity Compensation

Most robotic devices use one of the modalities of training, passive, active-assisted, or active-resisted, in combination with gravity compensation. Until recently it was unknown what the effect of solely gravity compensation is on the arm and hand function of stroke survivors. A device providing solely gravity compensation is the Freebal (Stienen 2007), see Figure 10.1. Research to the effect of providing gravity compensation has shown an instantaneously increase of the range of motion of the

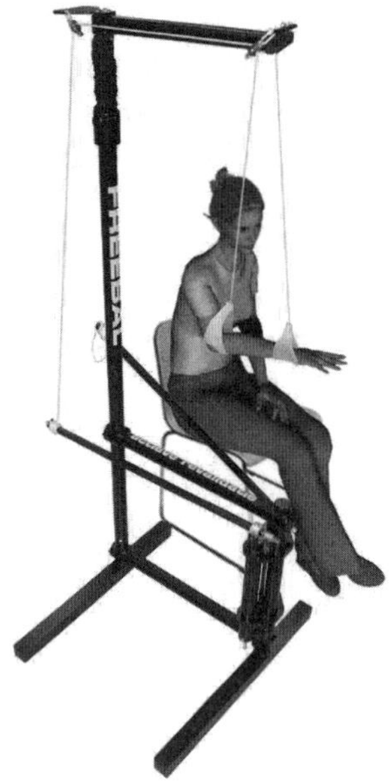

Figure 10.1 Gravity compensation system Freebal. For color reference, see page 219.

paretic arm (Beer 2007, Stienen 2007, Prange 2007). Also muscle activation levels during reach and retrieval movements with gravity compensation were lower than during movements without gravity compensation (Prange 2009a). These results can be explained, due to the reduced activation level of shoulder abductors, by arm support. As a result, the amount of coupled, involuntary elbow flexion is reduced, which facilitates elbow extension. Increased individual joint control can result in an increased range of motion.

Similar results are observed in a training study, where stroke survivors trained for 6 weeks in a gravity compensated environment. Improvements in unsupported reaching distance (3.6% of arm length) were observed, accompanied by increased shoulder elevation angle (up to 17.6 degrees) throughout the reaching movement and a larger range of elbow extension (up to 24.7 degrees) (Prange 2009b, Housman 2009). Application of gravity compensation is a promising tool for rehabili-tation therapy.

10.5 AUGMENTED FEEDBACK

Another way of stimulating motor relearning is providing augmented feedback. Addition of augmented feedback to (robotic therapy) exercises can stimulate the learning process by making patients more aware of their performance (Winstein 2006).

Augmented feedback is given in addition to intrinsic feedback. Intrinsic feedback is the sensory-perceptual information from internal sensory processes that is available as a result of the execution of a movement, such as vision, proprioception, and audition (Schmidt and Lee 2005). In stroke survivors intrinsic feedback mechanisms are often disturbed. By providing additional augmented feedback from an external source in therapy, motor relearning can be enhanced (van Vliet 2006).

Augmented feedback has the advantage of having the opportunity of incorporating several key elements (intensity, task-specificity, active-initiation, motivation, and feedback) in an environment which can be adjusted to the personal abilities of the patients. There are different possibilities of providing the desired augmented feedback. Two main categories exist in providing augmented feedback: aspects and types.

10.5.1 Aspects

An aspect of augmented feedback is defined as a more fundamental way of providing feedback. Aspects of augmented feedback are related to information about the movement performance or how many times the feedback is provided.

10.5.1.1 Nature

The nature of providing augmented feedback can be either knowledge of performance (KP), or knowledge of results (KR). KP feedback concerns information about the movement itself, such as information about the angle of the shoulder during execution of a movement. KR feedback concerns information about the outcome of the movement, such as information about the achievement of the goal.

Research in healthy subjects only gives inconclusive results about whether to provide KP or KR feedback. Studies investigating the effect of KP or KR on motor learning for stroke survivors are scarce (van Vliet 2006).

10.5.1.2 Timing

The timing of providing augmented feedback can be either concurrent or terminal. Concurrent feedback is delivered during movement execution. Terminal feedback can be given after completion of the movement.

In healthy subjects some research into the effectiveness of providing either concurrent or terminal feedback is performed. It has been demonstrated that the sooner after movement execution the augmented feedback was provided the better (Schmidt 1997). On the other hand, when concurrent feedback was provided during practice in healthy subjects, it enhanced the performance at that moment. But in post measurement tests without concurrent feedback, it resulted in performance decrements (Schmidt 1997). This indicates that caution needs to be taken about when to provide feedback, as this could cause a reliance of the person on the feedback during movement execution.

Research to the effectiveness of providing either concurrent or terminal feedback for stroke survivors is scarce. Therefore more insight in the influence of the timing of augmented feedback on motor learning for stroke survivors is necessary.

10.5.1.3 Frequency

The frequency of providing augmented feedback can be either summary or faded. An example of summary feedback is when after every 10th trial feedback is provided. An example of faded feedback is when feedback is provided in a certain schedule, after the 5th, 15th, 30th trial and so on (Schmidt and Lee 2005). Several studies in healthy subjects demonstrated that learning improved more when augmented feedback with a faded scheme was provided, than when feedback after every trial (summary) was provided (Wulf 1989, 1993, Winstein 1990). However, research into motor learning in stroke survivors shows no favorable effect of either summary or faded feedback (Winstein 1990).

10.5.2 Types

The type of augmented feedback reflects the source of feedback, which originates from an external source providing extra information to the internal sensors (ears, skin, and eyes) of the body.

10.5.2.1 Auditory Feedback

Auditory feedback can include verbal encouragements and sound beeps. Mostly auditory feedback is provided by means of verbal encouragements by physiotherapists in therapy (Molier 2009a).

Rehabilitation therapy for stroke survivors by means of auditory cueing has shown to be beneficial. In a study of Whitall (2000) 14 patients trained by means of bilateral rhythmic reaching and retrieving actions using a metronome to cue the patients, also called BATRAC training. After 18 training sessions patients increased on average three points on the Fugl-Meyer scale (Whitall 2000).

Furthermore, little is known about the effect of the different ways of providing augmented auditory feedback in both healthy subjects and stroke survivors.

10.5.2.2 Sensory Feedback

Sensory feedback is widely used since the introduction of rehabilitation robotics. It includes force, tactile and positional feedback about the executed movement. Mostly sensory feedback is provided combined with different kinds of augmented feedback, such as augmented visual feedback (Molier 2009a).

Research into the ability of stroke survivors to learn from solely augmented sensory feedback in a robotic device is promising (Molier 2009b). In the study of Molier (2009b) patients performed reach and retrieval movements over a predefined path, see Figure 10.2. When deviating from this path, sensory feedback was provided to the shoulder and elbow joints by means of resistance. To determine

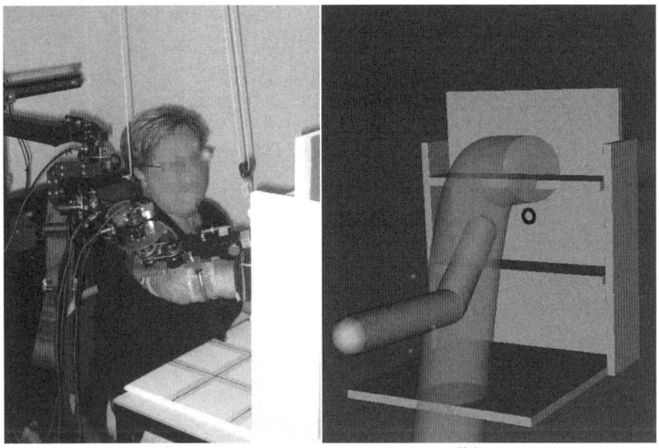

(a) (b)

Figure 10.2 (a) patient in exoskeleton with the table top in front of her (b) predefined path (in green), which was not shown to the stroke survivors. For color reference, see page 219.

if stroke survivors are able to learn from this sensory feedback, the number of collisions with the virtual tunnel wall was counted during a movement task with 15 repetitions. During several repeated movements patients were able to decrease the number of collisions with the virtual wall. These findings indicate that the patients were able to learn from sensory feedback when deviating from the predefined path, and adjust the movement to the imposed trajectory (Molier 2009b).

In a training study of Kahn (2006) robotically active-assisted exercises were compared with free reaching voluntary exercises (Kahn 2006). The robot constrained the subjects' movements, when it observed incorrect movement patterns, by forcing subjects to attempt to generate a more normal pattern. It was concluded that robotically assisting in reaching successfully improved arm movement ability. Nevertheless, there were no detectable, additional values beyond the free reaching movement practice (Kahn 2006).

Although provision of augmented sensory feedback seems to be a promising tool, the role of applied robotic forces to improve motor function is still unclear.

10.5.2.3 *Visual Feedback*

Another way of stimulating motor learning is providing augmented visual feedback, for example by means of Virtual Reality (VR). By means of augmented visual feedback several key elements of motor learning can be implemented in therapy, such as active, functional, and intensive exercises in a motivating environment. Also, multiple levels of difficulty can be presented for each exercise, allowing individually adjustable training programs (Holden 2005). Several applications of VR applied in stroke rehabilitation have shown a positive effect on motor function (Henderson 2007).

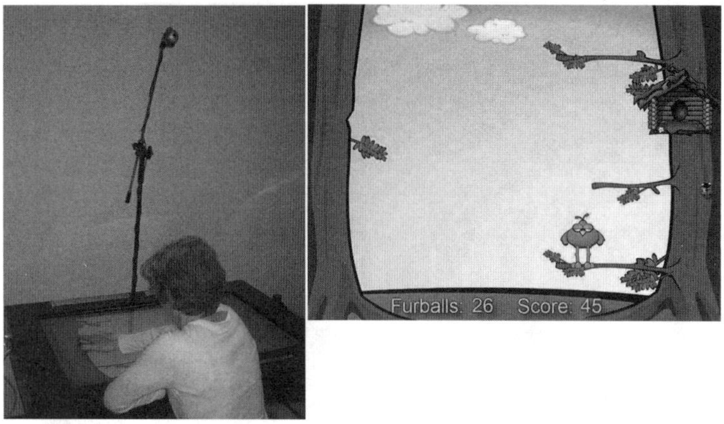

(a) (b)

Figure 10.3 Virtual environment (b) by means of motion capturing system (a). For color reference, see page 219.

Research into the ability of stroke survivors to transfer movements learned in a virtual environment to the real world, shows that motor tasks in most cases are transferred, and in some cases even generalized to other untrained tasks. In the studies that compared motor learning in real versus virtual environments, some advantage for VR training has been found (Holden 2005).

For the application of VR in rehabilitation therapy, different systems can be used, such as head mounted displays and motion capturing systems (see Figure 10.3). In the last system, movement of the arm is recorded by a camera and projected in the virtual environment on a screen. Stroke rehabilitation by means of motion capturing seems to be a promising therapy.

In a training study by Prange (2009b), patients performed goal-directed reaching movements within a virtual environment. In this virtual environment patients had to chase away birds from a tree branch by reaching for the bird with their hand, see Figure 10.3. The additional augmented visual feedback provided was a score on a screen, indicating the amount of chased away birds (knowledge of results). After six weeks of this training stroke patients improved on the Fugl-Meyer scale (on average 3.3 points) and increased their maximal reach distance (3.6% of arm length) (Prange 2009b).

Providing augmented visual feedback seems to be a promising tool for arm rehabilitation therapy for stroke survivors. However, more insight in the way (nature, timing, frequency) of providing augmented visual feedback is necessary.

10.6 FUTURE RESEARCH

Current robot-aided therapy focuses mainly on the proximal arm. To maximize independent use of the arm, not only proximal arm function is important, also functional use of the wrist and hand is essential. Information about the effectiveness or optimal application of simultaneous proximal and distal training using robotics is scarce at this point, and should be extended.

Since augmented feedback is closely related with the application of rehabilitation robotics, more extensive studies are needed to identify the added value and most optimal way of applying augmented feedback to complement technologically supported interventions.

10.7 CONCLUSIONS

A stroke may result in impaired arm and hand function which can cause serious limitations in activities of daily living. Optimal restoration of arm and hand motor function is essential for stroke survivors to independently perform activities of daily living. Several studies regarding underlying mechanisms of motor recovery have been performed. From these studies several key elements emerge; intensity, task-specificity, active-initiation, motivation and augmented feedback.

Current therapies, such as constraint-induced movement therapy, mirror-therapy, and therapeutic neuromuscular electrical stimulation, often implement few key elements in their therapy. With recent technological developments it is possible to implement more key elements in rehabilitation training. The effect of these innovative technologies, such as robotics and augmented feedback, on motor learning of stroke survivors is promising. By combining robotics and augmented feedback in one therapy, enhanced motor relearning can be expected.

References

Beer RF, Given JD, Dewald JPA, Task-dependent weakness at the elbow in patients with hemiparesis, *Arch. Phys. Med. Rehabil.* 1999;80:766–772.

Beer RF, Ellis MD, Holubar BG, Dewald JPA, Impact of gravity loading on post-stroke reaching and its relationship to weakness, *Muscle Nerve* 2007;36:242–250.

De Kroon JR, Van der Lee JH, IJzerman MJ, Lankhorst GJ, Therapeutic electrical stimulation to improve motor control and functional abilities of the upper extremity after stroke: A systematic review, *Clin. Rehab.* 2002;16(4):350–360.

Dewald JPA, Pope PS, Given JD, Buchanan TS, Rymer WZ, Abnormal muscle coactivation patterns during isometric torque generation at the elbow and shoulder in hemiparetic subjects, *Brain* 1995;118:495–510.

Ezendam D, Bongers RM, Jannink MJA, Systematic review of the effectiveness of mirror therapy in upper extremity function, *Disability & Rehabilitation*, 2009, 1464–5165.

Feys HM, De Weerdt WJ, Selz BE, Cox Steck GA, Spichiger R, Vereeck CE, Putman KD, Van Hoydonck GA, Effect of a therapeutic intervention for the hemiplegic upper limb in the acute phase after stroke, A single-blind, randomized, controlled multicenter trial, *Stroke* 1998; 29(4):785–92.

Fisher BE, Sullivan KJ, Activity-dependent factors affecting poststroke functional outcomes, *Top Stroke Rehabil.* 2001;8(3):31–44.

Henderson A, Korner-Bitensky N, and Levin M, Virtual reality in stroke rehabilitation: a systematic review of its effectiveness for upper limb motor recovery, *Top Stroke Rehabil.*, 2007;14: 52–61.

Holden MK,Virtual environments for motor rehabilitation: Review, *Cyberpsychol. Behav.* 2005 Jun;8(3):187–211; discussion 212–9.

Housman SJ, Scott KM, Reinkensmeyer DJ, A randomized controlled trial of gravity-supported, computer-enhanced arm exercise for individuals with severe hemiparesis, *Neurorehabil. Neural. Repair*, 2009 Jun;23(5):505–14.

Ijzerman MJ, Netwerk in beweging door technologische innovaties in de neurorevalidatie, Oration 17 november 2005, University of Twente, the Netherlands, 2005. http://www.utwente.nl/nieuws/wetenschapsnieuws/oratieteksten/oratieIJzerman-171105.pdf

Kahn LE, Zygman ML, Rymer WZ, Reinkensmeyer DJ, Robot-assisted reaching exercise promotes arm movement recovery in chronic hemiparetic stroke: A randomized controlled pilot study, *J. Neuroeng. Rehabil.* 2006 Jun 21;3:12.

Kaelin-Lang A, Sawaki L, Cohen LG, Role of voluntary drive in encoding an elementary motor memory, *J. Neurophysiol.* 2005 Feb;93(2):1099–103.

Krakauer JW, Arm function after stroke: from physiology to recovery, *Semin. Neurol.* 2005;25(4):384–395.

Kreisel SH, Bazner H, Hennerici MG, Pathophysiology of stroke rehabilitation: Temporal aspects of neuro-functional recovery, *Cerebrovasc. Dis.* 2006;21(1-2):6–17.

Kwakkel G, Wagenaar RC, Twisk JW, Lankhorst GJ, Koetsier JC, Intensity of leg and arm training after primary middle- cerebral-artery stroke: A randomized trial, *Lancet*, 1999;354(9174):191–96.

Kwakkel G, Kollen BJ, Van der Grond J, Prevo AJ, Probability of regaining dexterity in the flaccid upper limb: Impact of severity of paresis and time since onset in acute stroke, *Stroke* 2003;34 :2181-2186.

Kwakkel G, Kollen B, Lindeman E, Understanding the pattern of functional recovery after stroke: Facts and theories, *Restor. Neurol. Neurosci.* 2004;22:281–299.

Kwakkel G, Impact of intensity of practice after stroke: Issues for consideration, *Disabil. Rehabil.* 2006 Jul 15–30;28(13-14):823–30.

Kwakkel G, Kollen BJ, Krebs HI, Effects of robot-assisted therapy on upper limb recovery after stroke: A systematic review, *Neurorehabil Neural Repair* 2008 Mar-2008 Apr;22(2):111–21.

Lawrence ES, Coshall C, Dundas R, Estimates of the prevalence of acute stroke impairments and disability in a multiethnic population. *Stroke* 2001;32: 1279–1284.

Molier BI, van Asseldonk EHF, Hermens HJ, Jannink MJA, Effect of different types of augmented feedback in stroke rehabilitation training: A systematic review, *Conference Technically Assisted Rehabilitation* 2009, Berlin, Germany, March 18–19 2009a.

Molier BI, de Boer J, Prange GB, Jannink MJA, Error-enhanced augmented proprioceptive feedback in stroke rehabilitation training: a pilot study, *International Conference on Rehabilitation Robotics*, Kyoto, Japan, 23–26 June 2009b.

Nelles G, Jentzen W, Jueptner M, Müller S, Diener HC, Arm training induced brain plasticity in stroke studied with serial positron emission tomography, *Neuro Image* 2001;13:1146–1154.

Prange GB, Jannink MJ, Groothuis-Oudshoorn CG, Hermens HJ, Ijzerman MJ, Systematic review of the effect of robot-aided therapy on recovery of the hemiparetic arm after stroke, *J. Rehabil. Res. Dev.* 2006 Mar-2006 Apr;43(2):171–84.

Prange GB, Stienen AHA, Jannink MJA, Van der Kooij H, IJzerman MJ, and Hermens HJ, Increased range of motion and decreased muscle activity during maximal reach with gravity compensation in stroke patients, In: Proceedings of *the 10th International Conference on Rehabilitation Robotics (ICORR);* June 13–15, 2007, Noordwijk aan Zee, the Netherlands: 467–471.

Prange GB, Jannink MJ, Stienen AH, van der Kooij H, Ijzerman MJ, Hermens HJ, Influence of gravity compensation on muscle activation patterns during different temporal phases of arm movements of stroke patients, *Neurorehabil. Neural Repair.* 2009a Jun;23(5):478–85.

Prange GB, Krabben T, Renzenbrink GJ, Ijzerman MJ, Hermens HJ, Jannink MJA, Changes in muscle activation after reach training with gravity compensation in chronic stroke patients, Submitted 2009b.

Rosamond W, Flegal K, Furie K, Heart disease and stroke statistics 2008 update, *Circulation* 2008;117:e25–e146.

Schaechter JD, Motor rehabilitation and brain plasticity after hemiparetic stroke, *Prog. Neurobiol.* 2004 May;73(1):61–72.

Schmidt RA, Wulf G, Continuous concurrent feedback degrades skill learning: Implications for training and simulation, *Hum. Factors* 1997 Dec;39(4):509–25.

Schmidt RA, Lee TD, Motor control and Learning, a behavioral emphasis, 4th edition, *Human Kinetics* USA, 2005.

Speach DP, Dombovy ML, Recovery from stroke: Rehabilitation, *Baillieres Clin. Neurol.* 1995;4(2):317–338.

Stienen AHA, Hekman EEG, Van der Helm FCT, Prange GB, Jannink MJA, Aalsma AMM, Van der Kooij H, Freebal: Dedicated gravity compensation for het upper extremities, Proceedings of *the 10th International Conference on Rehabilitation Robotics*, June 13-15, 2007, Noordwijk aan Zee, the Netherlands: 804–808.

van Vliet PM, Wulf G, Extrinsic feedback for motor learning after stroke: What is the evidence? *Disabil Rehabil.* 2006 Jul;28(13-14):831–40.

Volpe BT, Ferraro M, Krebs HI, Hogan N, Robotics in the rehabilitation treatment of patients with stroke, *Curr. Atheroscler Rep.*, 2002;4(4):270–76.

Whitall J, McCombe Waller S, Silver KHC, Macko RF, Repetitive bilateral arm training with rhythmic auditory cueing improves motor function in chronic hemiparetic stroke, *Stroke* 2000;31;2390–2395.

Winstein C, Schmidt R, Reduced frequency of knowledge of results enhances motor learning, *Journal of Experimental Psychology: Learning, Memory and Cognition* 1990;16(4):677–91.

Winstein CJ, Campbell Stewart J, Conditions of task practice for individuals with neurologic impairments, In: Selzer M, Clarke S, Cohen L, Duncan P, Gage F, eds. Textbook of neural repair and rehabilitation, *Medical Neurorehabilitation* Volume II; Cambridge, UK, Cambridge University Press; 2006: 89–102.

Wolf SL, Blanton S, Baer H, Breshears J, Butler AJ, Repetitive task practice: A critical review of constraint-induced movement therapy in stroke, *Neurol.* 2002;8:325–338.

Wulf G, Schmidt R, The learning of generalized motor programs: reducing the relative frequency of knowledge of results enhances memory, *Journal of Experimental Psychology: Learning, Memory and Cognition* 1989;15(4):748–57.

Wulf G, Schmidt RA, Deubel H, Reduced feedback frequency enhances generalized motor program learning but not parameterization learning, *Journal of Experimental Psychology: Learning, Memory and Cognition* 1993 Sep;19(5):1134–50.

Chapter Eleven

Isokinetic Exercise Machine Using High Performance MR Fluid Brake and Iso-Contraction Exercise

Kunihiko Oda*, Takehito Kikuchi†, Shiro Isozumi‡ and Junji Furusho‡

*Department of Physical Therapy, Osaka Electro-Communication University, 1130-70 Kiyotaki, Shijonawate, Osaka 575-0063, Japan
†Graduate School of Science and Engineering, Yamagata University, 4-3-16 Jonan, Yonezawa 992-8510, Japan
‡Graduate School of Engineering, Osaka University, 2-1 Yamadaoka, Suita, Osaka 565-0871, Japan

Isokinetic exercises used in rehabilitation to strengthen muscles often require expensive exercise equipments. The safe isokinetic exercise system we developed uses only brakes with a magnetorheological (MR) fluid. Rapid fluid response gives this equipment good response and control. In this chapter, we give basic isokinetic exercise concepts using an MR fluid brake, focusing on high-speed controls up to 900 deg/s at the elbow. We also suggest a new training mode we call iso-contraction exercise.

11.1 INTRODUCTION

Clinicians use several types of muscle contraction, for example, isometric, isotonic and isokinetic contraction, in quantitative evaluation of muscle strength. In the isometric contraction, the angle of joints is fixed. A subject efforts to generate one's muscle strength at one's best. In this type of muscle contraction, we can measure maximal torque of muscles, but cannot measure dynamic properties. On the other hand, in the isotonic contraction, muscle lifts a constant load and a muscle tension is assumed to be constant. In this method, we can measure dynamic properties of muscles, but cannot measure maximal torque. In order to measure both maximal torque and dynamic properties of muscles, isokinetic contraction was suggested. In this method, we can measure maximal torque at any angle of joint dynamically, because subjects are required generating maximal torque during whole range of

Biomechatronics in Medicine and Healthcare by Le Li and Raymond Kai-Yu Tong

www.panstanford.com
978-981-4241-61-8

motion under restriction of constant angular velocity controlled by an isokinetic training machine.

In the isokinetic contraction, the constant velocity is not the velocity of the linear muscle contraction but joint angular velocity. This causes by the reason that the joint angular movements are affected of the length of the lever arm of the muscle origin and insertion. Little attention has been paid to these differences.

These days, isokinetic machines, for example, Cybex (Bohannon, 1991), Biodex (Kelli, 1996), are widely used in the rehabilitation medicine and sports medicine. Those machines are used in many researches for the relationship between the muscle strength and the contraction velocity. This contraction is based on the researches of Hill (Hill, 1938). However, those machines cost expensive depending on its actuation device (actuator is usually servomotor with high torque).

In order to develop an isokinetic exercise machine with low-cost, high safety and high performance, we have developed isokinetic and iso-contraction exercise machine by using a magnetorheological (MR) fluid brake. The primary purpose of this study is to make the mechanical model of the human joint movement on the consideration of the length of the lever arm effect. The secondary purpose is to develop the isokinetic machine to enable to evaluate the muscle strength in the constant linear velocity of the muscle contraction.

In this report, we describe development of the isokinetic and iso-contraction exercise machine. We use MR fluid as a working material of the brake. Because of the rapid response of the MR fluid, this brake performs superior response compared with conventional brakes. In other words, a simple and safe training machine with accurate velocity control can be realized with this brake. High-speed control (up to 900 [deg/s] at elbow joints) could be performed with this machine. Additionally, we suggest an iso-contraction exercise by using this machine and discuss experimental results.

11.2 CONVENTIONAL ISOKINETIC EXERCISE & PROPOSED ISO-CONTRACTION EXERCISE

11.2.1 Conventional Isokinetic Exercise

Muscle strengthening exercises are used for such purposes as medical rehabilitation, improving physical strength and athletic performance. A widely practiced exercise is isometric, in which persons with arthritis, for example, contract their muscles without joint movement while pushing an immovable wall. Recent emphasis is being placed, however, on isokinetic exercise rotating the joints at a certain speed with special training equipments to produce uniform movement applying appropriate reaction against autonomous movements by trainees. Isokinetic exercise has both advantages and disadvantages (Miura, 1992).
Advantages include:

(A) Sufficient muscle strengthening throughout the whole range of motion.
(B) Load is automatically set as needed for each angular velocity.

(C) Less potential for muscle damage.

(D) Muscle strength and torque of joints are easily determined

Disadvantages include:

(E) Expensive equipment.

(F) Acceleration properties of the system and artifacts during deceleration decrease reliability in muscle strength measurements, in terms of uniform speed and measurement results, when the reference speed for the exercise are set at 200 deg/s or more.

(G) Equipment must be prepared for individual muscle groups.

We can find from the above that isokinetic exercise is more effective than isotonic exercise and is superior in evaluating exercise results. Muscle contraction modes ensure replicable evaluation by maintaining constant muscle length in isometric contraction and load in isotonic contraction.

In isokinetic contraction based on A.V. Hill's theory (Hill, 1938) on the relationship between contractile speed of muscle and its tension, muscle contraction speed is not consistently controlled in practice because speed decreases at the start and finish of movement and increases in the middle, rather than because of kinetic joint structure.

11.2.2 Hill's equation

A.V. Hill formulated the relationship between force of muscle and its contraction speed as follows: (Hill, 1938.)

$$V = \frac{b(P_0 - P)}{P + a} \tag{11.1}$$

where P denotes force, V contraction speed, and P_0 maximum force at a speed of zero. a and b are experimental constants and determined in order that the experimental data fits to the formula (11.1). As shown in Fig. 11.1, the P-curve shows that the force decreases with increasing speed (Winter, 1990).

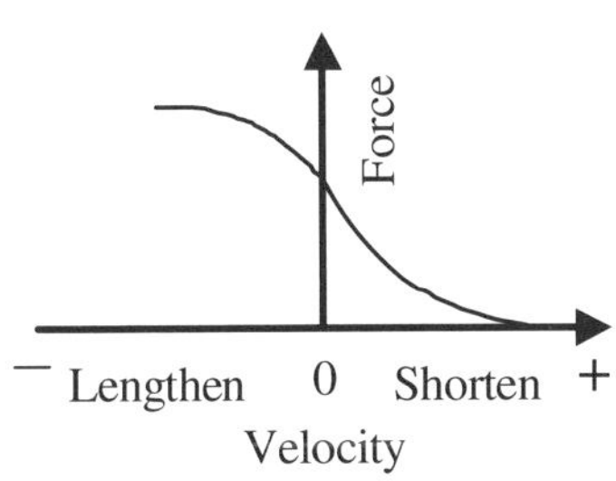

Figure 11.1 Hill's curve.

11.2.3 Proposal of Iso-contraction Exercise

Muscle contraction models proposed by A.V. Hill *et al.* present formulated linear muscle movement extracted from living examples. In conventional isokinetic training, joint rotation angles are constant and inner muscles are not contracted at a uniform speed. To evaluate the relationship between muscle speed and tension, we must model kinetic joint properties to adjust kinetic joint speed and maintain a constant muscle contraction speed.

Figure 11.2 models simple kinetic elbow flexion, called an elbow flexion model. The elbow is represented as two links of the forearm and upper arm, making a single axial rotation in most cases. We consider the biceps brachii and brachioradial muscles working in elbow flexion to be "working muscles" because they develop considerable power. These two muscles are symmetrically positioned anatomically around the elbow, so we use a single muscle model integrating the properties of both ("Biceps Brachii Muscle" in the figure). In the elbow flexion model, θ denotes angles [rad] and ω angular speed [rad/s] of the elbow. L denotes the length [m] of the biceps brachii muscle, R the length [m] from the elbow to the origin biceps brachii muscle, and r the length [m] of the lever arm. Based on this, L and ω are calculated as follows:

$$L = \sqrt{R^2 + r^2 + 2Rr\cos\theta} \tag{11.2}$$

$$\omega = \frac{-Rr\sin\theta}{\sqrt{R^2 + r^2 + 2Rr\cos\theta}}\frac{dL}{dt} \tag{11.3}$$

Expressing muscle-developed tension as P [N] and torque generated at the elbow as T [Nm] yields the following:

$$P = \frac{\sqrt{R^2 + r^2 + 2Rr\cos\theta}}{Rr\sin\theta}T \tag{11.4}$$

To evaluations muscle strength that better matches outcomes of conventional physiological research, we must maintain constant dL/dt rather than ω as in conventional isokinetic exercises, so we define constant dL/dt as an isokinetic muscle contraction exercise, or iso-contraction exercise.

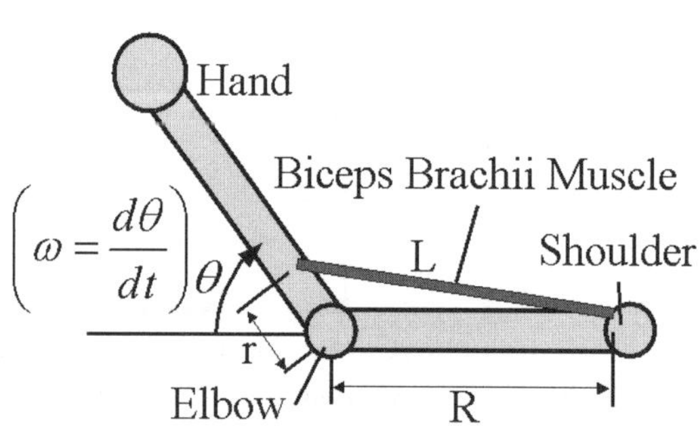

Figure 11.2 Simple model of the elbow flexion.

11.3 EXPERIMENTAL SETUP

11.3.1 MR Fluid Brake

Fluids whose properties vary with changes in external fields, called functional fluids, include electrorheological (ER) fluid) (Kikuchi, 2003), whose apparent viscosity changes in different electrical fields, and magnetorheological (MR) fluid (Carlson, 2000), whose viscosity changes in different magnetic fields. ER and MR fluid viscosity changes rapidly and reversibly, enabling application to clutches requiring rapid, highly accurate torque control (Furusho, 1999; Takesue, 2004).

The basic MR fluid brake structure, as shown in Fig. 11.3, involves MR fluid filled around a rotating disc. MR fluid viscosity varies with the magnetic field generated by the magnet coil, used as brake torque. Brake torque is rapidly reversibly controlled by supplying electricity to the magnet coil.

We use an MR fluid brake in which the rotational input of an MR clutch is fixed mechanically. Such an MR fluid brake with rapidly changing fluid viscosity should also respond rapidly as brake torque: its response time constant — the time until 63% of the constant is reached - is 3 to 5 milliseconds in both first and last transitions (Kikuchi, 2006).

Figure. 11.4 shows an experimental setup to determine the relationship between torque of the MR brake, in which MRF-132DG (Lord Inc., US) is used,

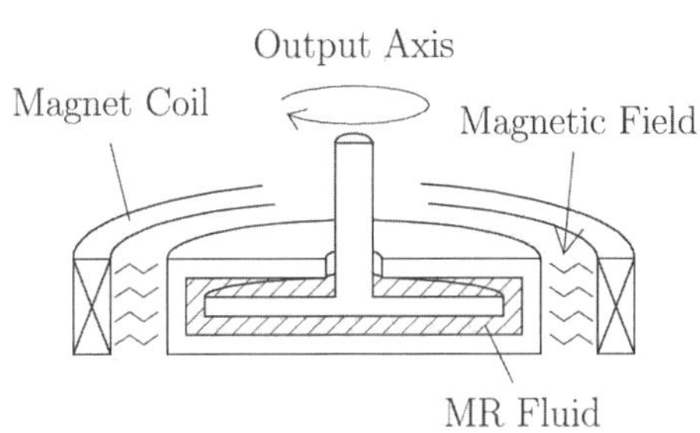

Figure 11.3 Basic structure of MR Fluid Break.

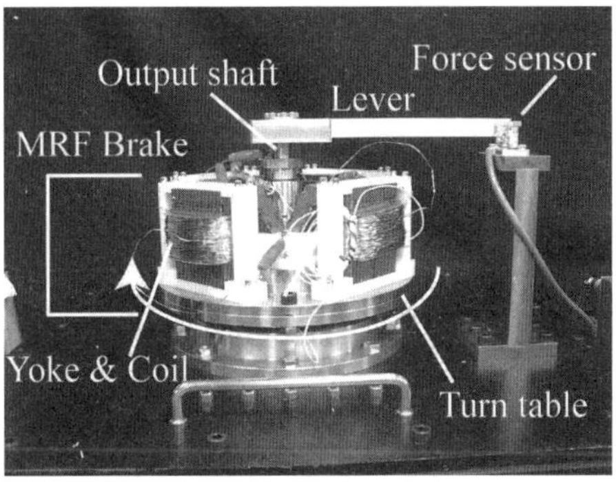

Figure 11.4 Experimental setup for MR Fluid Break.

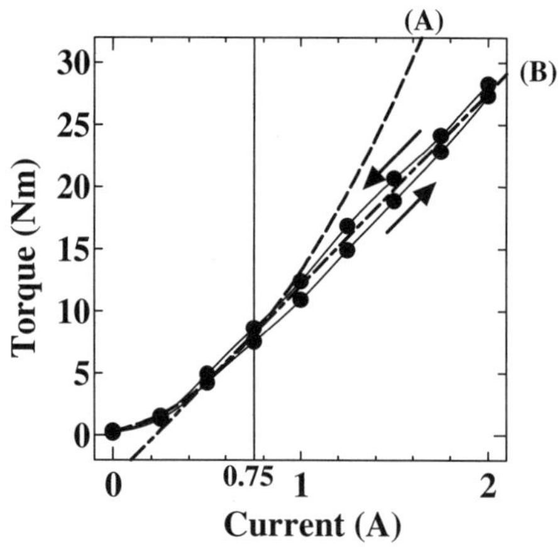

Figure 11.5 Torque vs.current of MR Fluid Break and its model.

and applied current. Torque is calculated from the load on the force sensor on the lever on the output shaft of the brake. The body of t brake is fixed to the turntable, which then rotates at a constant speed when output torque is measured from input current to the coil.

Figure. 11.5 shows the relationship between applied current and brake torque. Current is increased in steps of 0.25 A from 0.0 A to 2.0 A, then decreased the same way to 0.0 A. Turntable rotation is 1.0 rad/s. Black dots in Fig. 11.5 indicates measurement results. Although slight hysteresis exists in torque properties against input current, it is negligible and is ignored in this paper.

To unambiguously determine current corresponding to arbitrary brake torque, we must make an approximation model of torque properties, here using model curves (or straight lines) (A) and (B) in Fig. 11.5: Model (A) for current below 0.75 A and Model (B) for 0.75 A or more. Model (A) is given as follows:

$$T = 9.74I^2 + 3.25I + 0.26 \ (for\ I < 0.75) \tag{11.5}$$

where T denotes output torque [Nm] of the MR fluid brake and I coil current [A].

Model (B) is given as follows:

$$T = 15.5I - 3.44 \ (for\ I \geq 0.75) \tag{11.6}$$

Current corresponding to command torque is obtained using inverse functions of these model equations.

11.3.2 Muscle Strength Evaluation and Training using MR Fluid Brake

Figure 11.6 shows the system we developed and Fig. 11.7 a diagram of it (Kikuchi, 2009). The system is for isokinetic exercises for the upper arm. Users hold the grip with the left or right hand and exert maximum force to rotate it. With a belt-pulley reduction unit (reduction ratio: 1/3.63) between the handle and the brake rotation

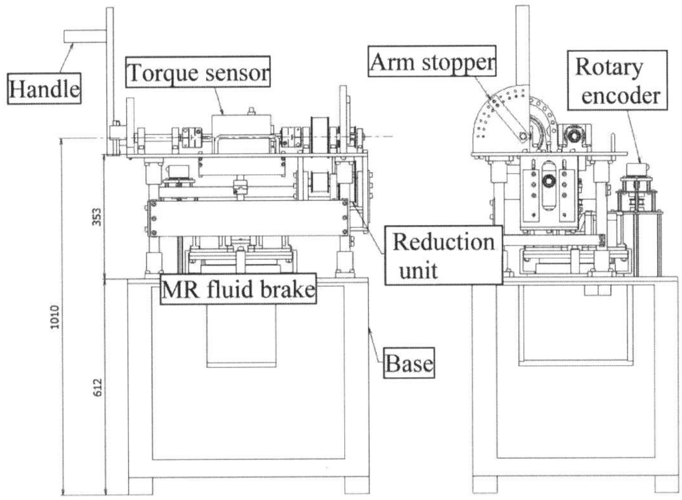

Figure 11.6 Isokinetic exercise machine with MR Fluid Break.

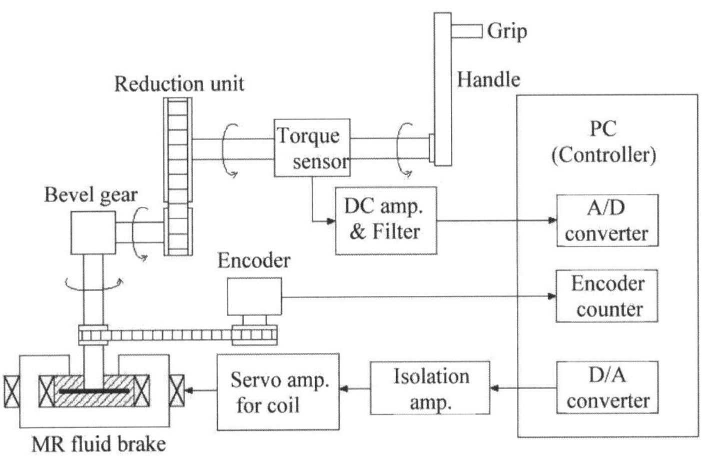

Figure 11.7 Systematic diagram of the equipment.

shaft, training controls up to 90 Nm given a maximum force of 27 Nm generated by the MR fluid brake, for which see Fig. 11.(5)

The MR fluid brake is activated by a servo-amplifier (SMCM10, Servoland Corp., Japan) based on commands from a PC via a digital/analog (DA) conversion board. Rotational angles of the brake output shaft are measured using an incremental rotary encoder that measures up to 20000 ppm resolutions (5000 ppr × 4) in one rotation, corresponding to resolutions of 0.005 deg at the handle via the reduction unit (reduction ratio: 1/3.63). The handle's operating torque is measured using a torque converter (TP-10KCB, Kyowa Dengyo, Japan) intercalated on the rotation shaft which is then input to the PC through the AD conversion board .

11.4 ISOKINETIC EXERCISE

11.4.1 Control Method

This system relies on the brake alone to control the angular velocity, ensuring high safety. The rotation velocity is controlled by commands given based on appropriate brake torque determined with the handle rotation torque operated by users. Such passive velocity control was used by Kikuchi*et al.* (Kikuchi, 2003) for an ER fluid brake.

This paper describes a proportional-integral (PI) velocity control, as shown in Fig. 11.8, and applied using the MR fluid brake. Symbols are defined in Table 11.1.

In control, operation torque given in training by the user is dealt with as disturbance. Only with the brake, the system cannot output torque in the same direction as that of rotation. Therefore, reference torque, either zero or negative, must be made zero when a positive value is commanded.

Control input ω_{ref} is arbitrarily set in a range from zero to the maximum speed the user develops. Control input remains constant from control start to end. Handle operation is started whenever the user likes. Brake control begins when handle rotation speed exceeds set value ω_{ref}. The integrator remain set at zero until handle rotation speed exceeds set value ω_{ref}.

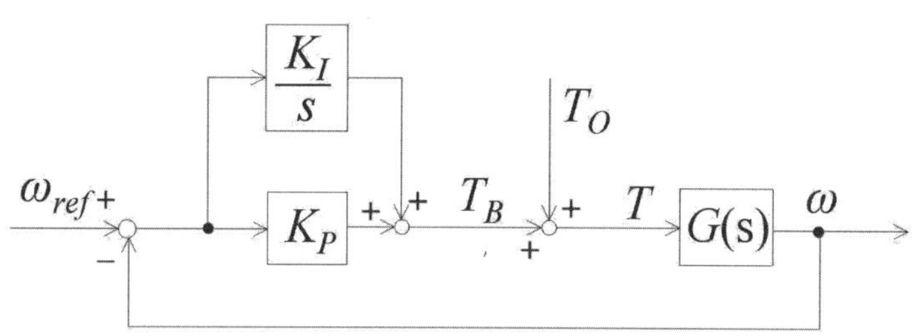

Figure 11.8 Block diagram for velocity control of MR Fluid Brake.

Table 11.1 Definitions of each parameter for velocity controller

ω_{ref}	:	Reference angular velocity [rad/s]
ω	:	Angular velocity [rad/s]
T_B	:	Reference torque [Nm]
T_O	:	Operation torque (disturbance) [Nm]
T	:	Torque [Nm]
K_P	:	Proportional gain [Nms/rad]
K_I	:	Integral gain [Nm/rad]

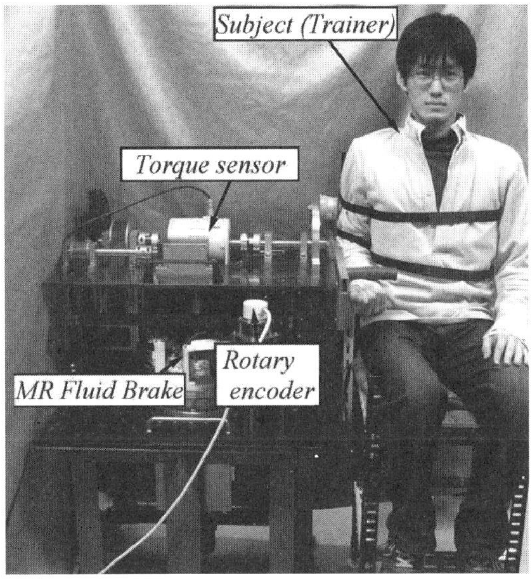

Figure 11.9 Muscle strengthening and evaluation machine.

Table 11.2 Definitions of each parameter for velocity controller.

K_P	:	0.5Nms/rad
K_I	:	100Nm/rad

11.4.2 Experimental Method

Figure 11.9 shows how experiments were conducted. In this paper, we will focus on the elbow flexion and fully extended elbow is defined as 0[deg]. The user, strapped in a chair, flexes an elbow at an initial angle of 45[deg] and a final angle of 140[deg]. The elbow can be flexed at any time when the user likes to maximize strength. Brake force is adjusted so that the system maintains a set speed.

Experiments were conducted by three subjects with different maximum developmental torque, as detailed for subjects A, B, and C in Table 2. Subjects all used their dominant hands in experiments.

11.4.3 Experimental Results

Reference velocity was increased in steps of 100deg/s from 0 to 900 deg/s. Figs. 10 and 11 show the experimental results for subjects A and B. Broken lines denote commanded values and solid lines measurement results indicating that stable, accurate control was achieved for references. When a brake is used for passive velocity control, drive torque is provided by the developmental torque of subjects. When the elbow is flexed in a range of angles between 45deg and 140deg, periods

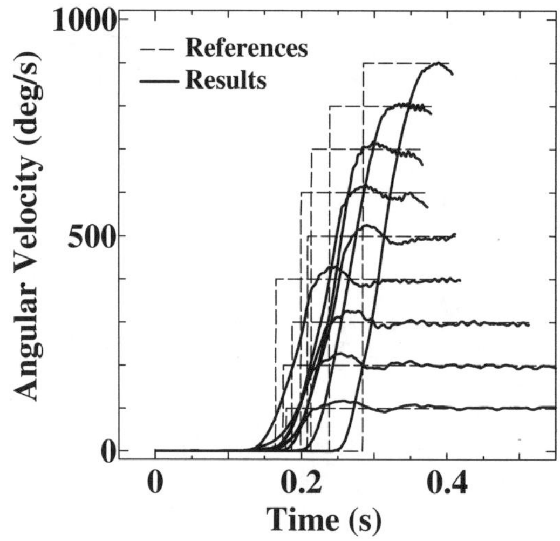

Figure 11.10 Experimental results for subject A.

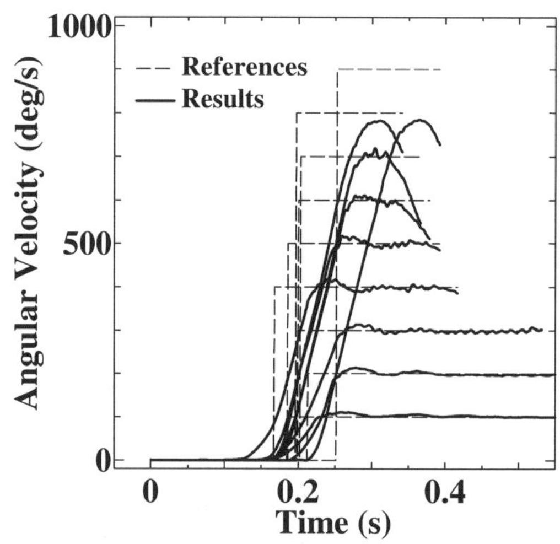

Figure 11.11 Experimental results for subject B.

of constant speed become shorter as speed increases: Subject A reached 900 deg/s. No conventional systems have, to our knowledge, recorded measurement results for such rapid movement areas, so low inertia properties appear to have produced such results. Although subject B failed to reach reference speed of 800 and 900deg/s, this brake-alone system helped complete experiments without forcing subjects to excess.

Figure 11.12 shows the relationship between exercise speed and operation torque in experiments. Operation torque was obtained by averaging the range of angles where normal and isokinetic control was achieved. Black circles indicate

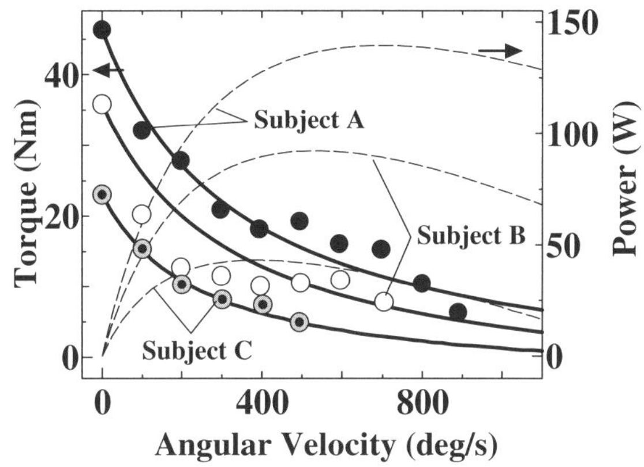

Figure 11.12 Experimental results for subject B.

results for subject A, white circles for subject B, and double circles for subject C. Solid lines indicate Hill's curves and broken lines power curves. In obtaining Hill's curves, parameters a and b in Eq.(1), where P denotes operation torque [Nm] and V exercise velocity [deg/s], were determined by applying the least squares method. In obtaining power curves, the product of P and V was converted to watts (W). The power curve peak represents the speed and power at which the subject exercises most efficiently: 139 W (700 deg/s) for subject A, 93 W (525 deg/s) for subject B, and 43 W (375 deg/s) for subject C. References (Fuchimoto, 1981) report 141 W as the maximum power developed in elbow flexion by 19-year-old men, so experimental results appear to be valid.

Isokinetic exercises thus enable muscles of subjects to be evaluated from different points, including maximum muscle power, maximum exercise efficiency, and speed in most efficient exercise.

11.5 ISO-CONTRACTION EXERCISE

11.5.1 Control Method

As discussed in Section 4.1, unlike in isokinetic exercises, input command speed ω_{ref} is not constant but changes with the angle, and dL/dt in Eq. (11.3) becomes constant. Fig. 11.13 shows examples of reference angular velocity curves (control input): angles in Eq. (11.2) are plotted on the horizontal axis, and angular velocity on the vertical axis. To draw up these reference curves, we must determine R and r in Eq.(11.3). In fact, however, it is difficult to determine actual *in vivo* R and r. These values are determined in relation to subject height H [m].

Based on references, we set the average bicep length at 0.18 times subject height (Kouchi, 2000). The origin biceps brachii muscle, attached to the shoulder blade and a bit shorter than the biceps, is determined as follows:

$$R = 0.18 \times 0.95 \times H \tag{11.7}$$

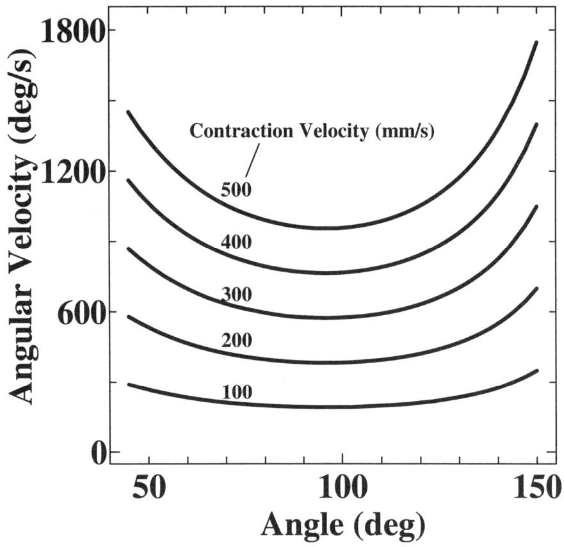

Figure 11.13 Examples of reference angular velocity curve for iso-contractile mode (H = 177 m).

Table 11.3 Information of subjects

Subject	Maximum torque	Dominant hand	Height
A	45N m	Left	177 m
B	35N m	Right	163 m
C	23N m	Right	172 m

Assuming r as 10% of R,

$$r = 0.1 \times H \tag{11.8}$$

11.5.2 Experimental Method

Experiments and subjects are the same as in Section 4.2. Control input for subjects was calculated from heights in Table 11.3 and Eqs. (11.3), (11.7), and (11.8).

11.5.3 Experimental Results

Our proposal on isokinetic contraction exercises was tried on training equipment with the MR fluid brake. Results for subject A are shown in Fig. 11.14, with time on the horizontal axis and muscle contraction velocity on the vertical axis, and in Fig. 11.15, with angles on the horizontal axis and contraction velocity on the vertical axis. Reference velocity is given from 0mm/s to the maximum speed

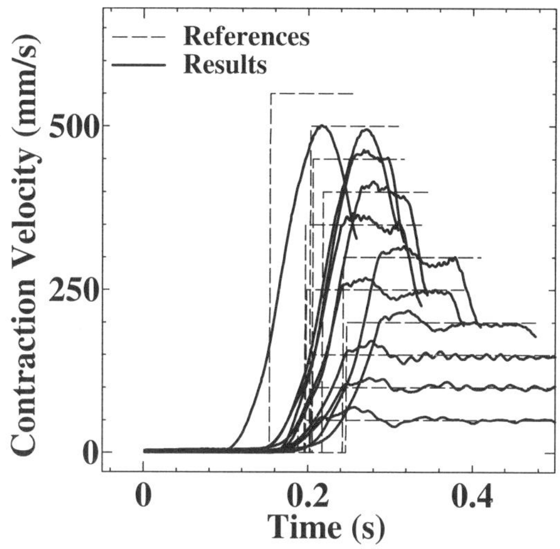

Figure 11.14 Experimental results of iso-contraction exercise (time vs. contraction velocity for subject A).

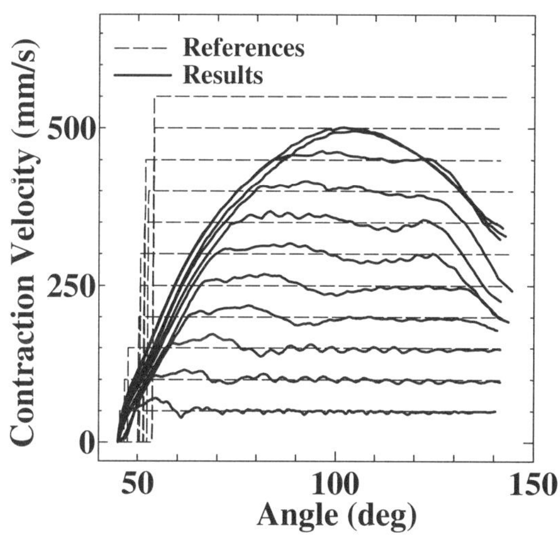

Figure 11.15 Experimental results of iso-contraction exercise (angle vs. contraction velocity for subject A.

subjects attained, in increments of 50 mm/s. The maximum velocity attained by subject A was 500 mm/s.

Subjects B and C underwent similar experiments to determine average muscle contraction in isokinetic contraction time. Muscle contraction is calculated from Eq.(11.4), using torque measured with the torque sensor in the system. Fig. 11.16 shows the relationship between average tension in muscle contraction and contraction velocity. Symbols are the same as in Fig. 11.12.

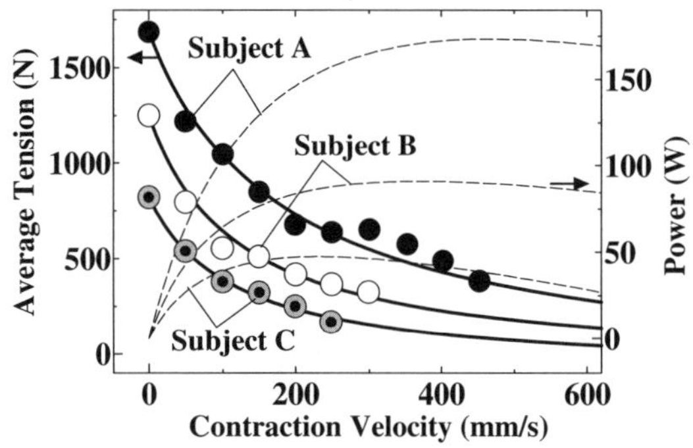

Figure 11.16 Hill's curve in iso-contraction exercise

Results show that the power curve of subject A peaks at 173 W (450 deg/s), of subject B at 93 W (350 deg/s), and of subject C at 47 W (230 deg/s).

11.6 CONCLUSIONS

The isokinetic exercise machine that we developed by using rapid response of the MR fluid brake was effective in solving problems in which the isokinetic contraction area narrows as contraction speed increases. We also attempted to the iso-contraction exercises, taking advantage of the rapid response. As a result, the system has come closer to the theoretical basis of isokinetic contraction, and isokinetic contraction area is made wider for rapid exercises than in conventional isokinetic contraction. This enables us to elaborate power-speed properties of human more accurately.

References

Bohannon R. W., Correlation of knee extension force and torque with gait speed in patients with stroke, *Physiotherapy Theory and Practice*, **7**(3): 185–190,(1991).

Carlson J. D., and Jolly M. R., MR fluid, foam and elastomer devices, *Mechatronics*, **10**: 555–569,(2000).

Fuchimoto T. and Kaneko M., Force, velocity and power relationships in different age groups, *Research of Physical Education*, **25**(4): 273–279, (in Japanese), (1981).

Furusho J. and Sakaguchi M., New actuators using er fluid and their applications to force display devices in virtual reality and medical treatments, *Int. Journal of Modern Physics B.*, **13–14/16**: 2151–2159,(1999).

Hill A. V., The heat of shortening and the dynamic constants of muscle, *Proc. Roy. Soc. B.* **126**: 136–195,(1938).

Miura A. and Ooi Y., Muscle strengthen-Isokinetic Exercise, *Sogo-rehabilitation* **20**(9): 940–944 (in Japanese),(1992).

Kelli E. and Baltzopoulos V., Agonist and antagonist moment and EMB-angle relationship during isokinetic eccentric and concentric exercise, *Isokinetics and Exercise Science*, **6**(2): pp.79–87,(1996).

Kikuchi T, Furusho J. and Oda K., Development of Isokinetic Exercise Machine Using ER Brake, *Proceedings of the 2003 IEEE International Conference on Robotics & Automation (ICRA 2003)*, 214–219,(2003).

Kikuchi T, Furusho J, Yamaguchi Y and Kimura S., Design of the high-performance MR brake and its characteristics, *Proceedings of the 10th International Conference on ER Fluids and MR Suspensions*, bf 132,(2006).

Kikuchi T, Oda K, Ohyama Y, Isozumi S. and Furusho J., Development of Isokinetic Exercise System Using High Performance MR Fluid Brake, *Proceedings of the 5th IEEE International Conference on Mechatronics*, We3A.1,(2009).

Kouchi M, Mochimaru M, Iwasawa H. and Mitani S., Japanese Body Dimension Data, 1997–98, Japanese Industrial Standards Center, National Institute of Advanced Industrial Science and Technology, (2000).

Takesue N, Furusho J. and Kiyota Y., Fast Response MR-Fluid Actuator," :*JSME International Journal, Series C*, **47**(3): 783–791,(2004).

Winter D. A., *Biomechanics and Motor Control of Human Movement, Second Edition*, John Wiley & Sons, 177–179,(1990).

Chapter Twelve

Robotic-Assisted Technology for Medical Training Purposes

Jorge Solis[*,†] and Atsuo Takanishi[*,†]

[*] *Faculty of Science and Engineering, Waseda University, Tokyo, Japan*
[†] *Humanoid Robotics Institute, Waseda University, Tokyo, Japan*

In recent years, thanks to the introduction of Robotic Technology (RT) in the medical field, advanced surgical tools have been developed to support surgeons in order to enhance their skills to assure the consistency and reliability while performing surgical tasks. More recently, several researchers have been developing medical training systems designed to transfer motor skills to unskilled subjects. As a result of this research field, robotic-assisted training devices (referred as *Active Training*) are capable of providing objective assessment and multimodal feedback while the conventional training devices (referred as *Passive Training*) are limited in providing subjective assessment and unimodal feedback.

12.1 MOTOR CONTROL AND LEARNING

Humans are capable of performing an impressive variety of movements that range from simple movements, such as looking at an object of interest by turning the head and eyes, to complex and intricate series of movements, such as executing a triple axel on ice. These movements are improved over an extensive period of practice. This iterative process, known as motor learning involves executing movements, identifying errors, and correcting those errors in subsequent movements. Motor learning affects many different components of sensory and motor processing. Motor control involves both simple movement trajectories and complex series of movements in which multiple muscles and joints need to be controlled in a precise manner.

To behaviorists such as Skinner (1938), motor control is an environmental stimulus followed by a resulting response. Several models of classical information processing have been proposed to describe how this process occurs. Psychologists have broken down stimulus-response into three stages (Wickens, 1984). Perceptual

Biomechatronics in Medicine and Healthcare by Le Li and Raymond Kai-Yu Tong

www.panstanford.com
978-981-4241-61-8

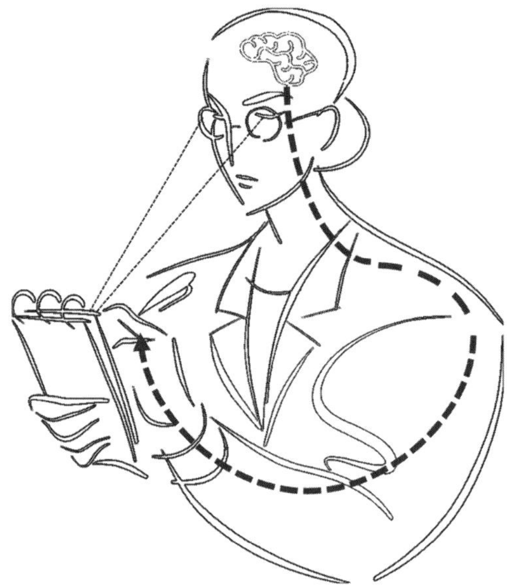

Figure 12.1 The existence in brain of "internal models" can mimic the input/output characteristics, or their inverses, of the motor apparatus (Kawato, Wolpert, 1998).

encoding is the meaning of the sensation, from the neural transmission coming from sensory receptors to our brain, this is also analyzed. This requires the application of information from long-term memory to organize, classify and interpret our sensations. In other words, perception changes sensation data into perceived information or meaning. The Central Processing tasks are to make the decision on the kind of movement to respond. It could use past experiences, also by using the long-term memory, in order to formulate a course or action. Responding is an action plan, step-by-step sequence of events that make up the planned movement.

On the other hand, the motor theory of perception illustrated by Berthoz (1997), presented the concept that perception is not a passive mechanism for receiving and interpreting sensory data, but that is the active process of anticipating the sensory consequences of an action, and thereby binding the sensory and motor patterns in a coherent framework. In computational terms, it implies the existence in the brain of some kind of "internal models" as a bridge between action and perception (Figure 12.1). The recent control learning models are based on the idea that instructions generated by the brain for controlling a movement are utilized by the brain to interpret the sensory consequences of the movement (Kawato, 1992).

From the above introduction of the literature on motor control, a high complexity of understanding processes has been briefly outlined (Solis, 2004). Motor skills are extremely complex, involving sensory and motor operations in a highly interactive way. Even the "simplest" motor action, like clicking a button, requires an enormous number of cerebral connections. Furthermore, the motor learning

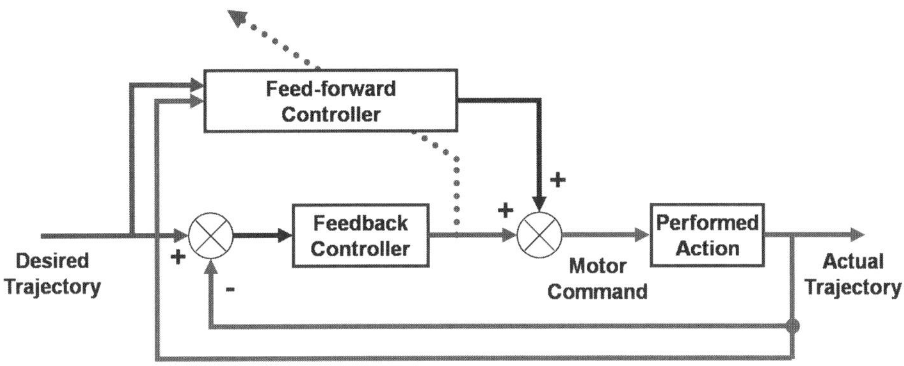

Figure 12.2 Feed back-error learning model (Kawato and Wolpert, 1998).

process, which is supposed to be activated by the formation of some kind of internal maps, cannot be observed directly, but can only be inferred from the observation of subject's performance. Such internal models seem to be created and reinforced through the repetitive execution of the task for understanding the relationships between the action outcome and the motor control parameters required (Figure 12.2). In fact, such relationships cannot be necessarily found in the same way for all humans, which mean that each person learns in a different manner and different learning experiences to draw from.

Even if the study of motor learning which analyzes behavioral, neurophysiological, and imaging data has demonstrated interesting results, the unobservability of the brain's internal processes makes it difficult to assess the validity of the theories. Therefore, the existence of a widely accepted theory describing all the learning processes is still unproven. Notwithstanding this, several approaches can be formulated in order to strengthen theories related to specific aspects of motor learning. Hence, it becomes necessary to find additional tools that may help us to understand these specific aspects of the learning process under repetitive controlled circumstances.

From this purpose, RT can be seen as powerful tools not only for understanding how the skill transfer occurs but also to enhance learners' performances. Such systems offer the possibility of controlling accurately the conditions of the learning process (Solis, 2004; Solis *et al.*, 2007) and moreover, meanwhile subjects are practicing the skill to be learned, their performances can be measured and analyzed by means of different performance indexes (Solis *et al.*, 2007; Solis *et al.* 2008).

It is worth to mention that in order to conduct effective learning experiments; the robotic system must actively interact with humans at the same logical/perceptual level through all the stages of the learning process. This means that robots should analyze the exchanged information between human and robot to evaluate learner's performance and furthermore, to provide some kind of feedback which may promote the creation of the internal models by the active training of learner on the task so that subjects can reconstruct accurately the motor skill. On the other hand, there is the possibility of studying which parameters (i.e. which feedback modality is provided, complexity of the skill) of the learning process may lead or break down the acquisition of the motor skill by modifying the conditions of the experiments.

12.2 RECENT ADVANCES IN MEDICAL TRAINING

It appears that current medical education approaches fall short of embracing the idea that every learner is unique. As an adjunct to the traditional apprenticeship training model, use of computer technology and educational innovations, such as simulation and bench model training are all factors influencing how future clinicians will practice the technical aspects of medical procedures (Ryan, 2008). In particular, the advances in Information Technology (IT) have revolutionized methods of educational delivery. In this era of knowledge-building, educational media and web-based learning are proving to be true enabling technologies transforming the possibilities of self-study and distance education (George, 2007). .

On the other hand, the emerging field of medical robotics aims to introduce intelligent tools as a support during the learning process. The principal challenges for developing efficient medical robotic training systems are simulating real-world conditions of the task and assuring training effectiveness (high anatomic fidelity has been achieved in conventional training systems, but they are limited to provide merely subjective assessments of the training progress). Thanks to the introduction of RT, surgeons are able to perform with higher accuracy minimally invasive surgery that could not be conceived by means of conventional techniques. More recently, several researchers have been particularly focused on developing novel medical training tools (Rosen, Hannaford, *et al.*, 2006; Mayrose *et al.*, 2003; Sewell, Salisbury, *et al.*, 2008; Noh, Solis *et al.*, 2008; etc.) as well as advanced measurement devices for the assessment of medical competence (Delson *et al.*, 2003; Chang, Pellegrini *et al.*, 2007; Solis *et al.*, 2009; Aggarwal, Darzi, *et al.*, 2009; etc.)

From the current state-of-art on robotic-assisted technology for medical training purposes, we may observe the importance on the introduction of more advanced methods of assessment of clinical competence as an approach to provide more objective information about the skill improvement and the reproduction of the real-world task conditions as an approach to provide multimodal feedback to trainees. In the next sections, an overview of the current research approaches for the assessment of clinical competence and the reproduction of task conditions will be given. In particular, two cases of studies will be detailed: an objective evaluation method for the ligature training and an actuated human model for the airway management training.

12.3 ASSESSMENT OF CLINICAL COMPETENCE AS AN APPROACH TO PROVIDE QUANTITATIVE INFORMATION

Even though it is widely accepted that introducing advanced tools for medical education purposes is important; up to now, there is no definite accepted scientific methodology for the assessment of surgical skills (Moorthy, Darzi, *et al.*, 2003; Rosen, Hannaford, *et al.*, 2006; Solis *et al*, 2008; etc.). In recent decades, researchers from the medical field have been proposing different ways of measuring the clinical competence of trainees. In particular, clinical examinations have been proposed to perform practical exams to trainees while their performances are evaluated. However, examiners lack of information which cannot be obtained through the simple observation of the task (surgical performance is a complex operation involving a surgeon-specific mix of cognitive and technical components).

The methodology for assessing surgical skill as a subset of surgical ability, is gradually shifting from subjective scoring by an expert which may be a variably biased opinion using vague criteria, toward a more objective, quantitative analysis (Gallagher *et al.*, 2002). RT platforms to teach and evaluate the cognitive aspects of surgery have been developed and shown to be of value to surgical education; tools to assess the technical aspects of surgery that potentially lead to effective teaching are currently under development. Such tools can be resumed as: instrumented tools (Rosen *et al.*, 2006), motion-efficiency analysis from motion tracking devices (Datta, 2002; Moorthy, Darzi, *et al.*, 2003), physical simulators (Pugh and Youngblood, 2002; Solis *et al.*, 2008) etc.

12.3.1 *Case of Study: Suture Training System*

In recent decades, researchers from the medical field have proposed different ways of measuring the clinical competence of trainees. In particular, the Objective Structured Clinical Examination (OSCE) has been proposed as a way of measuring clinical competence that allowed control of many of the biases of conventional methods (Harden, 1975). However, OSCE may not be as valid in the assessment of some technical skills. This is because the binary checklist typically used in most of the OSCEs is insufficiently sensitive detecting some behavioral patterns while performing the task. Due to the limitations of conventional training devices, examinees may evaluate trainees' performance through the simple observation of the task. As a result, up to now, there is no widely accepted quantitative assessment scheme.

For this purpose, at Waseda University, we have developed a suture training system designed to provide quantitative information of the trainees' performance (Solis *et al.*, 2008). The proposed system is integrated by a personal computer, a web cam, a dummy skin model with embedded sensors (Figure 12.3). Arrays of embedded sensors are used to measure the motion the artificial skin (by sensing

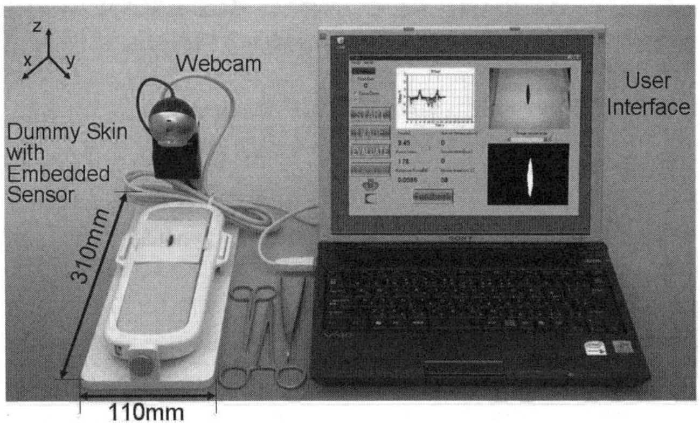

Figure 12.3 The proposed suture/ligature training system is composed by a personal computer, a dummy skin with embedded sensors and a webcam (Solis *et al.*, 2008). For color reference, see page 220.

the applied forces while performing the task). In addition, the web camera is used to capture a digital image of the suture just after the task is completed.

The reason why we have considered two different measurements methods is based on the principle that in order to provide objective assessments, we may require considering the following evaluation parameter categories which are integrated within an evaluation function (Solis, 2004):

- *Task Efficiency*: it refers to such parameters that measures the time trainees spend to complete the task.
- *Task Safety*: it refers to such task parameters that measures the applied forces exerted by trainees while doing the task.
- *Task Quality*: it refers to such parameters that measure how well trainees performed the task after concluding it.

In order to evaluate the suture/ligature task, we have proposed the following evaluation indexes which are mostly considered from OSCE examination's checklist. The below proposed evaluation indexes have been measured based on two sensing methods: dummy skin motion tracking and suture image processing.

- Time (I_T) : Conventionally, the time is measured from the starting up to the completion of the task.
- Force in Tissue (I_{FoT}) : If during the insertion of the needled, the trainee applies shear forces, the skin will be damaged.
- Judging Tension (I_{JuT}) : This evaluation parameter is related to the ligature phase. If ligature is done too tightly, it may be painful for the patient and may also provoke an infection.
- Equidistance (I_{EqD}) : The suture width is measured between the needle insertion point and the wound edge.

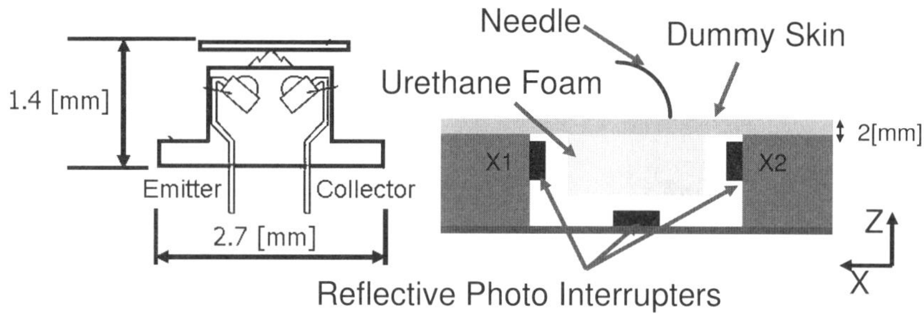

Figure 12.4 Detail of the proposed sensor mechanism to measure the movement of the skin dummy. An array of photo interrupters is placed in order to detect the deformation of the urethane foam.

- Distance between Sutures (I_{DbS}) : The suture distance is measured from one suture to another applied along the wounded area.
- Wound Dehiscence (I_{WoD}) : This parameter measures the open area of the wound just after the conclusion of the task.

The dummy skin motion tracking has been implemented by attaching urethane foam (10 mm of thickness) under a skin dummy made of polyurethane (Figure 12.4). The dummy skin movement can be determined by measuring the deformation of the urethane foam. For this purpose, arrays of photo interrupters are place around the foam. Each of the photo interrupters combines a gallium arsenideinfrared emitting diode (GaAs-IRED) with a high-sensitivity phototransistor. The principle is as follows. The light emitted from the GaAs-IRED is then reflected by the surface of the foam. The reflected light is then collected by phototransistor. When the distance between photo interrupter and urethane foam becomes closer, the volume of the reflected light becomes larger. Thus, the electric current that flows inside the phototransistor will increase in proportion to volume of the reflected light. As a result, we can sense the movement of skin dummy by embedding one photo interrupter under the skin dummy and four photo interrupters perpendicularly on the sideways.

On the other hand, we have implemented a suture image processing in order to measure the quality of the suture after the task is completed. For this purpose, a picture of the suture is taken and processed by using the APIs provided by the Open Source Computer Vision Library (OpenCV). As a first approach, we have considered the following physical parameters (Figure 12.5): *Equidistance*, *Distance between sutures*and *Wound Dehiscence*. In order to measure the distance between sutures, we perform the following steps: at first, we grabbed the image from the webcam and converted into HSV color space. This facilitates the search of suture thread (blue color) within the image frame just by scanning the thread blue color (threshold level) along the horizontal direction. When a blue color is detected on the HSV color space, the pixel is marked as part of the suture. In order to determine the suture dimensions and center of mass, the edge detection algorithm is performed to find the bounding box of the recognized object. By obtaining

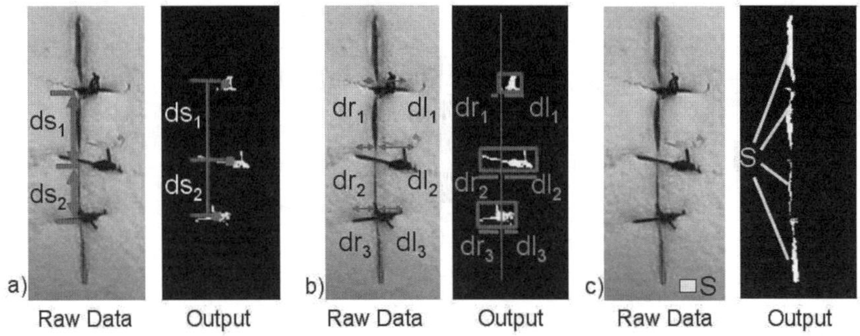

Figure 12.5 The physical parameters of the suture are automatically determined by using the proposed suture image processing: a) suture width, b) distance between sutures and c) open wound area.

the center of mass of each of the sutures performed, the *Equidistance* and *Distance between Sutures* are calculated. Finally, while computing the *Wound Dehiscence* after the conclusion of the task, we performed the same principle. In this case, we have marked the edges of the skin dummy with red color to be used as landmarks. By scanning the grabbed image from the webcam, we look for the red color. Therefore, the wound area can be easily computed.

By considering the parameters described above, the evaluation function can be defined as Eq. 12.1. As we may observe, it is required to determine the weighing coefficients of each of the proposed evaluation indexes. For this purpose, a discriminant analysis method has been applied to an experimental data from fifteen subjects (five surgeons, five medical students and five unskilled persons). Each subject performed the suture three times. The performance indexes were normalized by considering as reference point the average from surgeons and from unskilled persons. As a result, the following values were considered for the weight coefficients: ω_{Time}=0.843, ω_{FoT}=0.257, ω_{JuT}=1.367, ω_{EqD}=0.330, ω_{DbS}=1.072 and ω_{WoD}=0.746.

$$\begin{aligned} E_{Suture} &= \omega_T I_T + \omega_{FoT} I_{FoT} + \omega_{JuT} I_{JuT} \\ &+ \omega_{EqD} I_{EqD} + \omega_{DbS} I_{DbS} + I_{WoD}\omega_{WoD} \end{aligned} \tag{12.1}$$

By using (12.1), an experiment was proposed to verify and determine the differences among different kinds of *Teaching Methods* while using the proposed training system. In particular, three methods have been proposed: *No feedback, Medical Doctor's Feedback* and *Suture Training System's Feedback.* In particular, the last method was based on providing to trainees the information about their performance by showing the result of Eq. I.1 as well as presenting a pre-recorded movie. The pre-recorded movie contains specific advices from a medical doctor to unskilled persons. In fact, most of the beginners perform the task with common mistakes which can be easily determined from the collected data from the proposed training System.

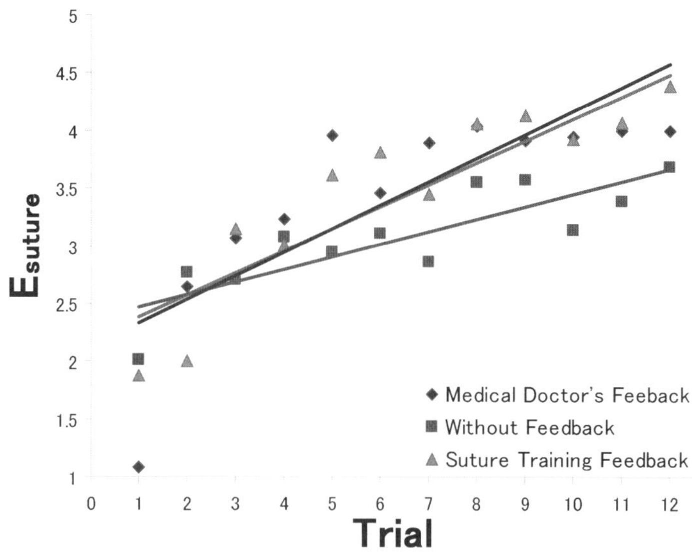

Figure 12.6 Experimental results while plotting the learning curve from E_{suture}.

For this experiment, we have asked eighteen unskilled subjects to perform the task (six for each group). All the subjects didn't have any previous experience in performing the task. In Fig. 12.6, we have plotted the learning curve by using the proposed evaluation function. In particular, the linear regression was performed to the collected data to observe their tendency. The coefficient of correlation for the groups with *No Feedback* and with *Suture Training System's feedback* was near to 1 (0.71 and 0.80 respectively). However, the correlation coefficient obtained in the case of the *Medical Doctor's Feedback* was lower (0.6266). In fact; as we may observe, the tendency of the performance between groups with *Suture Training System's Feedback* and *Medical Doctor's Feedback* is nearly similar. This may suggest a difference on the skills among the groups.

12.4 REPRODUCTION OF TASK CONDITIONS AS AN APPROACH TO PROVIDE MULTIMODAL FEEDBACK

The evolution of advanced computerized techniques technology, computer assisted surgery is revolutionizing the way doctors plan, perform, and follow-up of invasive surgical procedures. In contrast, the introduction of RT has been enabling doctors to perform with higher accuracy minimally invasive surgery that could not be conceived by means of conventional techniques. Up to know researchers and engineers have been particularly focused on developing novel surgical tools and training models. There is in fact, a significant amount of medical and surgical training is currently performed using actual patients, which can be costly to both patients and hospitals. For that purpose, engineers have been introducing novel approaches of training for medical students that potentially may reduce possible risks on patients and need for unnecessary follow-up treatments.

During last decades, computer based simulations have been introduced into medical training in the form of interactive software learning tools and anatomic instructional programs. Moreover, Virtual Reality (VR) techniques enhanced the complexity and realism of training simulators to new levels (Riva, 2003). VR is an advanced human-computer interface that goes far beyond existing interfaces. Such interfaces imply a three-dimensional computer-generated world that mimics the real world and allows trainees to interact with and navigate it, using components of their five senses in real time (immersion). However, these advanced simulators have been scarcely applied to training programs (Burt, 1995). In contrast, Augmented Reality (AR) is a relative new technology applied to medical applications. The idea of AR is placing virtual objects into the normal field of view. The main strength of AR compared to VR is the perception of the real scene (Sielhorst *et al.*, 2004). AR systems only overlay those pieces of information that are necessary. This eliminates the need for the trainee to immerse in a totally virtual environment and supports the intuitive integration of the information (Bajura *et al.*, 2002).

More recently, thanks to the introduction of Haptic Interfaces (HI), novel ways of medical and surgical training have been proposed. The research on HI is based on the study of the psychomotor touching experience and is an essential component if a meaningful surgical exercise is to be created. Haptic feedback is becoming an integral component of numerous training systems, particularly those designed for teaching motor skills (Solis, 2007; Sewell, Salisbury, 2008). Even the promising results of HI-based training systems, further analysis should be performed due to the complexity of understanding the processes involved during the learning process.

12.4.1 Case of Study: Airway Training System

Even though different kinds of active training systems have been proposed, most of them are designed to attach sensors to the medical instrument, which may affect the performance of trainees due to collisions between the tool and the patient model; as well as limit the surgical tool freedom of motion (Mayrose, 2003; Delson, 2003; Rose, Hannaford, 2006). Furthermore; trainees may have difficulties while performing the same task with real surgical tools because they are trained with a modified tool (different weight, dimensions, tool attachments, etc.).

For this purpose, at Waseda University, we proposed an airway management training system which embeds actuators in a patient model (mannequin) in order to reproduce the task conditions (Noh, Solis, *et al.*, 2009). The proposed airway training system has been designed to reproduce airway difficulties by embedding actuators into a conventional mannequin. In particular, the airway training system is composed of 12-DOFs that control the motion of sixteen wire driving mechanisms required to reproduce different kinds of airway difficulties.

The design concept of the proposed system aims to fulfill three requirements:

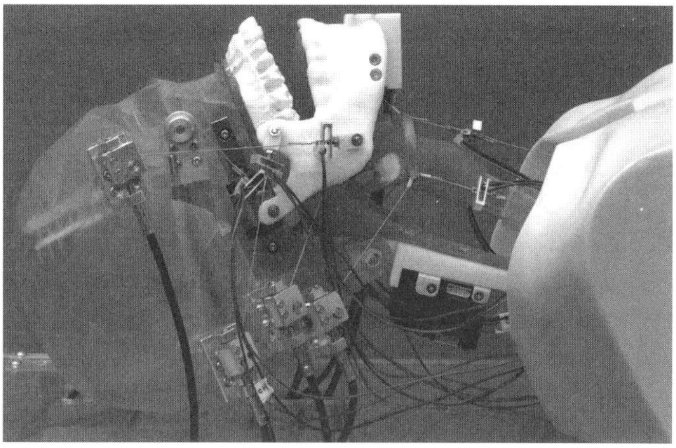

Figure 12.7 Detail of the mechanism of the Airway Training System: A wire driving mechanism has been designed to reproduce different kinds of airway difficulties (Noh, Solis, *et al.*, 2009). For color reference, see page 220.

at first, the proposed systems should reproduce the physiology and anatomy of the organs involved during the airway management. The second principle is that the proposed airway training system should be capable of reproducing various cases of difficult airway. Finally, an accurate positioning control should be implemented to simulate as much as possible the task conditions.

As a result of our research, the proposed system is composed of twelve active and one passive degree of freedom (Figure 12.7). Such actuation system has been designed to control the position of sixteen wire driving mechanism that reproduces the airway difficulties (i.e. mandible dental protusion, restricted opening mouth, etc.). In particular, the wire driving mechanisms was designed to control the motion of the following muscles: pterygoideus lateralis, masseter, genioglossus, anterior belly of digastrics, temporalis, styloglossus, and posterior belly of digastric muscle. In order to reproduce the various cases of difficult airway, we have designed the artificial organs by considering the range of motion of human organs. In particular, we reproduced the motion range of the head, neck, mandible, and hyoid bone as similar as possible to the human. For this purpose, we have collected information from the medical literature as well as from MRI's images.

The actuation system is based on a wire drive system to fit into the size of the human model. The wire drive system consists of the sixteen Teflon coated wires (low friction coefficient), pulleys and RC servo motors. Basically, the actuation system controls the motion of the mandible, tongue and oral cavity (Figure 12.8a). The details of such mechanisms are detailed as follows (Figure 12.8b). During the opening motion of the mouth, with respect with kinetic axis, human have 3-DOFs. In order to simplify the design, we have implemented 2-DOFs which represent the rotational motion (θ) and translational one (L). In order to control the motion of the mandible, we have attached six wires to the mandible. In addition, three common

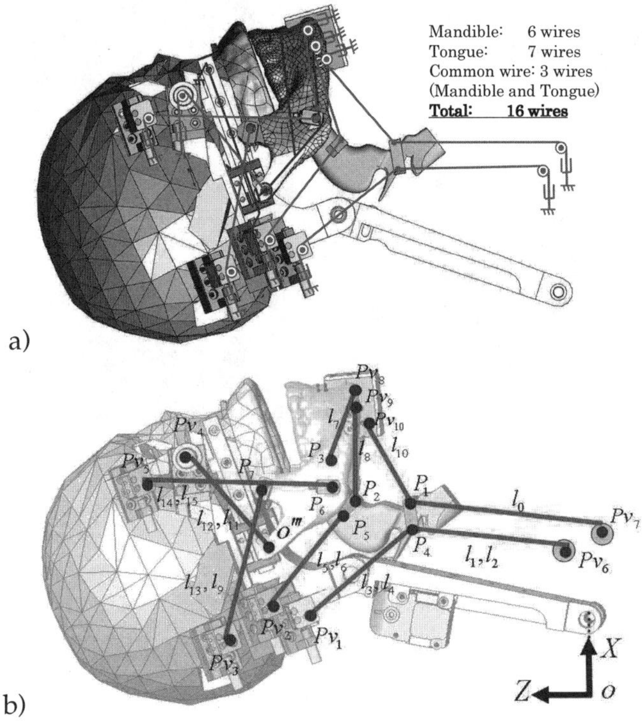

Figure 12.8 Detail of the proposed Airway Management Training System: (a) wiring mechanism; (b) kinematic analysis. For color reference, see page 221.

wires were connected between the mandible and tongue. For the kinetic axis, we attached two linear guides. On the linear guide, we also attached a rotational axis.

Regarding the control positioning of the tongue, we considered three points: tongue bone, center point of tongue, and tip of the tongue. The actuation mechanism of the tongue is composed by six wires attached to the tongue bone (three on the center point of the tongue and one on the tip of the tongue). As we have previously mentioned, three of those wires are common to the mandible, so the motion of the tongue and mandible are dependent. On the other hand, the control positioning of the tongue is done by controlling the position of the tongue bone. Therefore, the shape of the tongue was implemented by controlling the center point and tip. Of course, the control positioning of the center point and the tip of the tongue are dependent on the position of the tongue bone. As a result, by modifying the shape of the tongue, we may reproduce the space area of the oral cavity. By defining the position of the mandible, head and tongue; as it is shown in Fig. 12b, we may compute the length of each wire l_0 to l_{16} as follows (Eqs. 12.2–12.11):

$$l_0 = \sqrt{(Pv_{7x} - P_{1x})^2 + (Pv_{7y} - P_{1y})^2 + (Pv_{7z} - P_{1z})^2} \tag{12.2}$$

$$l_1, l_2 = \sqrt{(Pv_{6x} - P_{4x})^2 + (Pv_{6y} - P_{4y})^2 + (Pv_{6z} - P_{4z})^2} \tag{12.3}$$

$$l_3, l_4 = \sqrt{(Pv_{1x} - P_{4x})^2 + (Pv_{1y} - P_{4y})^2 + (Pv_{1z} - P_{4z})^2} \tag{12.4}$$

$$l_5, l_6 = \sqrt{(Pv_{2x} - P_{5x})^2 + (Pv_{2y} - P_{5y})^2 + (Pv_{2z} - P_{5z})^2} \tag{12.5}$$

$$l_7 = \sqrt{(Pv_{8x} - P_{3x})^2 + (Pv_{8y} - P_{3y})^2 + (Pv_{8z} - P_{3z})^2} \tag{12.6}$$

$$l_8 = \sqrt{(Pv_{9x} - P_{2x})^2 + (Pv_{9y} - P_{2y})^2 + (Pv_{9z} - P_{2z})^2} \tag{12.7}$$

$$l_10 = \sqrt{(Pv_{10x} - P_{1x})^2 + (Pv_{10y} - P_{1y})^2 + (Pv_{10z} - P_{1z})^2} \tag{12.8}$$

$$l_{11}, l_{12} = \sqrt{(Pv_{4x} - P_{o^m x})^2 + (Pv_{4y} - P_{o^m y})^2 + (Pv_{4z} - P_{o^m z})^2} \tag{12.9}$$

$$l_9, l_{13} = \sqrt{(Pv_{3x} - P_{7x})^2 + (Pv_{3y} - P_{7y})^2 + (Pv_{3z} - P_{7z})^2} \tag{12.10}$$

$$l_{14}, l_{15} = \sqrt{(Pv_{5x} - P_{6x})^2 + (Pv_{5y} - P_{6y})^2 + (Pv_{5z} - P_{6z})^2} \tag{12.11}$$

An experiment was proposed to verify the accuracy of the reproduction of the airway difficulties by using Eqs. 12.2–12.11. For this purpose, we performed an experiment to determine the differences between the kinematic results and the real ones. Thus, we compare the lengths of each of the wires which are obtained by the kinematic analysis, and the real length of each of wires by measuring them using a caliper (0.05mm of resolution). For this experiment; as a first approach, we have considered two kinds of cases of patients for the airway management training. The first case is the normal patient condition with its mouth closed (L=0 mm, θ=0°), and second case is the restricted mouth opening on patients with temporomandibular joint disorders (L=0 mm, θ=13°). For this purpose, we have adjusted the angle of mandible and the position of translational axis based on the each of the proposed cases by controlling the sixteen actuators.

The experimental results are shown in Table 12.1; where an average error of 3 mm was found. As we may observe, the wires connected to the mandible and the ones connected on the tongue have bigger length errors. Regarding the three tongue bones attached on the tongue, a total of ten wires were attached to them to control the tongue's position. In order to determine the initial position of the tongue, we used the tongue-offset device. With three bones fixed with the tongue-offset device, each of the actuators pulls the wires to determine an initial position of the tongue. However, the tongue which has high elastic coefficient makes it return to original shape, and the tensioned wires which are connected on the three bones make their positions change when the calibration device is removed from the mandible.

Table 12.1 Experimental results to compute the positioning error.

Wire	Normal Patient without restricted mouth opening Absolute Error Length (mm)	Patient with restricted mouth opening Absolute Error Length (mm)
l_0	1.44	0.7
l_1	3.86	4.66
l_2	6.36	5.16
l_3	6.12	5.23
l_4	5.62	4.73
l_5	3.35	4.07
l_6	3.35	4.57
l_9	1.97	0.84
l_{11}	0.7	0.77
l_{12}	0.7	0.27
l_{13}	1.47	1.34
l_{14}	1.69	2.03
l_{15}	1.69	2.53

12.5 CONCLUSIONS

The current advances on the research approaches towards implementing more efficient medical training systems were detailed. In particular, a suture training system (designed to provide assessment of the task) and an airway training system (designed to provide feedback by reproducing real-task conditions) were described. As it has been detailed, it becomes necessary to develop more effective training systems that contribute not only in improving the motor skills of trainees, but it also aim in understanding better specific aspects of the motor learning process under repetitive controlled circumstances. In particular, an effective training system should be designed to fulfill at least three basic principles: reproducing the real-world conditions of the task to be learnt, providing objective assessments of the training progress to trainees and providing multimodal feedback information to trainees about how their motor skills. It is important to provide stimuli to the five senses during the training.

The added value of using the Robot Technology for medical training purposes has been demonstrated by several researchers. However, still several research efforts should be carried out to improve the accuracy for providing more objective assessment of clinical competence as well as for providing more effective feedback to trainees.

References

Aggarwal R, Darzi A., Sullivan P., *et al.* (2009). Skills acquisition and assessment after a microsurgical skills course for ophthalmology residents, *Ophthalmology*, Vol. 116(2), pp. 257–62.

Bajura, M., Fuchs, H., Ohbuchi, R. (1992). Merging virtual objects with the real world: seeing ultrasound imagery within the patient, *Proc. of the 19th Annual Conference on Computer Graphics and Interactive Techniques*, pp.203–210.

Berthoz, A. (1997). *Le sens du mouvement*, Paris: Odile Jacob.

Burt, D. E. (1995). Virtual reality in anaethesia, *British Journal of Anaesthesia*, Vol. 75(4), pp. 472–480.

Chang L., Satava, R. M., Pellegrini, C. A., Sinanan, M. N. (2003). Robotic surgery Identifying the learning curve through objective measurement of skill, *Surgical Endoscopy*, pp. 1744–1748.

Datta V, Chang A, Mackay S, *et al*. (2002). The relationship between motion analysis and surgical technical assessments, *American Journal of Surgery*, Vol. 184, pp. 70–73.

Delson, N., Koussa, N., Tejani, N., (2003). Measuring 3D force and motion trajectories of a laryngoscope in the operating room, *Journal of Clinical Engineering*, Vol. 28(4), pp. 211–217.

Kawato, M, Gomi, H. (1992). A computational model of four regions of the cerebellum based on feedback error learning, *Biological Cybernetics*, 69, 95–103.

Kawato, M., Wolpert, D. (1998). Internal models for motor control, Novartis Foundation Symposium, 218, 291–304.

Gallagher, A. G, and Satava, R. M. (2002). Virtual reality as a metric for the assessment of laparoscopic psychomotor skills: Learning curves and reliability measures, *Surgical Endoscopy*, Vol. 16(12), pp. 1746–1752.

George, J.X., Dubrowski, A., (2007). Teaching suturing and knot-tying skills to medical students: A randomized controlled study comparing computer-based video instruction and (concurrent and summary) expert feedback, *Surgery*, Vol. 141, pp. 442–449.

Harden RM, *et al*. (1975). Assessment of clinical competence using objective structured clinical examination, *British Medical Journal*, pp. 447–451.

Mayrose, J., Kesavadas, T., Chugh, K., Dhananjay, J., Ellis, D.E. (2003). Utilization of virtual reality for endotracheal intubation training, *Resuscitation*, Vol. 59(1), pp. 133–138.

Moorthy, K., Munz, Y., Sarker, S. K., Darzi, A. (2003). Objective assessment of technical skills in surgery, *British Medical Journal*, Vol. 327, pp. 1032–1037.

Noh Y., Solis J., Takanishi, A., *et al*., (2009). Development of the airway management training system WKA-2 which can reproduce the cases of difficult airway, *Proc. of the International Conference on Robotics and Automation*, pp. 3843–3838.

Pugh, C. M., Youngblood, P. (2002). Development and validation of assessment measures for a newly developed physical examination simulator, *Journal of the American Medical Informatics Association*, Vol. 9(5), pp. 448–460.

Riva, G. (2003). Medical applications of virtual environments, Yearbook of Medical Informatics.

Rosen, J., Hannaford, B., *et al*. (2006). Generalized approach for modeling minimally invasive surgery as a stochastic process using a discrete markov model, *IEEE Transactions on Biomedical Engineering*, Vol. 53(3), pp. 399–413.

Ryan, B. R., Kurahashi, A., Brümmer, V., Satterthwaite, L., Classen, R., Dubrowski, A. (2008) Developing criteria for proficiency-based training of surgical technical skills using simulation: Changes in performances as a function of training year, *Journal of the American College of Surgeons*, pp. 205–211.

Sewell, C, Morris, D, Blevins, H, Dutta, S, Agrawal, S, Barbagli, F, Salisbury, K. (2008). Providing Metrics and Performance Feedback in a Surgical Simulator, *Computer Aided Surgery*, Vol. 13(2), pp. 63–81.

Sielhorst, *et al.* (2004). An augmented reality delivery simulator for medical training, *Proc. of the Augmented Environments for Medical Imaging Workshop*, pp. 11–20.

Skinner, B. F. (1938). *The Behavior of Organisms*. New York: Appleton-Century-Crofts.

Solis, J., (2004). Robotic Control Systems for Learning and Teaching Human Skills, Ph.D. dissertation, Perceptual Robotics Laboratory, Scuola Superiore Sant'Anna, Pisa, Italy.

Solis, J., Bergamasco, M, *et al.* (2007). Reactive Robots System: An active human/robot interaction for transferring skills from robot to unskilled persons, *Advanced Robotics Journal*, Vol. 21(3/4), pp. 267–291.

Solis, J., Takanishi, A., *et al.* (2008). Towards understanding the suture/ligature skills during the training process by using the WKS-2RII, *International Journal of Computer Assisted Radiology and Surgery*, Vol. 3(3-4), pp. 231–239.

Wickens, C. (1984). *Engineering Psychology and Human Performance*. Columbus, OH: Charles E. Merrill Publishing Company.

Chapter Thirteen

Wireless Active Capsule Endoscope: State-of-the-Art and Challenges

Xiaona Wang and Max Q.-H. Meng
Department of Electronic Engineering, The Chinese University of Hong Kong

This chapter introduces the state-of-the-art wireless capsule endoscopy in terms of commercially available products and prototypes currently under development in research labs worldwide. Challenges facing us in designing and manufacturing active wireless capsule endoscopes are outlined, together with potential methods to tackle them.

13.1 INTRODUCTION

Gastrointestinal (GI) disorder, such as stomach and colon cancers and ulcerative colitis, is one of the most common diseases in human body. According to recent statistics of the Hong Kong Cancer Registry in November 2008, the GI cancer rate is getting higher and higher each year since 1983 and the average age of the patients is getting younger. In 2006, 4,936 individuals newly developed cancers in the colorectum and stomach, which were among 10 most common cancers (Cancer statstics). The GI cancer rate and death rate are approaching that of the lung cancer, which is currently ranked the No. 1 killer.

Most GI cancers can be cured in the early stage. Regular checkup is an effective way to reduce the occurrence and mortality. There are several methods to detect diseases of GI tract without applying intrusive devices into the human body, such as stool test, double-contrast barium enema and more recently genetic analysis just among many others. However, conventional GI endoscopy is irreplaceable because it enables diagnosis based on analysis of real images and biopsy samples. Many research institutions and industries have embarked on the effort to improve conventional GI endoscopy procedures. Phee *et al.* (2002) presented thorough surveys of the related results.

Biomechatronics in Medicine and Healthcare by Le Li and Raymond Kai-Yu Tong

www.panstanford.com
978-981-4241-61-8

Current GI endoscopes can be categorized into two major groups: wired active endoscopes and wireless passive capsule endoscopes. Much work has been reported in the former category (Kassin *et al.* 2003). Modern fiber-optic based endoscopy made visualization of the whole stomach, upper small intestine and colon possible. Unfortunately, the procedures used for the examination, namely gastroscopy, push enteroscopy and colonoscopy, respectively, cause discomfort and pain to the patients because they require flexible, relatively bulky cables to be pushed into the GI tract. These cables are necessary to carry light by fiber-optic bundles, provide power and transmit video signals. Push enteroscopy in particular is severely constrained by limitations of how far it can be advanced into the small intestine. There is always some 15 – 20 feet of small intestine below the reach of push enteroscope and above the reach of colonoscope. Despite all the drawbacks, wired active GI endoscopy is still the most effective and widely used diagnostic and therapeutic procedure in dealing with diseases of the GI tract.

The wireless passive capsule endoscope is represented by a commercial product developed by Given Imaging Ltd (Givenimaging). The capsule contains a miniature camera for imaging, a wireless transmitter to send out the colored images of the GI tract to a portable recording device, and is self-powered by a battery cell without any externally connected wires or cables. The working principle of the wireless passive capsule endoscope is rather straightforward. During the examination, the patients just swallow the capsule and the capsule takes photos and transmits the images to the data recorder outside of the human body while going through the GI tract from mouth to anus by natural peristalsis, which takes about 8 to 24 hours.

Wireless capsule endoscopy has been proved to be a convenient, painless and effective diagnostic procedure, especially for the small intestine. However, the capsule endoscope depends on the peristalsis for moving passively in the GI tract; hence they are forced to go forward without the possibility of stopping, turning, going back or speeding during their journey, which causes a series of limitations in the diagnosis. Firstly, the long examination time (at least 8 hours) usually exhausts the battery power before the excretion of the capsule, which results in that the distal small intestine, where most ileum inflammatory diseases occur, is unreachable for over 25% of the capsules (Kornbluth *et al.* 2004). Secondly, the passive capsule may miss some interesting spots. Medical reports show that 75% of the second swallow of the passive capsules have new findings, and 62.5% of the new findings lead to the change of the final decision Rondonotti 2005. Multiple swallows may reduce the rate of missing diseases, nevertheless, the cost increases accordingly.

Next generation of active capsule endoscope, which is equipped with a locomotion mechanism, would allow interactive endoscopy in a totally controlled manner, enabling the surgeon to steer the capsule towards the more interesting pathological areas, with future potential to accomplish other related medical tasks such as biopsy and drug delivery in situ. An active capsule endoscope is a world-wide perception shared by the endoscopists and bio-robotic engineers (Kornbluth *et al.* 2004; Rondonotti *et al.* 2005; Meng *et al.* 2004). In this chapter, we introduce the state-of-the-art of wireless capsule endoscope. After a description of the current status, we discuss the promising solutions for a wireless active capsule endoscope.

13.2 MAJOR WORK IN WIRELESS CAPSULE ENDOSCOPE

The invention of the transistor made it possible to design swallowable electronic radio telemetry capsules for the study of GI physiological parameters. These capsules were first reported in the 1950′*s* and were used to measure temperature, pressure and pH (Zworkin *et al.* 1957; Mackay *et al.* 1957). Although the clinical applications were limited for these radio transmitting capsules, they did give inspirations for the invention of the video capsule endoscope. In the early 1990′*s*, complementary metal oxide semiconductor (CMOS) technology for imaging, along with progresses in application specific integrated circuit (ASIC) for control system and light emitting diode (LED) for illumination, paved the way for the advent of wireless capsule endoscope. In May 2000, the first video-telemetry capsule endoscope was released by an Israeli company Given Imaging. The device, which was named *M2A*™ (Iddan *et al.* 2000) and renamed to *PillCam*™ later, received marketing clearance from Food and Drug Administration (FDA) in 2001.

The wireless capsule endoscopy is a breakthrough in GI diagnosis. It releases the patients from the discomfort caused by conventional GI endoscopy and allows a direct visualization of the entire small intestine. Clinical practices have proved capsule endoscopy an effective tool in diagnosis of the diseases of the small intestine, such as obscure GI bleeding (Gossum *et al.* 2002); Crohn's diseases (Chermesh *et al.* 2008), Non-steroidal anti-inflammatory drugs (NSAIDs) induced damage, and other indications (Rondonotti *et al.* 2007). The device quickly attracted widespread interest within endoscopists and researchers. Following the emergence of *M2A*™, other companies and groups, such as Olympus, ChongQing JinShan, and IntroMedic have developed their own capsule endoscopy systems, which operate on the same principle as *M2A*™ with more or less improvements.

13.2.1 Products of Given Imaging

13.2.1.1 M2A™ and PillCam™ SB

The first capsule endoscopy system, *Given*™ Diagnostic System, was developed by Given Imaging, which consisted of the first passive wireless capsule endoscope M2A, the *Given*™ Data Recording Kit, and the *RAPID*™ Workstation (Fig. 13.1).

M2A™ capsule endoscope is a disposable, swallowable capsule, which has a dimension of 11 mm × 26 mm with a weight of 3.7 g. As shown in Fig. 13.2, it contains a miniature camera with a CMOS imager designed specifically for direct imaging within the GI tract, LED lighting system for illumination, and two silver oxide batteries. Different from the conventional endoscopes, the capsule also contains an integrated circuit and an RF transmitter for transmitting the images.

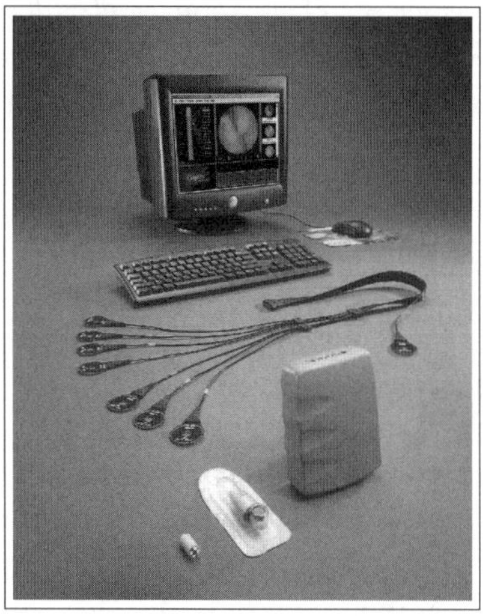

Figure 13.1 $M2A^{TM}$ Capsule Endoscopy $Given^{TM}$ Diagnostic System, including a wireless capsule endoscope (lower left), sensors for receiving data (middle), a portable data recorder(lower right), and a workstation (upper) for viewing the images. (From www.givenimaing.com). For color reference, see page 221.

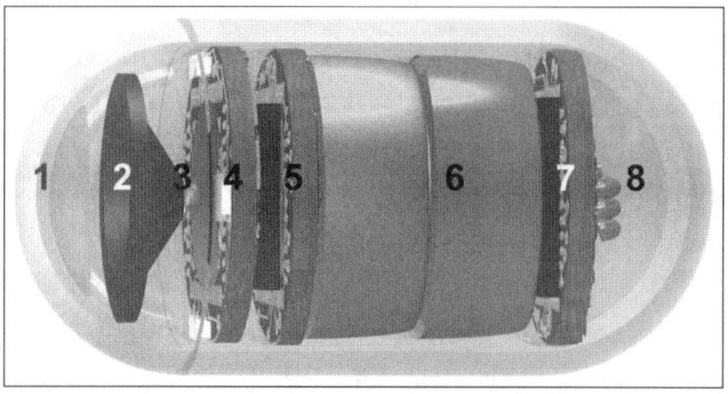

Figure 13.2 Schematic drawing of components inside the capsule endoscope. 1-optical dome, 2-lens holder, 3-lens, 4-illuminating LEDs, 5-CMOS image sensor, 6-battery, 7-ASIC transmitter, 8-antenna. For color reference, see page 221.

Prior to undergoing wireless capsule endoscopy, the patient is required to have a 10-hour fast. The procedure begins after the capsule is ingested with a sip of water. Then the capsule moves through the GI tract passively by natural peristalsis and captures 2 images per second. During the procedure, the sensor array is attached to the patient's skin in the abdominal region, and the other end is connected to the data recorder, which is worn by the patient on a belt around the waist. Images transmitted by the capsule at 433.10 MHz through the built-in antenna are picked up by the sensor array and then sent to the recorder.

The procedure usually takes about 8 hours, during which more than 55,000 images are acquired. At the conclusion of the examination, the patient returns the belt and the recording unit to the physician. Then the physician can download, view, edit and archive data images on the workstation, which is a computer

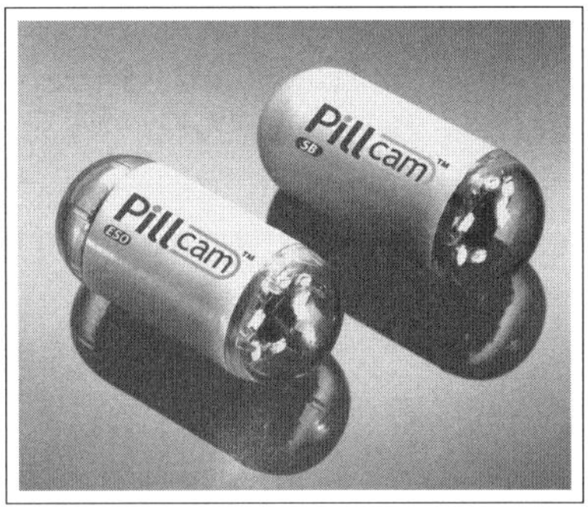

Figure 13.3 View of *PillCam*^{TM} ESO and *PillCam*^{TM} SB capsules. The main difference lies in the setting of cameras.

equipped with *RAPID*^{TM} software. It may take 30 minutes to 2 hours to evaluate the video, which mainly depends on the experience of the reader (Cave 2004, 2006).

In 2002, Given Imaging introduced *M2A*^{TM} PLUS featuring a localization system (Jacob *et al.* 2002), which allows physicians to locate small intestine diseases with increased precision. This function is achieved by a triangulation process of the signal strength received by three adjacent sensors. The accuracy is about $\pm$ 3 cm (Swain 2003).

The capsule endoscope was initially designed to diagnose disorders of the small intestine, such as Crohn's disease, Celiac disease, benign and cancerous tumors, ulcerative colitis, and etc. In 2004, the capsule was renamed to *PillCam*^{TM} and the company started to release capsules to examine other parts of GI tract. *PillCam*^{TM} SB was addressed specifically for small intestine video capsule.

In May 2007, *PillCam*^{TM} SB 2 was cleared for marketing by FDA. The new capsule is the same size as the previous version with superior performances, which include doubling the frame rate from two to four images per second, enlarging the view angle from 140° to 156°, incorporating a three-lens system and automatic light control, and increasing the capsule's operational time from eight to nine hours. Clinical studies showed that the overall image quality of *PillCam*^{TM} SB 2 was significantly superior, yet it did not produce a statistically greater diagnostic yield than the former version (Metzger *et al.* 2009).

13.2.1.2 *PillCam*^{TM} ESO

The *PillCam*^{TM} ESO video capsule is quipped with two miniature cameras on both ends. It is designed to view the inner lining of the esophagus for diagnosis of the disorders such as esophageal varices, esophagitis and Barrett's esophagus. The capsule measures 11 mm × 26 mm and weighs less than 4*g*. It was approved by FDA in 2004. Fig. 13.3 shows a comparison of outward appearance between *PillCam*^{TM} SB and *PillCam*^{TM} ESO.

No fasting or sedation is required prior to the endoscopy procedure. The patient swallows the capsule in a supine position, followed by two minutes at a 30° angle, another two minutes at a 60° angle, and the last two minutes at fully upright. The *PillCam*™ ESO travels through the esophagus by normal peristaltic waves, capturing 14 images per second. The images are transmitted to three sensor arrays placed on the patient's chest and connected to a data recorder. The pill is later excreted naturally after dropping into the stomach. It takes 20 minutes to complete the procedure and 2,600 color images are acquired. Then the physician views and assesses the results just like using *PillCam*™ SB.

The first clinical trial on *PillCam*™ ESO concerned gastroesophageal reflux disease (GERD) (Eliakim *et al.* 2004), which may develop Barrett's esophagus and in turn lead to esophageal adenocarcinoma. In 2007, *PillCam*™ ESO 2 gained FDA approval and was put into clinical use. The improvements of the new capsule are similar to *PillCam*™ SB 2, which include: increased capture rate of 18 frames per second, better image quality, wider angle of view and additional Automatic Light Control (ALC) to provide optimal illumination for each image.

13.2.1.3 *PillCam*™ Colon

The *PillCam*™ Colon capsule measures 11 mm × 31 mm. It has one micro camera at each end which captures 4 images a second for up to 10 hours. The platform for *PillCam*™ COLON includes the same components as *PillCam*™ SB, i.e., a sensor array, a data recorder and a *RAPID*™ workstation. But the procedure is different in two aspects. One is that a prep, as well as additional prokinetic agents to enhance capsule propulsion, are needed beforehand. Besides, the capsule takes pictures for three minutes after being swallowed, providing images of the esophagus and stomach. Then it turns itself off for 105 minutes to preserve the battery while it passes through most of the small intestine on its way to the large bowel.

PillCam™ COLON has received European CE Mark in 2006 and a medical device licence from Health Canada in 2007, but was rejected by FDA in 2008 for commercial distribution in the USA. The company claimed that they were accelerating development of a next generation colon capsule.

13.2.1.4 *Agile*™ Patency System

Capsule retention has been an area of significant controversy and concern amongst capsule users. As defined by 2005 International Conference on Capsule Endoscopy, this complication means the capsule remaining in the GI tract for at least two weeks and needing surgical, endoscopic or medical therapy to help to extract. The frequency of capsule retention depends on the clinical indication for capsule endoscopy, ranging from 0% in healthy subjects, 6.7% in patients with Crohn's disease (Buchman *et al.* 2004) and as high as 21% in patients with intestinal obstruction (Pennazio 2006). The overall incidence is about 1 − 2%. It also represents a risk for the patients with a history of dysphagia, i.e. a difficulty to swallow, while undergoing esophageal capsule endoscopy. Therefore, Given Imaging has put forward the *Agile*™ Patency System (Spada *et al.* 2005) as an accessory to the *PillCam*™ video capsule, which was approved by FDA in 2006.

The device is an 11 mm × 26 mm ingestible and dissolvable capsule made of a lactose body surrounded by dissolvable plugs at each end and containing an internal radiofrequency identification (RFID) tag. Its presence in the intestinal tract can be determined by an external scanner. The timer plugs at each end are designed to erode after about 30 hours resulting in disintegration and passage of the capsule if retained longer.

The *Agile*™ capsule is intended to verify adequate patency of the gastrointestinal tract in patients with known or suspected strictures prior to administration of the *PillCam*™ video capsule. If softening or any deformation of the body is observed, patency would be considered highly suspect and capsule endoscopy should probably be avoided. The clinical reports show that the patency system is a safe and useful predictive tool in high risk contraindicated patients (Radwin 2009).

13.2.2 Olympus Capsule Endoscope

Olympus Corporation launched EndoCapsule in Europe in 2005 Olympus. It's a 11 mm × 26 mm disposable and passive capsule with a CCD sensor camera for small intestine endoscopy. The lighting system contains 6 LEDs and automatic brightness control to adjust the illumination. An antenna sends two images per second to the recorder. An interesting feature is that physicians can view real-time images and estimate the capsule position thanks to the Real Time Viewer (Fig. 13.4).

The EndoCapsule Software owns some extra functions in addition to the management of the acquired data, which include: a multi display function for optimal observation, structure enhancement and enlargement display function to highlight the tiniest details, red colour detection function to highlight suspected bleeding symptoms, and auto speed adjustment function to optimize the review speed. The EndoCapsule has received marketing clearance from the FDA in September, 2007.

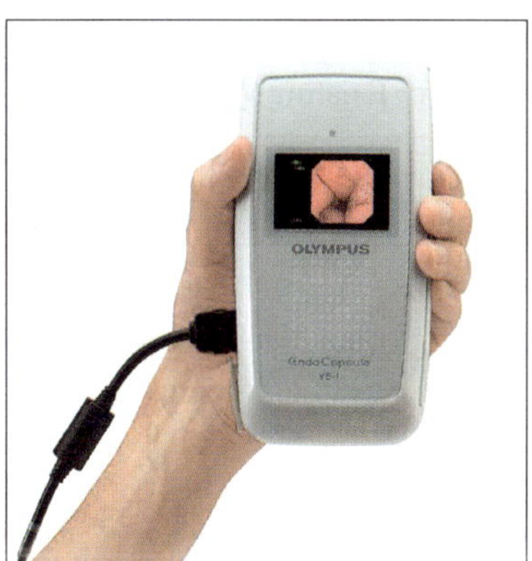

Figure 13.4 Olympus EndoCapsule Real Time Viewer. (From www.olympus-europa.com)

13.2.3 Other Capsules

Since the emergence of PillCam, other companies and groups would like to share the market of capsule endoscopy by putting forward their own systems. Competition is likely to stimulate new technical developments which may make capsule endoscopy cheaper.

Besides Endocapsule by Olympus company, ChongQing JinShan Science & Technology Co. Ltd developed OMOM Capsule Endoscopy System OMOM. The system has gone through three technical design changes with improved image quality and lower cost than other systems. It has obtained CE Mark from European Union and permission for marketing in China. MiRoCam implemented by IntroMedic Co. Ltd MiRoCam includes a novel transmission technology of electric-field propagation to take the place of radiofrequency (RF) data transmission, and results in saving power. The capsule is currently under clinical trial (Bang *et al.* 2009).

Table 13.1 and 13.2 list the major specifications of the capsules from different companies, including both approved products and those under clinical trial.

Table 13.1 Comparison of Existing Wireless Capsule Endoscope.

Company	Given Imaging *PillCam*™		
Model	SB/SB2	ESO/ESO2	COLON
Dimension ($D \times L$)	11 mm× 26 mm	11 mm× 26 mm	11 mm× 31 mm
Weight (g)	3.7	3.7	2.9
Camera	One-sided	Double-sided	Double-sided
Target Organ	Small Intestine	Esophagus	Colon
Image Sensor	CMOS	CMOS	CMOS
Frame Rate (fps)	2	14/18	4
View Angle (*degree*)	140/156	140/156	156
Image Display	Offline	Offline	Offline
Operating Time	8 *hours*	20 *minutes*	Up to 10 *hours*
Approval	FDA 2001/2007	FDA 2004/2007	CE Mark 2006

Table 13.2 Comparison of Existing Wireless Capsule Endoscope(cont.).

Company	Olympus	Jinshan	IntroMedic
Model	EndoCapsule	OMOM	MiRo#1
Dimension ($D \times L$)	11 mm× 26 mm	13 mm× 27.9 mm	10.8 mm× 24 mm
Weight (g)	3.8	5.0	3.3
Camera	One-sided	One-sided	One-sided
Target Organ	Small Intestine	Small Intestine	Small Intestine
Image Sensor	CCD	CCD	CMOS
Frame Rate (fps)	2	2	2
View Angle (*degree*)	145	140	150
Image Display	Real-time	Real-time	Offline
Operating Time	8 *hours*	6 – 8 *hours*	9 – 11 *hours*
Approval	FDA 2007	CE Mark 2007	In clinical trial

13.2.4 Technical limitations

The technique of capsule endoscopy has revolutionized the study of the small intestine; however, the same technical characteristics can represents, from a certain point of view, limitations of capsule endoscopy. One technical problem reported is a poor charge of the battery, resulting in short battery life and incompleteness of examination. There is also concern of the potential toxicity brought by the batteries. The problem of capsule retention is one of the main complications of the capsule endoscopy, as mentioned in section 13.1.2.4, and the $Agile^{TM}$ Patency Capsule may be used to provide an early warning of the intestinal stricture (ElMatary 2008, Rondonotti *et al.* 2007).

At present capsule endoscopy is a diagnostic tool and one major limitation is the absence of a remote control and the inability to take biopsies or perform any therapeutic procedure. It is also impossible for the capsule to stay in specific areas of the small intestine for repeated examinations. Sometimes double-balloon enteroscopy should be employed as a complimentary technique after initial imaging using capsule endoscopy (Yamamoto 2001, Heine 2006).

To overcome the obstacles, the capsule needs an active locomotion mechanism to vary its speed and reduce the transit time, and a braking mechanism to hold the movement of capsule for a prolonged time, together with a orienting mechanism to view around different directions. This would enable a more thorough analysis, at wherever interesting. A more precise localization system is necessary for both the actuation and the diagnosis (Wang *et al.* 2005, Rondonotti *et al.* 2007). Besides, the integration of sensors for detection of blood, white blood cells, pH, temperature and pressure measurement, and so forth are also needed to make other diagnostic and therapeutic tasks feasible. As a successful attempt to fulfill this requirement, a wireless ingestible capsule endowed with pH, temperature and pressure sensors developed by SmartPill Corporation and named Bravo (Dickman *et al.* 2006, Gonzalez *et al.* 2007), has been approved by FDA in 2006.

13.3 WIRELESS ACTIVE CAPSULE ENDOSCOPE

There has been continuous development and improvement of the wireless capsule endoscope. Gong *et al.* (2000) introduced a conceptual interactive system, which included a joystick to communicate with the wireless endoscope, controlling the light, image capture and transmission of the capsule. Although methods of propulsion have not been proposed in this paper, the authors did emphasize on the need of some innovative and intriguing ideas about propulsion for the next generation of wireless capsule endoscopy. The Intelligent Microsystem Center (IMC), Seoul, Korea, has launched a project on designing of a multi-functional capsule endoscope (Kim *et al.* 2005). The conceptional capsule will be loaded with moving mechanism, detecting sensors, medical information acquisition and treatment system, telemetry and power source. With this device, not only video based diagnosis but also physiological tests will be feasible in real time manner.

Because the prospective multiple functions of the capsule endoscope are based on the controllable motion of the capsule, it is a key point to equip the capsule with a specific locomotion mechanism, so that the robotic capsule can be guided to any interesting spots in the GI tract and can move through unimportant areas in a much faster pace than the natural peristaltic movement (Meng *et al.* 2004; Fireman *et al.* 2004). In addition, such a robotic capsule endoscope can work as a platform for further operations such as biopsy, drug delivery, and so on.

There are two major possible approaches to the development of a locomotion system for the capsule endoscope: the external approach and the internal approach. An internal approach implies integration of the locomotion mechanism completely onto the capsule. The external approach is generally achieved by magnetic field manipulation and the control system is worn by the patient or to be put around him/her. In the following, some typical locomotion mechanisms proposed for an active capsule endoscope will be introduced.

13.3.1 Electrical stimulation

The first locomotion mechanism for capsule endoscope was proposed by Mosse *et al.* (2001). They used an acrylic ovoid-shaped endoscope with two stainless steel electrodes mounted on the tapered section, which apply electro-stimulation to the intestinal wall. The stimulation caused circular muscle contraction when the devices were in contact with the intestinal wall, resulting in forward propulsion of the device. Fig. 13.5 shows a schematic view of the working principle. The tests in the small intestine and esophagus of an anaesthetized pig produced encouraging results: the ovoid advanced up and down in the esophagus at $6mm/s$; and moved in the small intestine at up to $4.5mm/s$ with the ability to negotiate tight curves.

P Swain *et al.* (2002) reported more investigations on the device. The ovoid was equipped with bipolar electrodes at both the rear and the front so that it can exert a forward or backward force. The tests in pigs showed that controlled bidirectional movement of the device was feasible in esophagus, small intestine and colon. This

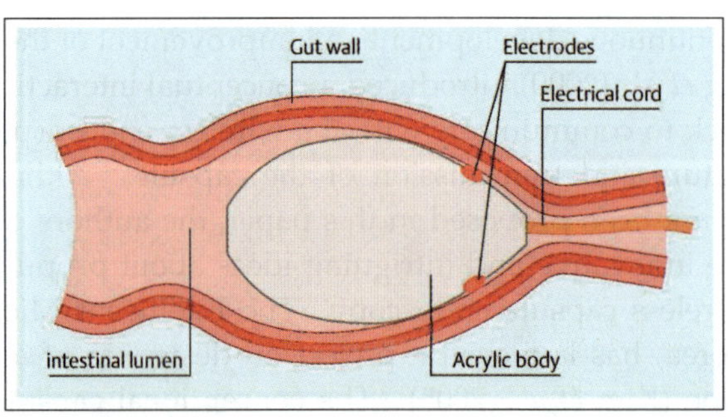

Figure 13.5 Schematic diagram of ovoid-shaped device as it moves through the intestine via electrical stimulation of the intestinal wall. (Reproduced according to Mosse *et al.* (2001).)

technology has also been tested in humans (Swain 2008) and got positive results. It is a promising solution for the propulsion of wireless capsule endoscopes if the design of the device is further optimized, and the safety and controllability of the mechanism are stringently assessed.

13.3.2 Mechatronic locomotion mechanisms

Engineers are seeking bio-inspired mechatronic solutions for the locomotion of the wireless capsule endoscope. The research team of CRIM Lab developed a series of active locomotion mechanisms based on bio-inspired legs (Menciassi *et al.* 2004; Quirini *et al.* 2008; Valdastri *et al.* 2009). The legs were made of superelastic shape memory alloy (SMA) ending with 200 micron high hooks to provide friction. In the initial version each leg was driven by a SMA actuator independently, and later brushless micro DC motors were used to actuate several sets of legs. The number of legs in the prototypes varied from four to twelve. Fig. 13.6 shows the outward appearance of a 12-legged robotic capsule. A human machine interface (HMI) was responsible for control of the movement. In-vitro and in-vivo tests proved that the mechanism could proceed and stop in the small intestine.

Glass *et al.* (2008) also studied on the legged feature for the actuation of capsule endoscope. Yet they put particular emphasis on enhancing the friction between the leg and the wall of the intestine. Micro-patterned adhesives inspired by gecko and beetle foot hairs were applied to the robotic legs so as to anchor the device at a fixed location. It was supposed to reduce the actuation force significantly by using micro-pillars coated with a thin silicone oil layer.

Kim *et al.* (2005) developed a capsule prototype with two-way linear actuators using four pairs of SMA springs. Biomimetic micro-hooks acted as clamping

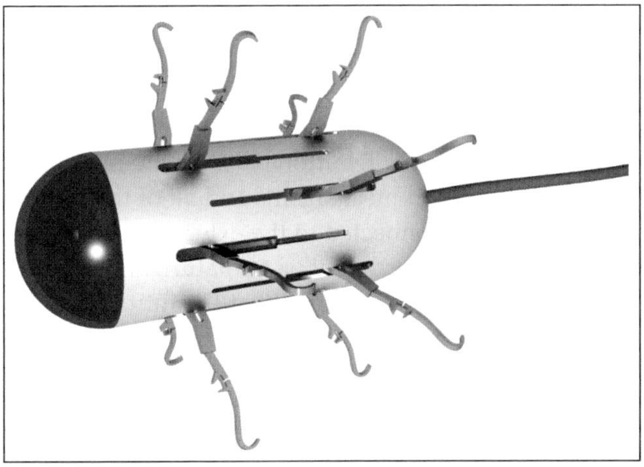

Figure 13.6 The outward appearance of a 12-legged endoscopic capsular robot. (Reproduced from Valdastri *et al.* (2009)).

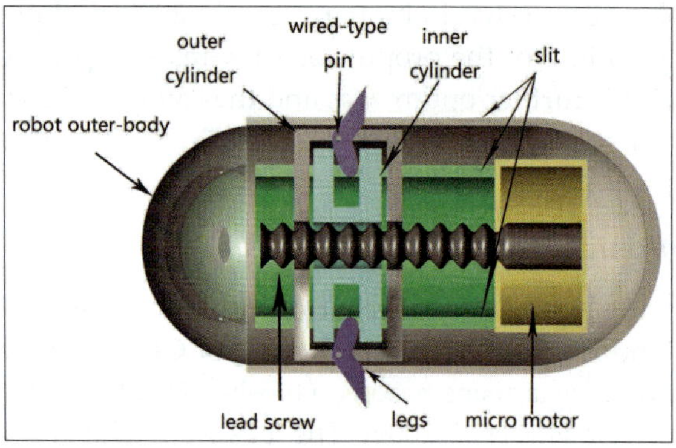

Figure 13.7 Schematic view of a paddling based microrobot for capsule endoscope. (Reproduced according to Park *et al.* (2007).)

devices to ensure the unidirectional movement. The prototype was 13mm in diameter and 33mm in total length, leaving a hollow space of 7.6mm in diameter to hold other parts needed for endoscopy, such as a camera, an RF modules and batteries. An average speed up to 14.7mm/min was measured on the surface of porcine colons during in-vitro experiments. The characteristic of SMAs is the ability of deformation according to temperature change; unfortunately, the environment in the living body is hostile for heat dissipation of the SMA and will lower the efficiency of in-vivo test. Moreover, the local temperature rise of the intestinal wall at the contact point should be guaranteed to be of no harm.

Park and colleagues Park *et al.* (2007) proposed a paddling based locomotive mechanism for the capsule endoscope. The 13mm $\times$ 30mm capsule-type microrobot achieved movement by the six legs driven by a stepper micromotor together with two mobile cylinders inside. Fig. 13.7 shows the structure of the design. A moving speed up to 6.42 mm/s was obtained during in-vitro experiments in porcine small intestine.

The internal locomotion mechanism is usually integrated on board the capsule and may offer better flexibility and dexterity. However, power constraint and size limitation are two bottlenecks in the development of a completely wireless active capsule endoscope. At present, button batteries are not powerful enough to supply energy for the locomotion mechanisms and all of the mechatronic designs introduced above need a cord connected to the external power supply. Moreover, the sizes of the active capsules need further miniaturization in order to be swallowable. Another aspect need to mention is that the introduced mechanisms can only make one-way movement due to the directional shapes of the clampers, e.g., the legs and hooks.

13.3.3 Magnetic actuation methods

Magnetic force is an appealing option for the actuation of an active capsule endoscope wirelessly because it can avoid internal power consumption by using

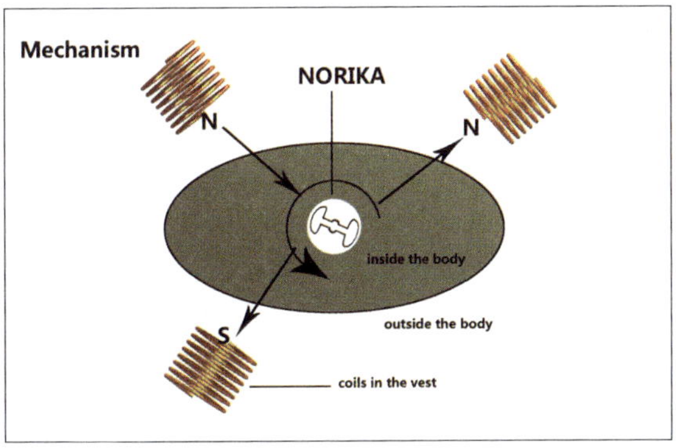

Figure 13.8 Conceptional description of external rotation mechanism for NORIKA capsule

permanent magnets. Many research groups and companies have been trying to incorporate the magnetic actuation mechanisms into the capsule design.

Since 1998, RF System Lab has been working on NORIKA capsule endoscope system (Uehara *et al.* 2003), which includes a 9 mm $\times$ 23 mm capsule, an external controller, a transmitter vest and a workstation. The capsule is externally powered by wireless power transmission. It integrates a CCD image sensor with the digital signal processor (DSP) separated from CCD by microwave and moved outside body, which can save 94% of the total internal power. NORIKA has a rotation feature to gain some level of control. A schematic drawing of the working principle is depicted in Fig. 13.8. Three coils are placed inside the capsule as rotor coils, while another three coils embedded in a vest-like jacket act as stators. When the charged energy in the capacitor is quickly released to the rotor coil, a strong magnetic force is generated within a short time so as to rotate the capsule. The rotation direction is decided by the stator's magnetic field direction.

Sayaka supersedes the basic technology of NORIKA. Its camera has been moved to the side of the capsule to provide a better view of the intestinal walls. In addition, the camera can spin as the capsule passes through the digestive tract, thanks to Sayaka's small permanent magnets and an electromagnet which causes "stepping rotation". The NORIKA/Sayaka capsule is still under development and may need more years before entering the market.

Besides the rotation of the cameras inside the capsule by magnetic force, the researchers are also endeavor to manipulate the body of the capsule magnetically. Sendoh *et al.* (2003) enclosed an axially magnetized permanent magnet inside a capsule with a spiral structure and rotated the capsule by applying an external rotational magnetic field; and thus the spiral shape generated a linear movement, as demonstrated in Fig. 13.9. Both forward and reverse motion could be achieved in this mechanism by control of the rotating direction. This idea has been one instance of Olympus's conceptual capsule navigation system, which could control the position, orientation and posture of the permanent magnets built in the capsule by an external magnetic field generator (Kusuda 2005).

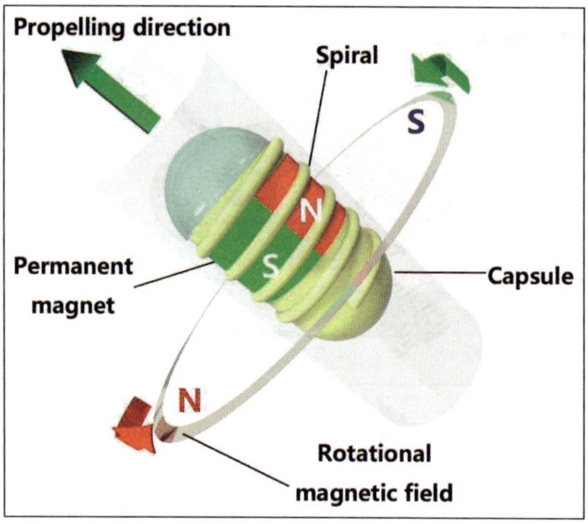

Figure 13.9 Working principle of Olympus magnetic guidance system. (Reproduced from Sendoh *et al.* (2003).)

Carpi *et al.* (2006); Carpi *et al.* (2007) carried out a series of experiments on the magnetic manoeuvring of endoscopic capsules. They fabricated magnetic shells made of a silicone elastomer mixed with magnetic particles to cover the central portion of the capsule (Fig. 13.10). The shells were capable of interacting with an imposed external magnetic field. Preliminary tests demonstrated translations, rotations and roto-translations of the capsule/shell complex onto pieces of bovine tissues and inside a human-sized plastic phantom as well. The external actuation system was a commercial system, Stereotaxis *Niobe*™ System Stereotaxis, which is for intrabody magnetic navigation of interventional catheters (Carpi *et al.* 2009).

G. Kosa Kosa *et al.* (2008) proposed a swimming capsule endoscope using MRI's magnetic fields for both propulsion and wireless energy delivery. Alternating current in the coils, which was contained in a swimming tail, acting on the

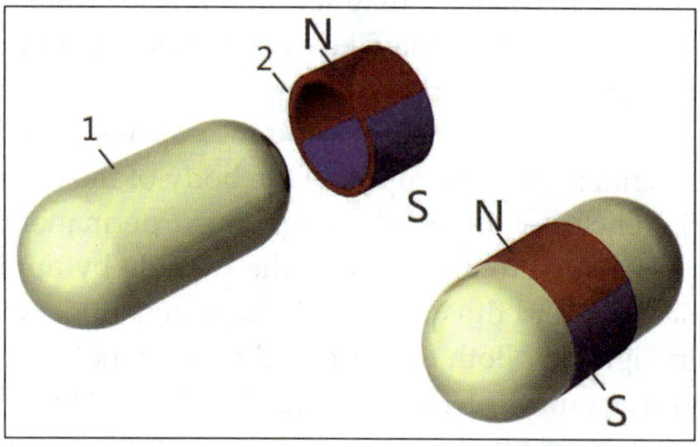

Figure 13.10 Elastic shell and capsule/shell complex. 1-capsule, 2-magnetic shell. (Reproduced from Carpi *et al.* (2006).)

static magnetic field of MRI, generated propulsion force, and RF magnetic field of MRI produced power for the coils. The numerical model predicted that a $10mm$ tail could produce a speed of 7.9 mm/s force up to $5.5mN$ in a 3T static magnetic field.

P. Valdastri *et al.* (2008) assessed the feasibility of using a swallowable wireless capsule to deploy a surgical clip under remote control. The $12.8mm \times 33.5mm$ capsule equipped with four permanent magnets was steered by means of the external magnetic guidance to a specific target successfully in an in vivo surgical experiment. This study paves a way to a new generation of capsule device able to perform both diagnostic and therapeutic tasks.

In all, the external magnetic actuation is capable of both propulsion and orientation of the capsule. It saves internal energy of the capsule compared with mechatronic mechanisms, which makes it possible to achieve wireless control. The deficiency is that the external system is usually quite complex and bulky, like the magnetic field generator of MRI. There is a trade-off between the internal and external power consumptions. One possible solution of the problem may be to combine the advantage of the two approaches by designing an internal locomotion mechanism which can interact with external magnetic system for part of control (Wang *et al.* 2007).

13.4 CONCLUSION AND FUTURE PROSPECT

Capsule endoscopy has opened up a new world of diagnostic and other possibilities for the gastroenterologist. It is remarkable to see images of small intestinal abnormalities in the small intestine, which was not possible until recently when development of wireless capsule endoscopy enabled a much less invasive and more complete examination of the small intestine.

In the future, the capsule endoscopy is likely to have a substantial impact on the management of small intestinal disease as well as other parts of the GI tract after it evolves from passive to active, i.e., it can make autonomous movement in the GI tract. Currently, the progress is hindered by power and size limitations inside the swallowable capsule since the device may require more power for movement, altering the view, spraying medicine, activating a biopsy and other features, and more space to embody the equipments.

Some attempts are being or to be considered to generate power within living body. These may include transcutaneous induction system, biologic batteries, rechargeable batteries, motion energy, wireless power transmission Wang *et al.* (2007) and etc. In respect of the size limitation, a possible solution may be combination of multiple robotic capsules. The tiny capsule robotic components are ingested and assembled by themselves to configure in the GI tract to perform precise interventions (Menciassi 2008, Harada 2009).

The invention of the capsule endoscope reminds people of the science fiction movie The Fantastic Voyage, which was considered a mere figment of the imagination years ago to have a miniature submarine into the human body. Now capsule endoscopy has become a well established tool for evaluating the entire GI tract even though it does not have the ability to carry out therapeutic tasks yet. Nevertheless, future always comes soon enough. We can expect the next generation of active capsule endoscope comes into reality in the future, maybe in the near future.

ACKNOWLEDGMENT

The authors would like to thank Mr. Xijun Chen for reproducing the relevant images in the chapter.

References

Bang, S., Park, J., Jeong, S., Kim, Y., Shim, H., Kim, T., Lee, D. and Song, S. First clinical trial of the MiRo capsule endoscope by using a novel transmission technology: Electric-field propagation, *Gastrointestinal Endoscopy* **69**(2), 253–259 (2009).

Buchman, A., Miller, F., Wallin, A., Chowdhry, A. and Ahn, C. Videocapsule endoscopy versus barium contrast studies for the diagnosis of crohns disease recurrence involving the small intestine, *The American Journal of Gastroenterology* **99**, 2171–2177 (2004).

Cancer statistics (2008). Published by the Hong Kong Registry, Hospital Authority of Hong Kong.

Carpi, F., Galbiati, S. and Carpi, A. Magnetic shells for gastrointestinal endoscopic capsules as a means to control their motion, *Biomedicine & Pharmacotherapy* **60**, 370–374 (2006).

Carpi, F., Galbiati, S. and Carpi, A. Controlled navigati on of endoscopic capsules: Concept and preliminary experimental investigations, *IEEE Transactions on Biomedical Engineering* **54**(11), 2028–2036 (2007).

Carpi, F. and Pappone, C. Magnetic maneuvering of endoscopic capsules by means of a robotic navigation system, *IEEE Transactions on Biomedical Engineering* **56**(5), 1482–1490 (2009).

Cave, D. R. Reading wireless video capsule endoscopy, *Gastrointestinal Endoscopy Clinics of North America* **14**(1), 17–24 (2004).

Cave, D. R. Technology insight: current status of video capsule endoscopy, *Nature Clinical Practice Gastroenterology & Hepatology* **3**, 158–164 (2006).

Chermesh, I. and Eliakim, R. Capsule endoscopy in crohns disease — Indications and reservations 2008, *Journal of Crohns and Colitis* **2**, 107–113 (2008).

Dickman, R. and Fass, R. Ambulatory esophageal ph monitoring: New directions, *Digestive Diseases* **24**, 313–318 (2006).

El-Matary, W. Wireless capsule endoscopy: Indications, limitations, and future challenges, *Journal of Pediatric Gastroenterology and Nutrition* **46**, 1 (2008).

Eliakim, R., Yassin, K., Shlomi, I., Suissa, A. and Eisen, G. A novel diagnostic tool for detecting oesophageal pathology: The pillcam oesophageal video capsule, *Alimentary Pharmacology & Therapeutics* **20**, 1083–1089 (2004).

EndoCapsule (on line). http://www.olympus-europa.com/endoscopy/. Fireman, Z., Glukhovsky, A. and Scapa, E. Future of capsule endoscopy, Gastrointestinal Endoscopy Clinics of North America **14**(1), 219–227 (2004).

Givenimaging (on line). http://www.givenimaging.com.

Glass, P., Cheung, E. and Sitti, M. A legged anchoring mechanism for capsule endoscopes using micropatterned adhesives, *IEEE Transactions on Biomedical Engineering* **55**(12), 2759–2766 (2008).

Gong, F., Swain, P. and Mills, T. Wireless endoscopy, *Gastrointestinal Endoscopy* **51**(6), 725–729 (2000).

Gonzalez-Guillaumin, J., Sadowski, D., Kaler, K. and Mintchev, M. Ingestible capsule for impedance and ph monitoring in the esophagus, *IEEE Transactions on Biomedical Engineering* **54**(12), 2231–2236 (2007).

Gossum, A. V., Francois, E., Hittelet, A., Schmit, A. and Deviere, J. A prospective comparative study between push-enteroscopy and wireless video capsule in patients with obscure digestive bleeding, *Gastrointestinal Endoscopy* **55**, AB88 (2002).

Harada, K., Susilo, E., Menciassi, A. and Dario, P. Wireless reconfigurable modules for robotic endoluminal surgery, in *Proceedings of 2009 IEEE International Conference on Robotics and Automation*, 2699–2704 (2009).

Heine, G., Hadithi, M., Groenen, M., Kuipers, E., Jacobs, M. and Mulder, C. Double-balloon enteroscopy : Indications, diagnostic yield, and complications in a series of 275 patients with suspected small-bowel disease, *Endoscopy* **38**(1), 42–48 (2006).

Iddan, G., Meron, G., Glukhovsky, A. and Swain, P. Wireless capsule endoscopy, *Nature* **405**, 717 (2000).

Jacob, H., Levy, D., Shreiber, R., Glukhovsky, A. and Fischer, D. Localization of the given m2a ingestible capsule in the given diagnostic imaging system, *Gastrointestinal Endoscopy* **55**, AB135 (2002).

Kassin, I., Ng, W., Feng, G. and Phee, S. Review of locomotion techniques for robotic colonoscopy, in *Proceedings of IEEE International Conference on Robotics and Automation*, 1086–1091 (2003).

Kim, B., Lee, S., Park, J. and Park, J.-O. Design and fabrication of a locomotive mechanism for capsule-type endoscopes using shape memory alloys (smas), *IEEE/ASME Transactions on Mechatronics* **10**(1), 77–86 (2005a).

Kim, B., Park, S., Jee, C. and Yoon, S. An earthworm-like locomotive mechanism for capsule endoscopes, in *Proceedings of 2005 IEEE/RSJ International Conference on Intelligent Robots and Systems*, 2997–3002 (2005b).

Kornbluth, A., Legnani, P. and Lewis, B. S. Video capsule endoscopy in inflammatory bowel disease–past, present, and future, *Inflammatory Bowel Diseases* **10**(3), 278–285 (2004).

Kosa, G., Jakab, P., Jolesz, F. and Hata, N. Swimming capsule endoscope using static and RF magnetic field of MRI for propulsion, in *Proceedings of 2008 IEEE International Conference on Robotics and Automation*, 2922–2927 (2008).

Kusuda, Y. A further step beyond wireless capsule endoscopy, *Sensor Review* **25**(4), 259–260 (2005).

Mackay, R. and Jacobson, B. Endoradiosonde, *Nature* **179**, 1239–1240 (1957).

Menciassi, A., Stefanini, C., Gorini, S., Pernorio, G., Kim, B., Park, J. and Dario, P. Locomotion of a legged capsule in the gastrointestinal tract: Theoretical study and preliminary technological results, in *Proceedings of the 26th International Conference of the IEEE Engineering in Medicine and Biology Society*, 2767–2770 (2004).

Menciassi, A., Valdastri, P., Harada, K. and Dario, P. Single and multiplerobotic capsules for endoluminal diagnosis and surgery, in *Proceedings of the 2nd IEEE/RAS-EMBS International Conference on Biomedical and Biomechatronics*, 238–242 (2008).

Meng, M. Q.-H., Mei, T., Pu, J., Hu, C., Wang, X. and Chan, Y. Wireless robotic capsule endoscopy: State-of-the-art and challenges, in *Proceedings of 5th World Congress on Intelligent Control and Automation (WCICA04)*, 5561– 5565 (2004).

Metzger, Y., Adler, S., Shitrit, A., Koslowsky, B. and Bjarnason, I. Comparision of a new pillcam sb2 video capsule versus the standard pillcam sb for detection of small bowel disease, *Reports in Medical Imaging* **2**, 7–11 (2009).

MiRoCam (on line). http://www.intromedic.com/.

Mosse, A., Mills, T., Appleyard, M., Kadirkamanathan, S. and Swain, P. Electrical stimulation for propelling endoscope, *Gastrointestinal Endoscopy* **54**(1), 79–83 (2001).

OMOM (on line). http://www.cqjs.net/.

Park, H., Park, S., Yoon, E., Kim, B., Park, J. and Park, S. Paddling based microrobot for capsule endosocpe, in *Proceedings of IEEE International Conference on Robotics and Automation*, 3377–3382 (2007).

Pennazio, M. Capsule endoscopy: where are we after 6 years of clinical use? *Digestive and Liver Disease* **38**(12), 867–878 (2006).

Phee, L., Accoto, D., Menciassi, A., Stefanini, C., M.Carrozza and Dario, P. Analysis and development of locomotion devices for the gastrointestinal tract, *IEEE Transactions on Biomedical Engineering* **49**(6), 613–616 (2002).

Quirini, M., Menciassi, A., Scapellato, S., Stefanini, C. and Dario, P. Design and fabrication of a motor legged capsule for the active exploration of the gastrointestinal tract, *IEEE/ASME Transactions on Mechatronics* **13**(2), 169–179 (2008).

Radwin, M. (2009). NSAID enteropathy and capsule retention; complication or guide to therapy? *Visible Human Journal of Endoscopy* **8**(2), 9–14.

Rondonotti, E., Herrerias, J., Pennazio, M., Caunedo, A., Mascarenhas-Saraiva, M. and de Franchis, R. Complications, limitations, and failures of capsule endoscopy: A review of 733 cases, *Gastrointestinal Endoscopy* 62, 5, 712–716 (2005).

Rondonotti, E., Villa, F., Mulder, C., Jacobs, M. and Franchis, R. Small bowel capsule endoscopy in 2007: Indications, risks and limitations, *Journal of Gastroenterology* **13**(46), 6140–6149 (2007).

Sayaka (on line). http://www.rfamerica.com/sayaka/index.html.

Sendoh, M., Ishiyama, K. and Arai, K.-I. Fabrication of magnetic actuator for use in a capsule endoscope, *IEEE Transactions on Magnetics* **39**(5), 3232– 3234 (2003).

Spada, C., Spera, G., Riccioni, M., Biancone, L., Petruzziello, L., Tringali, A., Familiari, P., Marchese, M., Onder, G., Mutignani, M., Perri, V., Petruzziello, C., Pallone, F. and Costamagna, G. A novel diagnostic tool for detecting functional patency of the small bowel: The given patency capsule, *Endoscopy* **37**(9), 793–800 (2005).

Stereotaxis (on line). http://www.stereotaxis.com.Swain, P. (2003).Wireless capsule endoscope, Gut 52, 4, 48–50.

Swain, P. The future of wireless capsule endoscopy, *World Journal of Gastroenterology* **14**(26), 4142–4145 (2008).

Swain, P., Mosse, A., Burke, P., Fritscher-Ravens, A., Lewkovicz, S., Kraizer, Y. and Mills, T. Remote propulsion of wireless capsule endoscopes, *Gastrointestinal Endoscopy* **55**(5), AB88 (2002).

Uehara, A. and Hoshina, K. Capsule endoscope norika system, *Minimally Invasive Therapy and Allied Technologies* **12**(5), 227–234 (2003).

Valdastri, P., Quaglia, C., Susilo, E., Menciassi, A., Dario, P., Ho, C., Anhoeck, G. and Schurr, M. Wireless therapeutic endoscopic capsule: *In vivo* experiment, *Endoscopy* **40**, 979–982 (2008).

Valdastri, P., Webster, R., Quaglia, C., Quirini, M., Menciassi, A. and Dario, P. A new mechanism for mesoscale legged locomotion in compliant tubular environments, *IEEE Transactions on Robotics* (2009)

Wang, L., Drysdale, T. and Cumming, D. In situ characterization of two wireless transmission schemes for ingestible capsules, *IEEE Transactions on Biomedical Engineering* **54**(11), 2020–2027 (2007).

Wang, X. and Meng, M. Q.-H. Study of a position and orientation tracking method for wireless capsule endoscope, *International Journal of Information Acquisition* **2**(2), 113–121 (2005).

Wang, X. and Meng, M. Q.-H. A magnetic stereo-actuation mechanism for active capsule endoscope, in *Proceedings of the 29th International Conference of the IEEE Engineering in Medicine and Biology Society* (2007)

Yamamoto, H., Sekine, Y., Sato, Y., Higashizawa, T., Miyata, T., Iino, S., Ido, K. and Sugano, K. Total enteroscopy with a nonsurgical steerable doubleballoon method, *Gastrointestinal Endoscopy* **53**(2), 216–220 (2001).

Zworkin, V. Radio pill, *Nature* **179**, 898 (1957).

Color Inserts

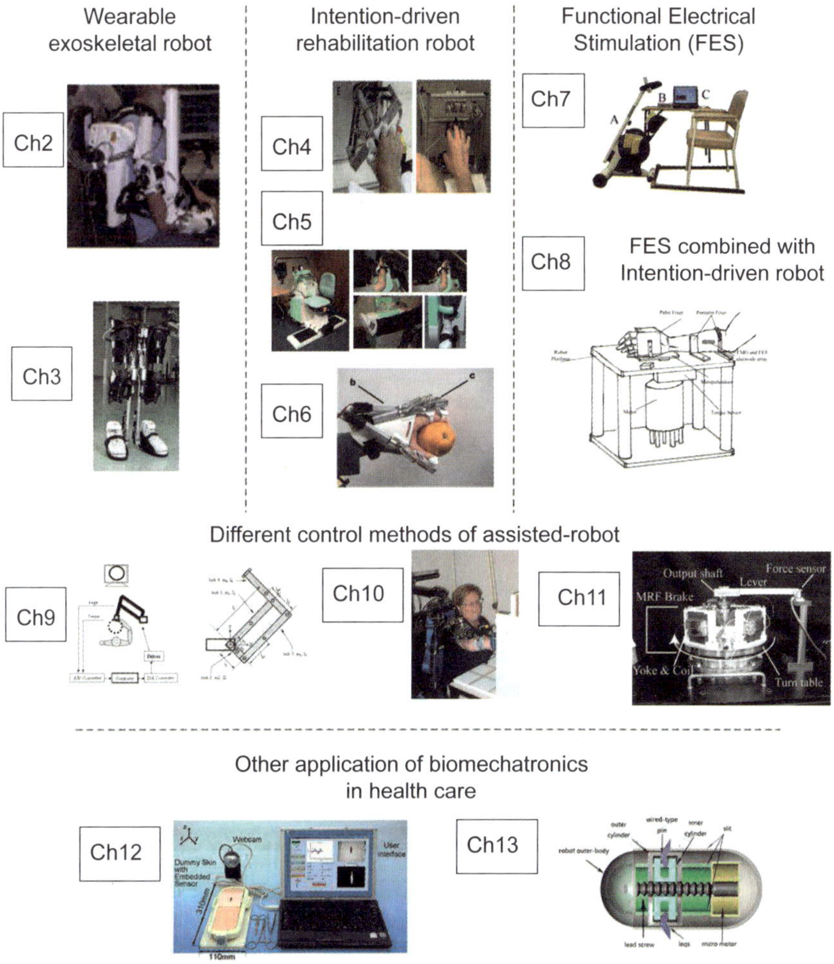

Figure 1.3 Structure of the book.

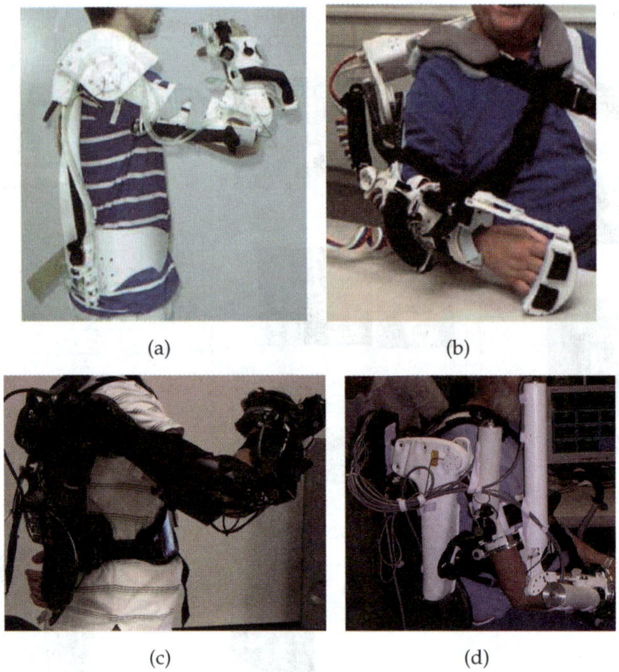

Figure 2.1 Pictures of the four versions of RUPERT depicting the changes in the device over the years. (a) RUPERT; (b) RUPERT II; (c) RUPERT III; (d) RUPERT IV.

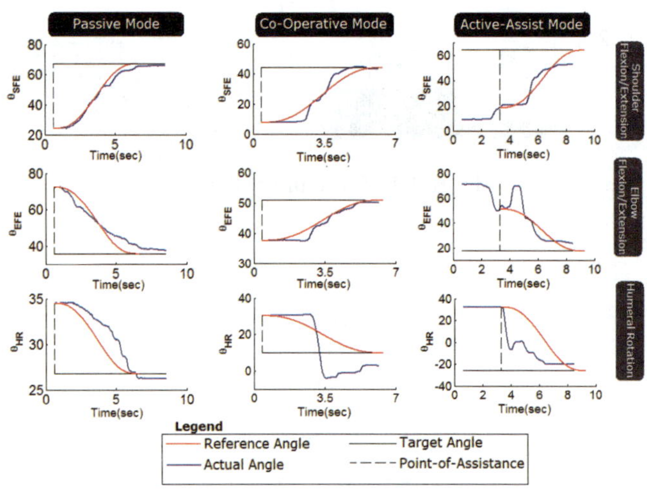

Figure 2.4 Plot of the joint angle profiles of the shoulder flexion/extension, elbow flexion/extension and humeral rotation DOFs for the three therapy modes developed for RUPERT.

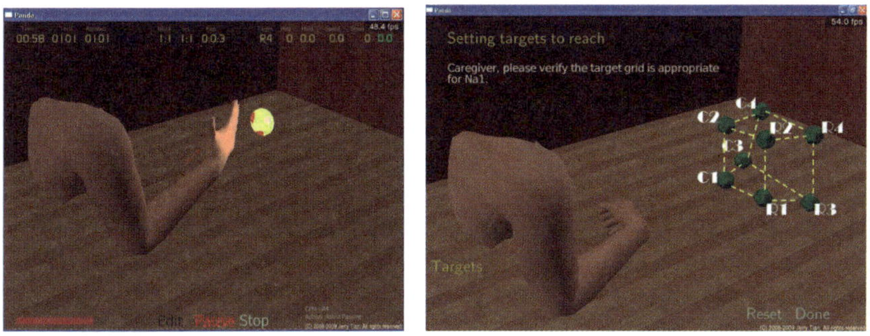

(a) (b)

Figure 2.5 Screen-shot of the virtual reality environment of the biofeedback interface (a) Screen short of subject performing a reaching task. (b) Screen-shot of the different targets used to practice reaching tasks.

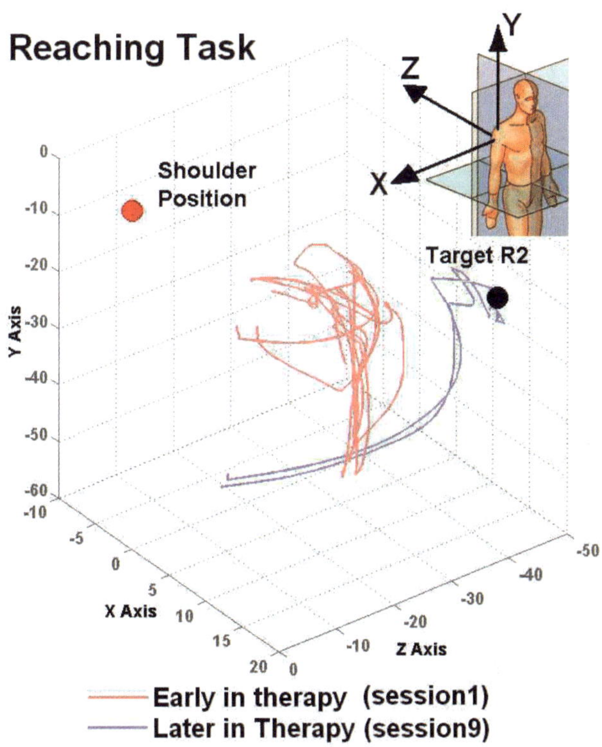

Figure 2.6 Endpoint trajectories of voluntary reaching movements to target R2. The figure shows the endpoint trajectories early (red trace) and late (blue trace) in therapy.

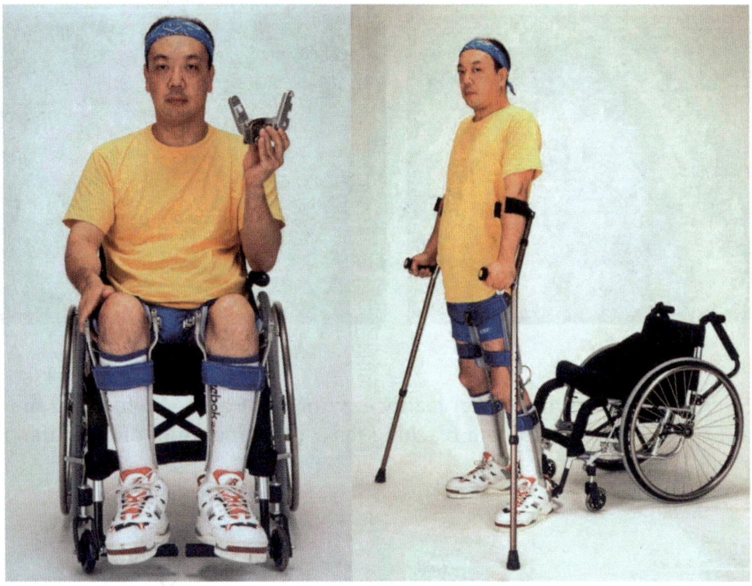

Figure 3.3 Primewalk System.

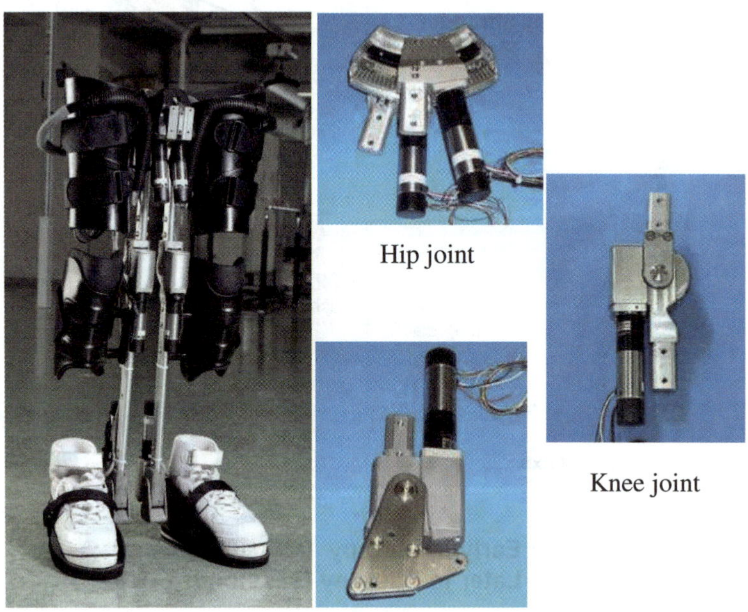

Figure 3.6 (WPAL) Wearable Power-Assist Locomotor.

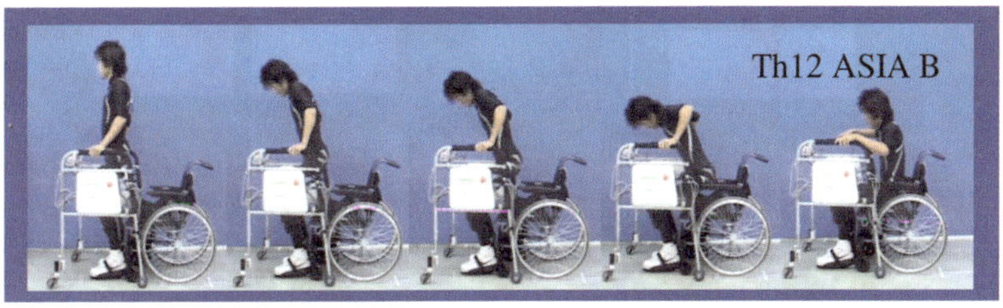

Figure 3.7 Standing up with WPAL.

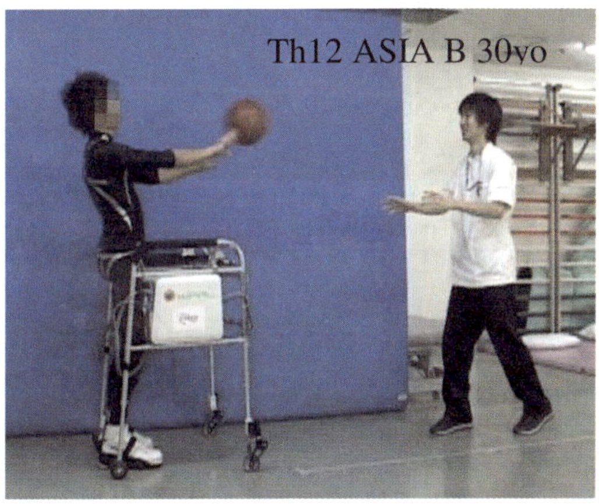

Figure 3.8 Standing balance with WPAL Th12 ASIA B 30 yo.

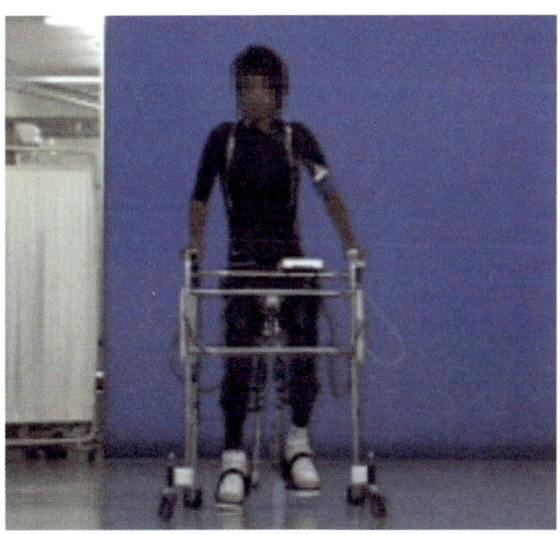

Figure 3.9 Gait with WPAL.

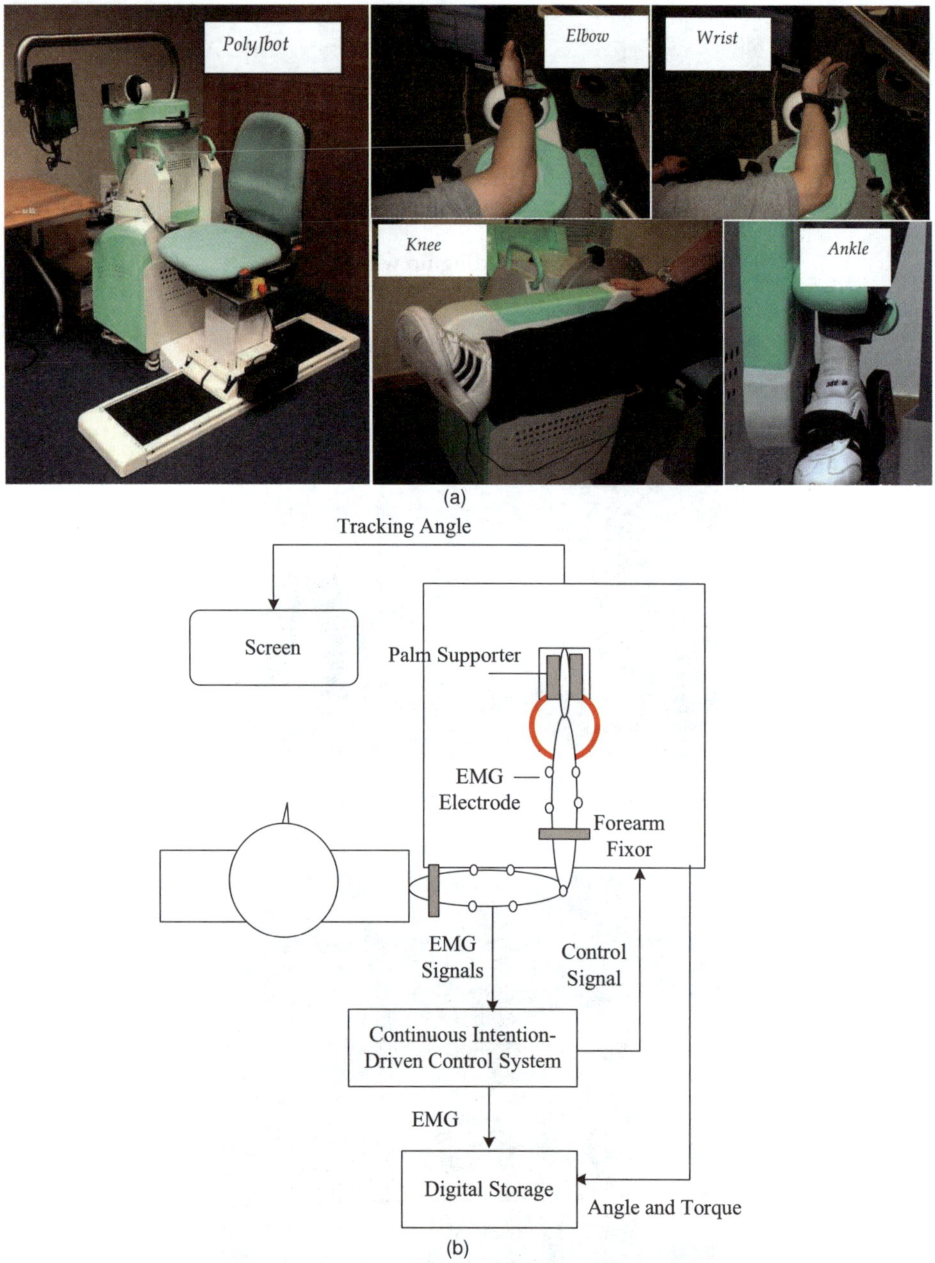

Figure 5.1 The rehabilitation robot (PolyJbot) with continuous intention-driven algorithm for multi-joint training (a), and the schematic diagram of the setup for the wrist training (b).

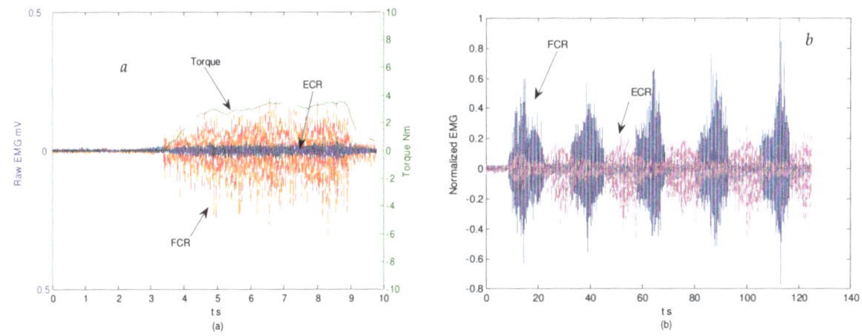

Figure 5.2 The representative EMG signals and torque signal obtained during isometric maximum voluntary flexion at wrist joint of 0° (a), and the representative EMG from the FCR and ECR in a wrist tracking trial (b).

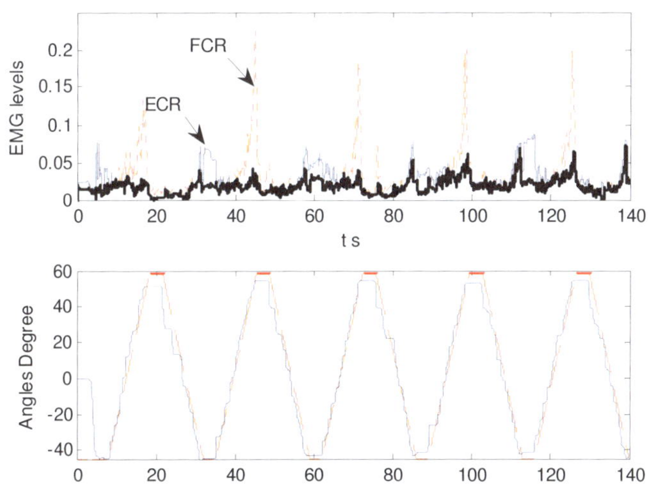

Figure 5.3 A representation of the EMG envelopes of the FCR (doted line), ECR (solid line) muscles, and their overlap (thick solid line) in a tracking trial (upper panel) and the tracking trajectory (lower panel) represented by the actual wrist angle (solid line) and the target angle (dashed line).

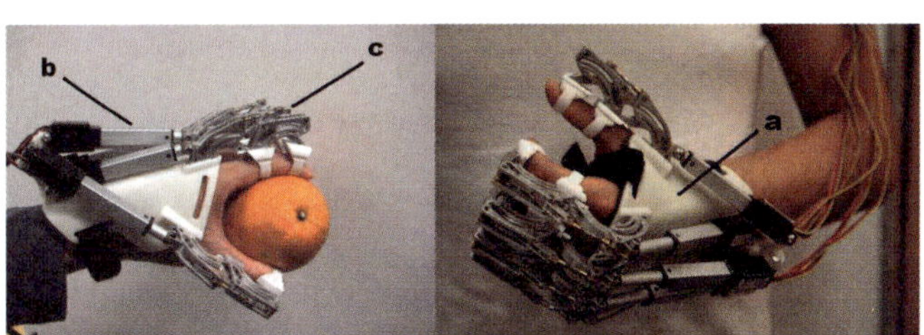

Figure 6.1 The task training hand system (a) actuators platform (b) linear actuator and (c) finger assembly.

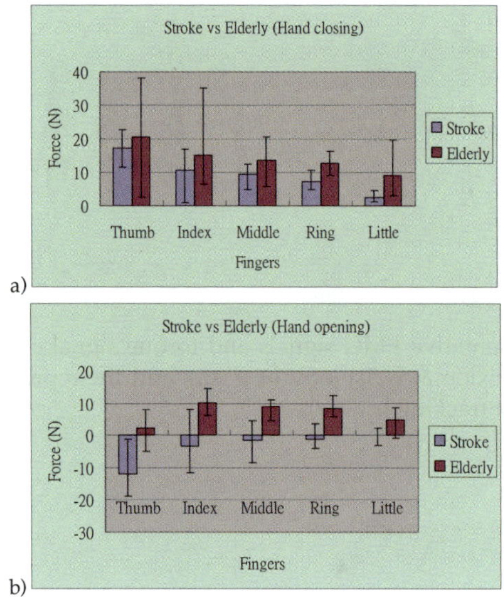

Figure 6.12 Maximum voluntary force between stroke and elderly groups during (a) hand grasp and (b) hand opening. The vertical bar is the maximum and minimum value within the group. The shaded bar is the mean value within the group.

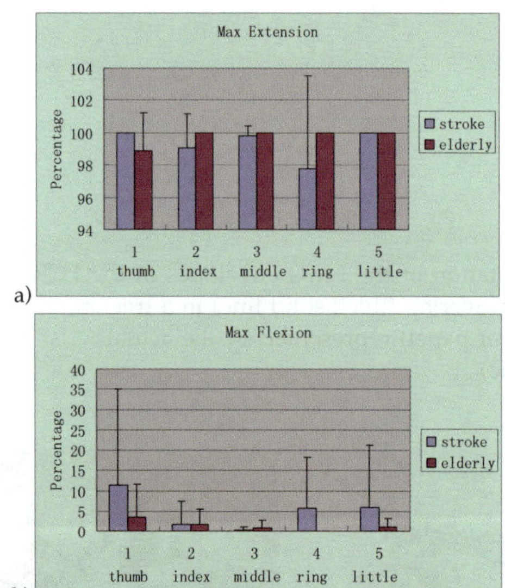

Figure 6.13 Comparison of the mean extension between 5 stroke and 5 elderly subjects during hand opening (extension). (a) Showing the maximum extension achieved in all cycles. Best result is 100% equals full extension. (b) Showing the maximum flexion achieved in all cycles. Best result is 0% equals complete hand grasp position. The vertical bar is the standard deviation and the shaded bar is the mean average.

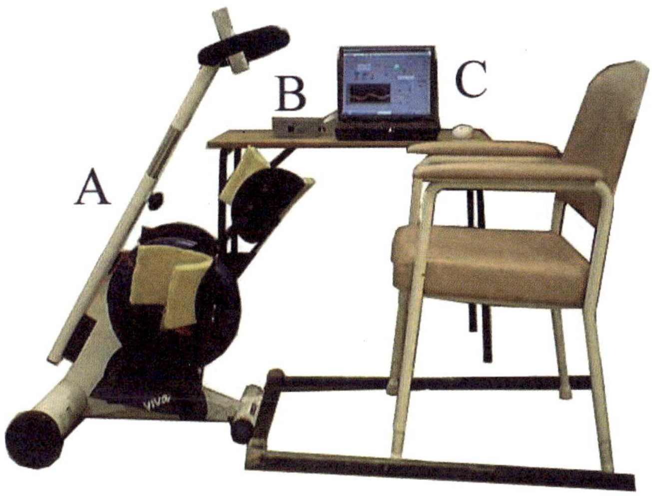

Figure 7.3 The iFES-LCE exercise system. Shown are a Motomed Viva® (A), the DS2000 neuromuscular stimulator (B), the control computer (C), and a chair for the subject.

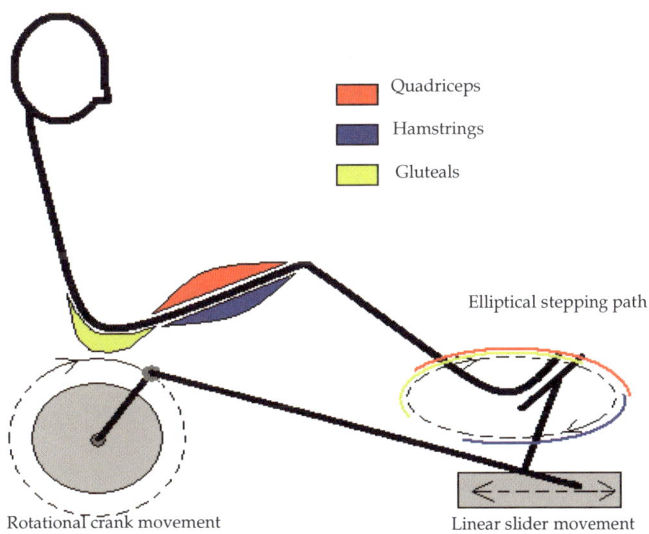

Figure 7.4 Joint and linkages of an elliptical stepper. Primary muscles and the muscle stimulation path is illustrated.

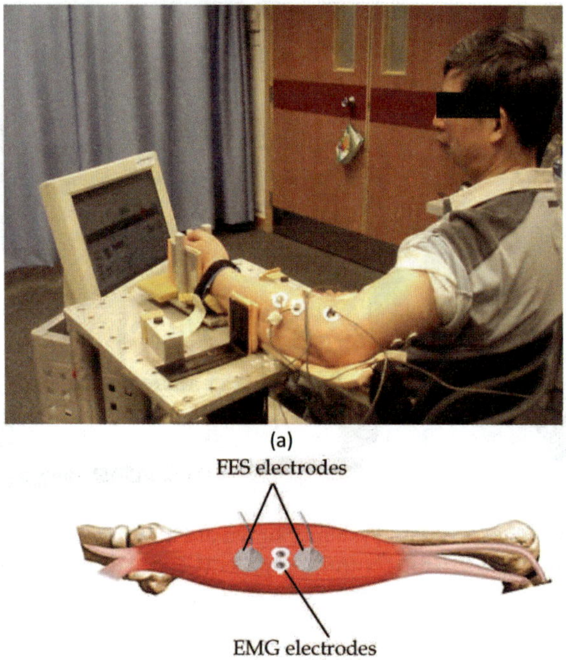

Figure 8.1 The FES-robot training experimental setup (a). The configuration of the FES electrodes and EMG electrodes on a muscle (b).

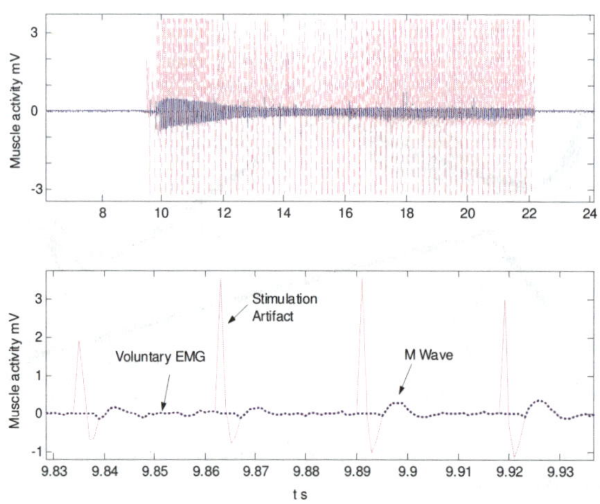

Figure 8.3 The captured EMG signals after the process of sample-and-hold. The upper panel shows the EMG signal before (dotted line) and after (solid line) the process of sample-and-hold. The lower panel shows the enlarged signals in the upper panel.

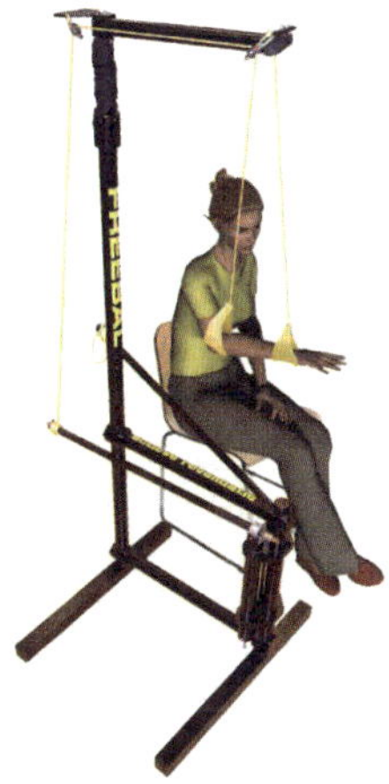

Figure 10.1 Gravity compensation system Freebal.

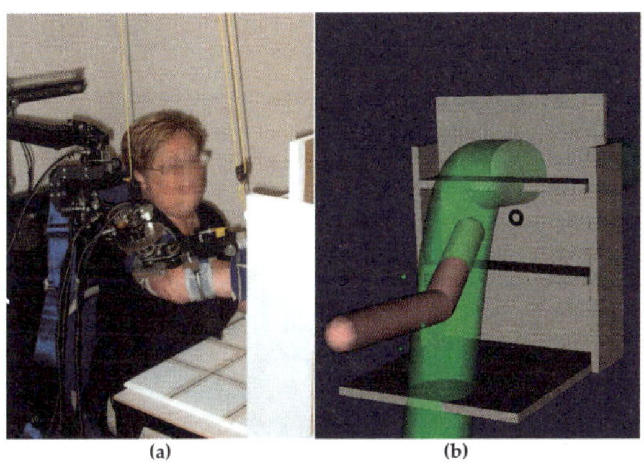

Figure 10.2 (a) Patient in exoskeleton with the table top in front of her (b) predefined path (in green), which was not shown to the stroke survivors.

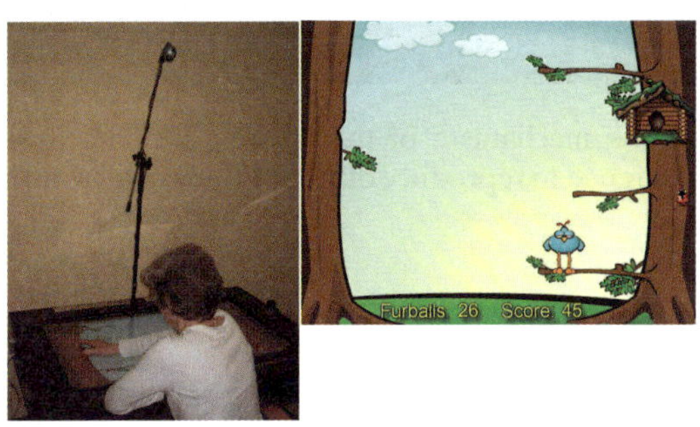

Figure 10.3 Virtual environment (b) by means of motion capturing system (a).

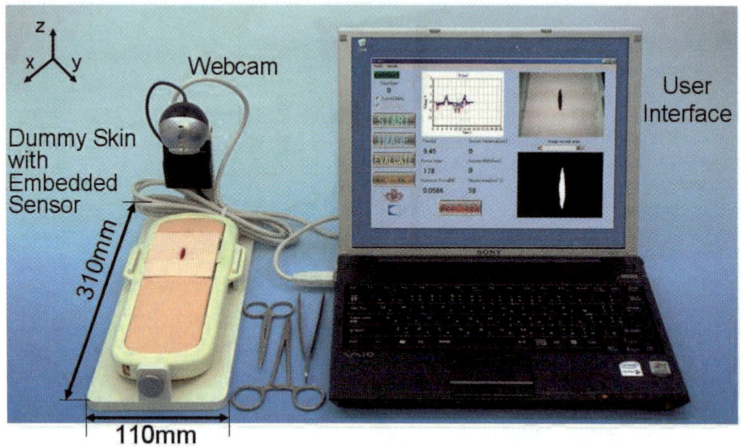

Figure 12.3 The proposed suture/ligature training system is composed by a personal computer, a dummy skin with embedded sensors and a webcam (Solis *et al.*, 2008).

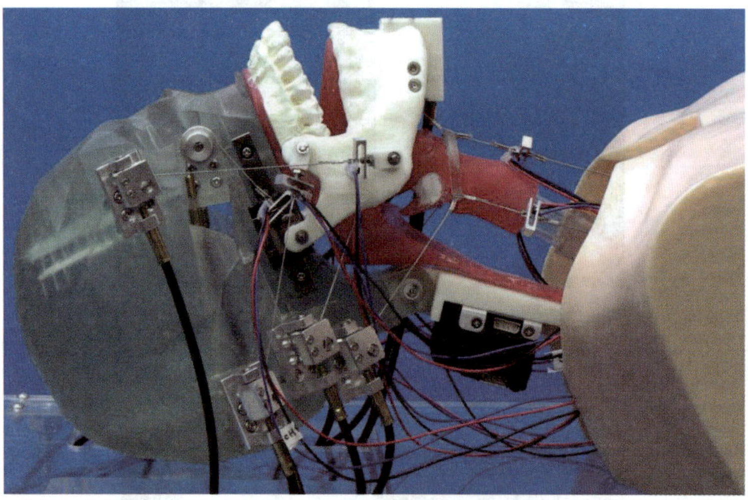

Figure 12.7 Detail of the mechanism of the Airway Training System: A wire driving mechanism has been designed to reproduce different kinds of airway difficulties (Noh, Solis, *et al.*, 2009).

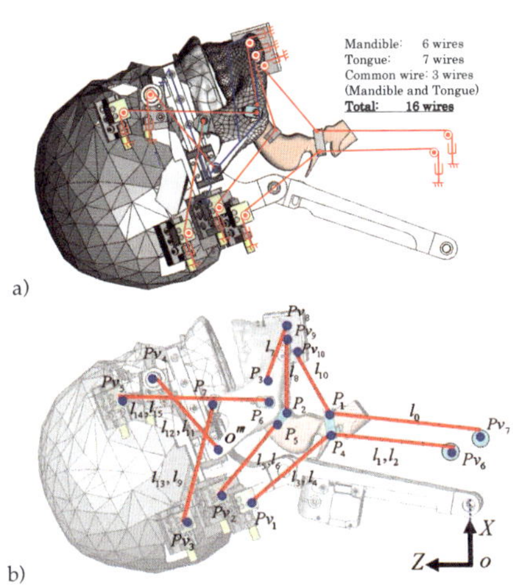

Figure 12.8 Detail of the proposed Airway Management Training System: (a) wiring mechanism; (b) kinematic analysis.

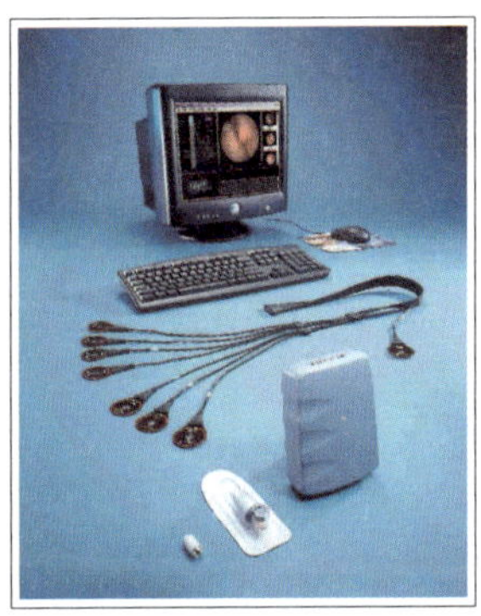

Figure 13.1 *M2A*™ Capsule Endoscopy *Given*™ Diagnostic System, including a wireless capsule endoscope (lower left), sensors for receiving data (middle), a portable data recorder(lower right), and a workstation (upper) for viewing the images. (From www.givenimaing.com).

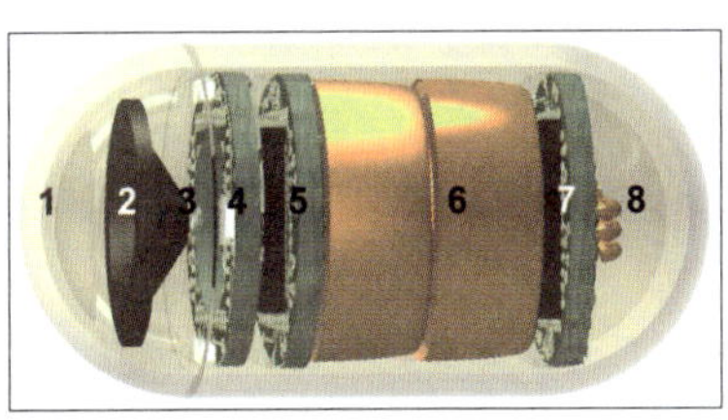

Figure 13.2 Schematic drawing of components inside the capsule endoscope. 1-optical dome, 2-lens holder, 3-lens, 4-illuminating LEDs, 5-CMOS image sensor, 6-battery, 7-ASIC transmitter, 8-antenna.

Index